Pediatric Otolaryngology for the Clinician

Ron B. Mitchell • Kevin D. Pereira
Editors

Pediatric Otolaryngology for the Clinician

Humana Press

Editors

Ron B. Mitchell, MD
Professor and Director of Pediatric Otolaryngology
Department of Otolaryngology – Head and Neck Surgery
Cardinal Glennon Children's Medical Center
Saint Louis University School of Medicine
St. Louis, MO
USA
rmitch11@slu.edu

Kevin D. Pereira, MD
Professor and Director of Pediatric Otolaryngology
Department of Otorhinolaryngology – Head and Neck Surgery
University of Maryland School of Medicine
Baltimore, MD
USA
kevindpereira@gmail.com

ISBN 978-1-62703-842-3 ISBN 978-1-60327-127-1 (eBook)
DOI 10.1007/978-1-60327-127-1
Springer Dordrecht Heidelberg London New York

Printed on acid-free paper

Springer is part of Springer Science+Business Media (www.springer.com)

Foreword

Since the early part of the 20th century there have been individuals with expertise and a very strong interest in pediatric otolaryngology, but the field has really emerged as a comprehensive specialty over the last 20 to 30 years. During this time we have seen the development of specialties within the general field of pediatric otolaryngology such as laryngotracheal reconstruction, hearing disorders, swallowing dysfunction, and sleep disorders in children.

There have been several pre-eminent textbooks written that address the field of pediatric otolaryngology; the current book, edited by Ron Mitchell and Kevin Pereira, brings the field together in a practical and accessible way for the clinician whether they be a pediatrician or an otolaryngologist. It provides practical clinical approaches to the treatment of external, middle ear and hearing disorders. In t e section on rhinology, the topics of trauma, epistaxis, nasal obstruction, allergic rhinitis, and acute and chronic rhinosinusitis are discussed. In a comprehensive section on the head and neck, a full range of disorders is covered from congenital neck masses, chronic cough, and adenotonsillar disease to evaluation of stridor. Treatment by tracheotomy and evaluation of sleep disordered breathing are also discussed in this section. The section on emergencies in pediatric otolaryngology includes chapters on foreign bodies, infections in the neck, acute complications of otitis media and complications of sinusitis.

We hope that this book will become a well-worn clinical resource for busy clinicians who see children with these disorders.

Robert W. Wilmott, MD
IMMUNO Professor and Chair
Saint Louis University
St. Louis, MO

Preface

Pediatric Otolaryngology for the Clinician is a user-friendly book directed at practicing general otolaryngologists, pediatricians, and family practice physicians. It will also be of interest to otolaryngology and pediatric residents, medical students, nurse practitioners, and physician assistants. However, all clinicians treating children with ear, nose, and throat disorders will find it a useful reference. The book is both comprehensive and easy to follow. It will provide an overview of the main aspects of pediatric otolaryngology and highlight the important clinical facets of care of a child with ear, nose, and throat problems.

Over the last 20 years, pediatric otolaryngology has become a recognized subspecialty within otolaryngology–head and neck surgery. The care of children with ear, nose, and throat problems has become more complex. The book is divided into five sections: general ENT topics, otology, rhinology, head and neck disorders, and emergencies. The chapters within each section were written by recognized experts in their respective fields. However, each chapter is short, informative, and self-contained. The book will act as a quick reference guide on a variety of topics such as antibiotic treatment of ear infections, sleep disorders in children, cochlear implantation, airway management, and many more topics. It was designed to be a source of succinct information for use in a busy pediatric clinic.

We would like to extend our thanks to the many authors who have devoted an extensive amount of time to the development of this book. Our thanks to Casey Critchlow of Saint Louis University and Cardinal Glennon Children's Medical Center for the endless hours she has spent in making this book a reality. We would also like to thank Humana Press/Springer for their commitment to publishing this book. This book would have remained an unfulfilled dream if not for the support of our spouses Lauren Mitchell and Iona Pereira and our children who allowed us the many nights and weekends spent writing and editing this book.

Ron B. Mitchell
St. Louis, MO

Kevin D. Pereira
Baltimore, MD

Contents

Contributors

Samantha Anne, M.D.
Fellow, Department of Otolaryngology, Division of Pediatric Otolaryngology, Children's Hospital of Pittsburgh, University of Pittsburgh School of Medicine, Pittsburgh, PA

Jean E. Ashland, PhD, CCC-SLP
Speech Language Pathologist, Department of Speech Language and Swallowing Disorders, Division of Patient Care Services, Massachusetts General Hospital, Harvard University, Boston, MA

Thomas J. Balkany, M.D. FACS, FAAP
Hotchkiss Professor and Chairman, Department of Otolaryngology, University of Miami Ear Institute, Miller School of Medicine, Miami, FL

Cherie L. Booth, M.D.
Resident, Department of Otolaryngology/Head and Neck Surgery, University of Texas Health Science Center at San Antonio, San Antonio, TX

David Brown, M.D.
Assistant Professor, Division of Pediatric Otolaryngology, Department of Otolaryngology–Head and Neck Surgery, Children's Hospital of Wisconsin, Medical College of Wisconsin, Milwaukee, WI.

Margaretha Casselbrant, M.D.
Professor and Chair, Division of Pediatric Otolaryngology, Children's Hospital of Pittsburgh, University of Pittsburgh School of Medicine, Pittsburg, PA

C.Y. Joseph Chang, M.D., F.A.C.S.
Clinical Professor and Director, Department of Otolaryngology Head & Neck Surgery, Texas Ear Center, University of Texas Houston Medical School, Houston, TX

David Darrow, M.D., D.D.S.
Professor of Otolaryngology and Pediatrics, Department of Pediatrics, Department of Otolaryngology–Head & Neck Surgery, Eastern Virginia Medical School, Norfolk, VA

Alessandro de Alarcon, M.D.
Fellow, Division of Pediatric Otolaryngology–Head and Neck Surgery, Cincinnati Children's Medical Center, Cincinnati, OH

Craig S. Derkay, M.D.
Professor of Otolaryngology and Pediatrics, Department of Otolaryngology Head and Neck Surgery, Eastern Virginia Medical School, Norfolk, VA

Paul Digoy, M.D.
Assistant Professor and Director of Pediatric Otorhinolaryngology, Department of Otorhinolaryngology, University of Oklahoma College of Medicine, Oklahoma City, OK

Kelley Dodson, M.D.
Assistant Professor of Otolaryngology–HNS, Department of Otolaryngology–HNS, Virginia Commonwealth University Medical Center, Richmond, VA.

Cindy Jon, M.D.
Assistant Professor of Pediatrics, Department of Pediatrics, Division of Pediatric Pulmonary and Critical Care Medicine, University of Texas Health Science Center at Houston, Houston, TX

Stanton Jones, AuD.
Director, Cochlear Implant Program, Department of Otolarynolgoy Head and Neck Surgery, Saint Louis University School of Medicine, St. Louis, MO

Nathan Kludt, M.D.
Resident, Department of Surgery, University of California, Davis, Davis, CA

Peter J. Koltai, M.D.
Professor, Stanford University School of Medicine, Department of Otolaryngology, Head and Neck Surgery, Division of Pediatric Otolaryngology, Head and Neck Surgery, Stanford, CA

Sandra Koterski, M.D.
Resident, Department of Otolaryngology–Head & Neck Surgery, Division of Pediatric Otolaryngology, Children's Memorial Hospital of Chicago, Northwestern University Feinberg School of Medicine, Chicago, IL

Rodney Lusk, M.D.
Director, Boys Town ENT Institute, Boys Town National Research Hospital, Omaha, NE

John P. Maddolozzo, M.D., FACS, FAAP
Associate Professor, Department of Otolaryngology–Head & Neck Surgery, Division of Pediatric Otolaryngology, Children's Memorial Hospital of Chicago, Northwestern University Feinberg School of Medicine, Chicago, IL

Ellen M. Mandel, M.D.
Associate Professor, Department of Otolaryngology, Division of Pediatric Otolaryngology, Children's Hospital of Pittsburgh, University of Pittsburgh School of Medicine, Pittsburgh, PA

Scott Manning, M.D.
Professor, Department of Otolaryngology, Chief, Division of Pediatric Otolaryngology, Children's Hospital and Regional Medical Center Seattle, University of Washington, Seattle, WA

K. Christopher McMains, M.D.
Assistant Professor, Department of Otolaryngology/Head and Neck Surgery, University of Texas Health Science Center at San Antonio, San Antonio, TX

Ron B. Mitchell, M.D.
Professor and Director of Pediatric Otolaryngology, Department of Otolaryngology Head & Neck Surgery, Division of Pediatric Otolaryngology, Cardinal Glennon Children's Medical Center, Saint Louis University School of Medicine, St. Louis, MO

Anthony Mikulec, M.D.
Associate Professor and Chief, Otologic and Neurotologic Surgery, Department of Otolaryngology–Head and Neck Surgery, Saint Louis University School of Medicine, St. Louis, MO

Harlan Muntz, M.D.
Professor of Surgery, Division of Otolaryngology, Chief of Pediatric Otolaryngology. The University of Utah School of Medicine, Salt Lake City, UT

Charles M. Myer, III, M.D.
Professor, Department of Otolaryngology–Head and Neck Surgery, Division of Pediatric Otolaryngology–Head and Neck Surgery, Cincinnati Children's Medical Center, University of Cincinnati College of Medicine, Cincinnati, OH

T.J. O-Lee, M.D.
Assistant Professor of Otolaryngology–Head and Neck Surgery, Department of Surgery, Division of Otolaryngology–Head and Neck Surgery, University of Nevada School of Medicine, Las Vegas, NV

Alexander J. Osborn, M.D.
Resident, Bobby Alford Department of Otolaryngology–Head and Neck Surgery, Baylor College of Medicine, Houston, TX

Angela Peng, M.D.
Resident, Department of Otolaryngology–HNS, Virginia Commonwealth University Medical Center, Richmond, VA

Kevin D. Pereira, M.D.
Professor and Director of Pediatric Otolaryngology, Department of Otorhinolaryngology–H&N Surgery, University of Maryland School of Medicine, Baltimore, MD

Jonathan A. Perkins, D.O.
Associate Professor, Department of Otolaryngology, Director, Vascular Anomalies Service, Children's Hospital and Regional Medical Center, University of Washington, Seattle, WA

Michael E. Pichichero, M.D.
Professor, Department of Microbiology and Immunology, University of Rochester Medical Center, Rochester, NY

Ryan Raju, M.D., MBA
Resident, Department of Otolaryngology, University of Oklahoma Health Sciences Center, Oklahoma City, OK

Peter S. Roland, M.D.
Arthur E. Meyerhoff Professor and Chairman, Department of Otolaryngology Head and Neck Surgery, University of Texas Southwestern Medical Center at Dallas, Dallas, TX

Emily Rudnick, M.D.
Assistant Professor, Department of Otolaryngology–Head and Neck Surgery, Division of Pediatric Otolaryngology, Johns Hopkins University School of Medicine, Baltimore, MD

Thomas Sanford, M.D.
Assistant Professor, Department of Otolaryngology–Head and Neck Surgery, Saint Louis University School of Medicine, St. Louis, MO

Zoukas Sargi, M.D.
Assistant Professor of Clinical Otolaryngology–Head and Neck Surgery and Reconstructive Surgery, Department of Otolaryngology, University of Miami Miller School of Medicine/Sylvester Comprehensive Cancer Center, Miami, FL

James W. Schroeder, Jr., M.D.
Clinical Instructor, Department of Otolaryngology–Head & Neck Surgery, Division of Pediatric Otolaryngology, Children's Memorial Hospital of Chicago, Northwestern University Feinberg School of Medicine, Chicago, IL

Tyler W. Scoresby, M.D.
Resident, Department of Otolaryngology–Head and Neck Surgery, University of Texas Southwestern Medical Center at Dallas, Dallas, TX

Yisgav Shapira, M.D.
Department of Otolaryngology–Head and Neck Surgery, Sheba Medical Center, Israel

James Sidman, M.D.
Associate Professor, Department of Otolaryngology, Children's Hospitals and Clinics, University of Minnesota, Minneapolis, MN

Stacey Leigh Smith, M.D.
Resident, Department of Otolaryngology
Head and Neck Surgery, University of Texas Health Science Center at San Antonio, San Antonio, TX

Marc C. Thorne, M.D.
Assistant Professor, Department of Otolaryngology–Head and Neck Surgery, Division of Pediatric Otolaryngology, University of Michigan, Ann Arbor, MI

Tulio Valdez, M.D.
Assistant Professor of Otolaryngology, Texas Children's Hospital, Baylor College of Medicine, Houston, TX

Kathleen Wasylik M.D.
Pediatric Otolaryngology Head and Neck Surgery Associates, St. Petersburg, FL

Ralph F. Wetmore, M.D.
E. M. Newlin Professor and Director of Pediatric Otolaryngology, Department of Otorhinolaryngology and Head and Neck Surgery, Division of Otolaryngology and Human Communication, University of Pennsylvania School of Medicine, The Children's Hospital of Philadelphia, Philadelphia, PA

Stephen M. Wold, M.D.
Resident, Department of Otolaryngology Head and Neck Surgery, Eastern Virginia Medical School, Norfolk, VA

Hau Sin Wong, M.D.
Assistant Professor, Children's Hospital of Orange County, University of California Irvine Medical Center, Orange, CA

Robert F. Yellon, M.D.
Associate Professor, Department of Otolaryngology, University of Pittsburgh School of Medicine, Division of Pediatric Otolaryngology, Children's Hospital of Pittsburgh, Pittsburgh, PA

Ramzi Younis, M.D.
Professor and Chief of Pediatric Otolaryngology, Department of Otolaryngology Head and Neck Surgery, University of Miami Miller School of Medicine, Miami, FL

General

Antibiotic Therapy for Acute Otitis, Rhinosinusitis, and Pharyngotonsillitis

Michael E. Pichichero

Key Points

- Classification of otitis media and bacterial rhinosinusitis into acute, recurrent and chronic impacts treatment decisions. Other variables of importance include the child's age, symptom severity, prior treatment history and daycare attendance.
- The etiology of both acute otitis media (AOM) and acute bacterial rhinosinusitis (ABRS) are similar, with the predominant pathogens being *Haemophilus influenzae*, *Streptococcus pneumoniae*, and *Moraxella catarrhalis*.
- Symptomatic and adjunctive therapies other than pain relievers are of limited value.
- Guidelines have been promulgated for antibiotic selection for both AOM and ABRS. Amoxicillin is recommended as first line. Amoxicillin/clavulanate, cefuroxime, cefpodoxime, and cefdinir are preferred as oral second-line agents. Duration of antibiotic therapy may be shortened to 5 days for many cases.
- Group A beta hemolytic streptococci (GABHS) are the major pathogens of the tonsillopharynx requiring antibiotic treatment.
- GABHS are sensitive in vitro to penicillins, macrolides, and cephalosporins. To eradicate GABHS, antibiotic concentrations in the throat must exceed minimum defined concentrations for time spans that vary with the drug.
- Penicillin is the treatment of choice endorsed by all guidelines. Cephalosporins produce better bacteriologic and clinical cure rates than penicillin; this superiority in outcomes has been increasing for over two decades.

Keywords: Otitis media • Sinusitis • Rhinosinusitis; Group A streptococci • Tonsillitis • Pharyngitis • Penicillin • Cephalosporin

Treatment Considerations

A first step in treatment decisions regarding otitis media must focus on accurate diagnosis to distinguish the normal examination from that of acute otitis media (AOM) from otitis media with effusion (OME) or a retracted tympanic membrane (TM) without middle ear effusion. Acute bacterial sinusitis is defined by an inflammation of the mucosa of the paranasal sinuses caused by bacterial overgrowth in a closed cavity; the disorder is also called acute bacterial rhinosinusitis (ABRS). Persistent AOM and ABRS are defined as the persistence of symptoms and signs during or shortly (<1 month) following antibiotic therapy. Recurrent AOM and ABRS are defined as three or more separate episodes in a 6-month time span or four or more episodes in a 12-month time span. Chronic OM and sinusitis occur when there is a persistence of symptoms and signs for 3 months or longer ***(1–6)***.

Antibiotic treatment of AOM and ABRS hastens recovery and reduces complications, but uncomplicated AOM and ABRS usually have a favorable natural history regardless of antibiotic therapy. Patients with persistent or recurrent AOM or ABRS more frequently have infections caused by antibiotic-resistant bacterial pathogens; a combination of host, pathogen, and environmental factors results in a markedly reduced spontaneous cure rate (approximately 50% in most studies).

M.E. Pichichero
Rochester General Hospital, Research Institute, 1425 Portland Avenue, Rochester, NY 14621
e-mail: Michael.pichichero@rochestergeneral.org

R.B. Mitchell and K.D. Pereira (eds.), *Pediatric Otolaryngology for the Clinician*,
DOI: 10.1007/978-1-60327-127-1_1, © Humana Press, a part of Springer Science + Business Media, LLC 2009

In the absence of appropriate treatment, chronic otitis media and chronic ABRS infrequently resolve without significant sequelae.

GABHS (Group A beta-hemolytic streptococci) infection produces a self-limited, localized inflammation of the tonsillopharynx generally lasting 3–6 days. Antibiotic treatment, if prompt and appropriate, reduces the duration of symptoms, shortens the period of contagion, and reduces the occurrence of localized spread and suppurative complications. A major objective of administering antibiotics is to prevent rheumatic fever *(7)*.

Additional Considerations in Antibiotic Selection

A number of factors can be implicated when initial empiric antibiotic treatment fails: (1) inadequate dosing, (2) poor absorption of orally administered antibiotics, (3) poor patient compliance, (4) poor tissue penetration, or (5) the presence of copathogens. Before prescribing an antibiotic, the clinician must consider several factors: (1) bacterial resistance patterns within the patient's community, (2) the severity and duration of the infection, (3) any recent antibiotic therapies, (4) patient age, (5) past drug response, (6) any risk factors that may preclude an agent from the decision-making process, (7) product cost, and (8) availability. Before prescribing an antibiotic, the clinician should also consider the likely susceptibility of the suspected pathogen, as well as the patient's allergy history.

Analgesics, decongestants, antihistamines, nasal sprays, and anti-inflammatory agents have been used to relieve symptoms, to treat, and to attempt to prevent the development of infections. None is particularly helpful. Systemic or local treatments (for example, topical analgesic ear drops for AOM) may reduce the pain associated with the infection, but this is perhaps only at the early stages of pathogenesis.

As noted in the guidelines, consideration should be given to comparative compliance features and duration of therapy in antibiotic selection in children. The main determinants of compliance are frequency of dosing, palatability of the agent, and duration of therapy. Less frequent doses (once or twice a day) are preferable to more frequent doses that interfere with daily routines. In many instances, palatability of the drug ultimately determines compliance in children.

Patients (and parents) prefer a shorter course of antibiotic therapy (5 days or less) rather than the traditional 10-day courses often used in the United States. Many patients and parents continue antibiotic therapy only while symptoms are present, perhaps followed by an additional 1 or 2 days; the remainder of the prescription may be saved for future use when similar symptoms arise. A 10-day treatment course with antibiotic has been standard in the United States although 3-, 5-, 7-, and 8-day regimens are frequently used in other countries. There is microbiologic and clinical evidence that shorter treatment regimens are effective in the majority of AOM and ABRS episodes.

Antibiotic cost is an interesting component of the treatment paradigm. Drug costs alone rarely reflect the total cost of treating an illness. For example, three office visits and three injections of intramuscular ceftriaxone would greatly escalate the cost of treatment. However, the cost of loss of work or school attendance as a result of treatment failure and repeat office visits for additional evaluation are also important yet often overlooked factors.

Antibiotic Treatment for AOM and ABRS

Factors favoring development of persistent and recurrent AOM and probably ABRS include: (1) an episode of infection in the first six months of life, (2) patient age less than 3 years, (3) parental smoking, and (4) day care attendance *(1–6)*. Treatment of AOM and ABRS should target the common pathogens. Various studies from the United States, Europe, and elsewhere over the past 40 years have been consistent in underscoring the importance of *Streptococcus pneumoniae* and nontypeable *Haemophilus influenzae* as the most important pathogens. *Moraxella catarrhalis*, Group A Streptococcus and *Staphylococcus aureus* are less common causes *(1–6)*.

Today, antibiotic choices should reflect pharmacokinetic/pharmacodynamic data and clinical trial results demonstrating effectiveness in eradication of the most likely pathogens based on tympanocentesis (and sinus) sampling and antibiotic-sensitivity testing. Thereafter, compliance factors (e.g., formulation, dosing schedule) and accessibility factors (e.g., availability, cost) should be taken into account. Studies from the early 1990s have described significant decreases in the susceptibility of upper respiratory bacteria to various antibiotics. After the introduction of a 7-valent pneumococcal conjugate vaccine in 2001 in the US, the prevalence in middle ear aspirates of *H. influenzae* increased and *S. pneumoniae* decreased.

The increasing prevalence of antibiotic resistance among upper respiratory bacterial pathogens and the changing susceptibility profiles of these bacteria should be considered in antibiotic selection. The prevalence of penicillin-resistant *S. pneumoniae* isolates causing AOM and ABRS has been increasing worldwide. At the same time, the increasing occurrence of beta-lactamase-producing *H. influenzae* and *M. catarrhalis* strains (from 8 to 65% and up to 98%, respectively) raises concerns about the choice of antibiotics for treatment of AOM. Some classes of antibiotics provide higher levels of antimicrobial activity against penicillin-resistant *S. pneumoniae* (e.g., second- and third-generation cephalosporins, clindamycin, macrolides, ketolides) and against beta-lactamase-producing *H. influenzae* and *M. catarrhalis* strains (e.g., amoxicillin/clavulanate, second- and third-generation cephalosporins). The finding of antibiotic-resistant strains is complicated by frequent concomitant multidrug resistance and by wide geographic variation in the prevalence of antibiotic resistance for the various bacterial species. More information is needed to understand the relationships between in vitro antibiotic susceptibility determinations and the factors affecting the rise in antibiotic-resistant pathogens ***(1–6)***.

Aminopenicillins

Amoxicillin has good activity against *S. pneumoniae* and nonbeta-lactamase-producing strains of *H. influenzae* and *M. catarrhalis*. It is recommended as first-line therapy for AOM and ABRS in every current guideline mainly due to low cost, minimal side effects, and reliance on frequent spontaneous resolution of infection.

Sulfonamides

Sulfonamide antibiotics have been used in the past in penicillin-allergic individuals. However, because of increasing resistance among *S. pneumoniae* and *H. influenzae*, trimethoprim/sulfamethoxazole is no longer guideline recommended.

Tetracyclines

Efficacy of tetracyclines is marginal in AOM and ABRS and these agents are not guideline-recommended.

Amoxicillin/Clavulanate (Augmentin)

The spectrum of activity of amoxicillin/clavulanate includes Gram-positive and Gram-negative bacteria that cause AOM and ABRS. This agent is usually efficacious and is recommended in every current guideline as a second-line agent but generally at an increased dose of 80–100 mg/kg/day of amoxicillin component.

Cephalosporins

Cephalexin and Cefadroxil are not recommended for the treatment of AOM or ABRS unless a specific bacterium has been isolated and shown to be susceptible. These cephalosporins come in good-tasting suspension formulations for children.

Cefaclor (Ceclor) has a spectrum of activity that is better than first-generation cephalosporins against Gram-positive organisms (but marginal against penicillin-intermediate and -resistant pneumococci), and with enhanced Gram-negative activity. However, the in vitro activity of Cefaclor against contemporary beta-lactamase-producing strains of *H. influenzae* and *M. catarrhalis* has been inconsistent, so it is not guideline-recommended.

Cefuroxime axetil (Ceftin) is a second-generation cephalosporin; it has broad-spectrum activity against both Gram-positive and Gram-negative organisms. Its in vitro activity suggests it would be effective in eradication of intermediate penicillin-resistant pneumococci. This is a particularly beta-lactamase stable drug and perhaps the most beta-lactamase stable among the second-generation cephalosporins. It is recommended in every current guideline as second-line therapy.

Cefprozil (Cefzil) has a spectrum of activity similar to that of cefuroxime axetil. In vitro susceptibility testing suggests this antimicrobial may not be as stable against some beta-lactamase-producing *H. influenzae* and *M. catarrhalis* as cefuroxime axetil or amoxicillin/clavulanate. Cefprozil is recommended in some guidelines as a second-line therapy.

Loracarbef (Lorabid) actually falls in a unique antimicrobial class called carbacephems; however, its antimicrobial activity is virtually identical to that of Cefaclor.

Cefixime (Suprax) has enhanced activity against Gram-negative organisms (*H. influenzae* and *M. catarrhalis*). Efficacy of cefixime against penicillin-resistant *S. pneumoniae* is not comparable to that achieved with amoxicillin, or second-generation cephalosporins. Therefore, it is not a guideline-recommended antimicrobial when pneumococci are suspected as probable pathogens but has been endorsed as an agent that could be used in combination with high-dose amoxicillin.

Cefpodoxime proxetil (Vantin) has broad-spectrum activity against Gram-negative bacteria and improved activity against Gram-positive organisms in comparison to cefixime. Cefpodoxime proxetil is an adequate therapy in the management of intermediate and some penicillin-resistant pneumococci. It is recommended in every guideline as second-line therapy.

Ceftibuten (Cedax) has an antimicrobial spectrum similar to that of cefixime. Clinical studies suggest that this agent could be substituted for cefixime and offer a lower likelihood of diarrhea as a combination agent with amoxicillin.

Cefdinir (Omnicef) has a spectrum of activity most similar to cefuroxime axetil and cefpodoxime proxetil. Cefdinir is recommended in all guidelines published since its licensure.

Macrolides/Azalides

Erythromycin is bacteriostatic and has moderate Gram-positive and poor Gram-negative activity. It is not guideline-recommended even in combination with a sulfonamide.

Clarithromycin (Biaxin) has a broad spectrum of activity that includes Gram-positive and Gram-negative organisms. It has additive/synergistic activity with its primary metabolite 14-hydroxy clarithromycin against *H. influenzae*. Clarithromycin is guideline-recommended in beta-lactam-allergic patients.

Azithromycin (Zithromax) has a spectrum of activity similar to clarithromycin. Recent trials suggest azithromycin probably is ineffective against *H. influenzae* in AOM and ABRS and is slower to eradicate *S. pneumoniae* than amoxicillin/clavulanate. Slower eradication may impact clinical outcome. Therefore, azithromycin is not recommended in any guideline except in beta-lactam-allergic patients.

Fluoroquinolones

Levofoxacin (Levaquin) has been studied to treat persistent and recurrent AOM. Its spectrum includes nearly all intermediate and fully penicillin-resistant *S. pneumoniae, H. influenzae*, and *M. catarrhalis*. Levofloxacin use in children, like all fluroquinolones, is restricted to very selective cases where the benefits outweigh theoretical risks of arthropathy and facilitation of antibiotic resistance in children.

Ciprofloxacin, ofloxacin, enoxacin, norfloxacin, and lomafloxacin have inconsistent activity against pneumococci and therefore will not be evaluated for AOM or ABRS in children.

Current Best Practice/Guidelines

Important elements in all current treatment guidelines include the recommendation to (1) start with amoxicillin for uncomplicated disease, (2) continue or switch to an alternative antibiotic based on clinical response after 48 h of therapy (on the third day) thereby giving the first-selected antibiotic enough time to work or fail, and (3) select second-line antibiotics as first-line choices when the patient has already been on an antibiotic within the previous month or is disease prone (Fig. 1). Table 1*(**4**)* shows recommendations from the American Academy of Pediatrics (AAP) for AOM treatment.

Antibiotic selection for persistent and recurrent AOM and ABRS for children under 2 years of age must be more precise because resistant organisms are more often involved and host defense has failed, clinically. Current best practice and guidelines for treatment of persistent and recurrent AOM give considerable weight to data on antibiotic concentrations achievable in middle ear fluid relative to the concentration necessary to kill the relevant pathogens, i.e., pharmacokinetics and pharmacodynamics. Two selection criteria have been universally recommended: (1) the antibiotic should be effective against most drug-resistant *S. pneumoniae* and (2) the antibiotic should be effective against beta-lactamase-producing *H. influenzae* and *M. catarrhalis (**8**)*.

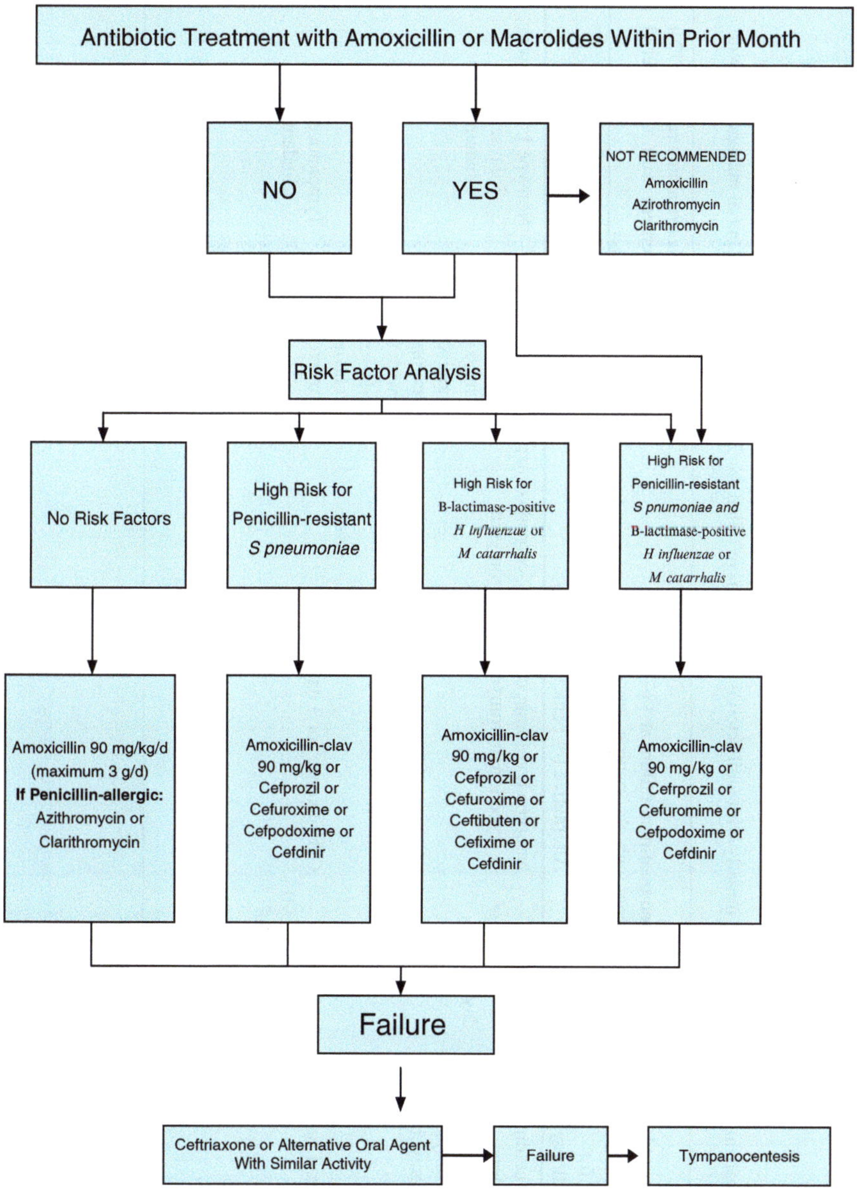

Fig. 1 Author's algorithm for treatment of persistent or recurrent acute otitis media *(1)*

Tympanocentesis

Tympanocentesis with a culture of middle ear fluid may be useful for patients in pain, those who appear toxic, or those with high fever. Diagnostic tympanocentesis is very helpful to guide the choice of therapy in persistent or recurrent AOM but not recommended in uncomplicated AOM. The Centers for Disease Control (CDC) and AAP have recommended that physicians learn the skills required to perform tympanocentesis or have a ready-referral source for patients who would benefit from the procedure. Evacuation (drainage) of the middle ear effusion may be beneficial in breaking the cycle of persistent and recurrent AOM. The information provided by the culture and susceptibility report may be valuable for treatment. If a bacterial pathogen is

Table 1 Recommended antibacterial agents for patients who are being treated initially with antibacterial agents or have failed 48–72 h of observation on initial management with antibacterial agents, 2004 *(4)*

Temperature ^{3} 39°C and/or severe otalgia	At diagnosis for patients being treated initially with antibacterial agents		Clinically defined treatment failure at 48–72 h after initial management with observation option		Clinically defined treatment failure at 48–72 h after initial management with antibacterial agents	
	Recommended	Alternative for penicillin allergy	Recommended	Alternative for penicillin allergy	Recommended	Alternative for penicillin allergy
No	Amoxicillin, 80–90 mg/kg/day	Nontype I: cefdinir, cefuroxime, cefpodoxime; type I: azithromycin, clarithromycin	Amoxicillin, 80–90 mg/kg/day	Nontype I: cefdinir, cefuroxime, cefpodoxime; type I: azithromycin, clarithromycin	Amoxicillin/clavulanate, 90 mg/kg/day of amoxicillin component, with 6.4 mg/kg/day of clavulanate	Nontype I: ceftriaxone, 3 days; type I: clindamycin
Yes	Amoxicillin/clavulanate, 90 mg/kg/day of amoxicillin, with 6.4 mg/kg/day of clavulanate	Ceftriaxone, 1 or 3 days	Amoxicillin/clavulanate, 90 mg/kg/day of amoxicillin, with 6.4 mg/kg/day of clavulanate	Ceftriaxone, 1or 3 days	Ceftriaxone, 3 days	Tympanocentesis, clindamycin

reported, selecting an appropriate antibiotic will reduce the likelihood of further treatment failure; if no bacterial pathogen is isolated, the patient will not require further antibiotic treatment.

Antibiotic Treatment for Group A Beta-Hemolytic Streptococci (GABHS) Pharyngotonsillitis

Group A beta-hemolytic streptococci (GABHS) are the major treatable pathogens of the tonsillopharynx. Prompt eradication shortens illness, eliminates contagion, and prevents complications *(9)*. GABHS are highly susceptible to penicillins and cephalosporins and are usually susceptible to erythromycin, clarithromycin, azithromycin, lincomycin, and clindamycin. However, GABHS resistance to the macrolides occurs and may develop in a community or country as a consequence of antibiotic pressure from their extensive use. Cross-resistance among macrolides is observed. Concurrent resistance to penicillin and cephalosporins does not occur. The minimal inhibitory concentration (MIC) of the aminoglycosides, sulfonamides, chloramphenicol, and tetracycline against most GABHS strains is consistent with the clinical observation that these agents are of limited value in the treatment of GABHS. Sulfadiazine is acceptable for secondary prophylaxis in rheumatic fever. This is reflective of the difference between antibiotic efficacy when bacterial colonization first begins (where prophylactic drugs might be effective) versus when active infection is established (when agents effective in treatment are required).

Tissue and Blood Levels

For penicillin and the cephalosporins, the duration of effective drug level is much more important than the height of the peak serum concentration. Once a concentration of penicillin is reached, that insures activity at the bacterial cell wall. Increased concentrations of the drug do not eradicate GABHS more effectively. Beta-lactam antibiotics work against actively growing bacteria. After initial bactericidal activity, there is a time span of treatment before active bacterial growth resumes in which the antibiotic is not essential. This makes intermittent oral therapy feasible as an alternative to the continuous levels of antibiotics achieved with injectable benzathine penicillin G.

Antibiotic Choices

Benzathine Penicillin G

To reduce the discomfort from injection, a preparation of injectable penicillin (CR Bicillin) combines the long-acting effect of benzathine with procaine penicillin. Procaine penicillin provides diminished injection-site pain and a rapid high level of penicillin in the bloodstream and tonsillopharynx. A combination of 900,000 units of benzathine penicillin G plus 300,000 units of procaine penicillin is superior to a variety of other regimens.

Oral Penicillin G and Penicillin V

Comparison of benzathine penicillin G and oral penicillin G were undertaken between 1953 and 1960 when oral therapy became available. Eradication rates were demonstrated to be similar with 10 days of oral penicillin G as with intramuscular penicillin.

Oral penicillin V was introduced in the early 1960s as an improvement over penicillin G; it is better absorbed and therefore produces higher blood and tonsillar tissue levels. Various dosing regimens with oral penicillin V have been assessed. A daily dose of 500–1,000 mg of penicillin V is preferable. Lower doses have lower eradication rates and higher doses are not beneficial. Twice-daily dosing with oral penicillin V may be adequate therapy for GABHS tonsillopharyngitis, whereas once-daily treatment is not.

Nafcillin, Cloxacillin, and Dicloxacillin

The efficacy of oral penicillin G has been compared with oral nafcillin and the latter is less effective. Cloxacillin and dicloxacillin are adequate therapy for GABHS eradication.

Ampicillin and Amoxicillin

Orally administered amoxicillin is equivalent and in some studies superior to penicillin in bacteriologic eradication of GABHS from the tonsillopharynx. Amoxicillin is more effective than penicillin against the common pathogens that cause otitis media and middle ear infections. These organisms are seen concurrently with GABHS tonsillopharyngitis in up to 15% of pediatric patients. In patients under 4 years of age, the incidence of concurrent GABHS tonsillopharyngitis and otitis media may reach 40%. There is a second issue with regard to oral amoxicillin; it tastes better than oral penicillin in suspension formulation, which is compliance-enhancing for children.

Erythromycin

For penicillin-allergic patients, erythromycin emerged in the 1960s as the suggested agent for GABHS tonsillopharyngitis. Erythromycin estolate and ethylsuccinate have been shown as more favorable with oral penicillin in bacteriologic eradication than erythromycin base or stearate. Dosing-frequency studies with various erythromycin preparations have shown two-, three-, or four-times-daily administration to produce equivalent bacteriologic eradication rates.

Amoxicillin/Clavulanate

Amoxicillin/clavulanate has been shown to improve outcomes compared to penicillin in several, but not all, comparative studies in the treatment of GABHS tonsillopharyngitis. Amoxicillin is bactericidal against GABHS and clavulanate is a potent inhibitor of beta-lactamase. Thus, amoxicillin/clavulanate would be effective if copathogens were co-colonizing the tonsillopharynx in a GABHS-infected patient.

Azithromycin and Clarithromycin

Azithromycin and clarithromycin have been assessed for treatment of GABHS tonsillopharyngitis and bacteriologic eradiation rates have been similar or superior to penicillin. The efficacy of roxithromycin is uncertain. A 5-day regimen of azithromycin treatment is necessary to produce an adequate antibiotic level for an adequate duration; shorter regimens are less effective in children ***(10)***.

Cephalosporins

Oral cephalosporins have been studied as alternative antibiotics for the treatment of GABHS tonsillopharyngitis since 1969. A consistent superior bacteriologic eradication rate, and in many cases clinical cure, has been observed with the cephalosporins compared to penicillins. In 2004, a meta-analysis was published comparing the bacteriologic and clinical cure rates achieved with various cephalosporins compared with oral penicillin ***(11)***. The meta-analysis included approximately 3,969 children prospectively and randomly assigned to receive one of several cephalosporin antibiotics in comparison with 3,156 children treated with oral penicillin. The mean bacteriologic failure rate was threefold higher in those treated with penicillin compared to those treated with cephalosporins ($p < 0.001$).

Duration of Therapy

Injections of benzathine penicillin provide bactericidal levels against GABHS for 21–28 days. The addition of procaine alleviates some of the discomfort associated with benzathine injections and may favorably influence the initial clinical response. The necessity for 10 days of oral penicillin and erythromycin therapy in order to achieve a maximum bacteriologic cure rate has been documented. Five to seven days of therapy with injectable penicillin or oral penicillin does not produce adequate GABHS eradication. Since compliance with 10 days of therapy is often problematic, a shorter course of therapy is an attractive option. A shortened course of 4–5 days of therapy with several cephalosporins, cefadroxil, cefuroxime axetil, cefpodoxime proxetil, and cefdinir has been shown to produce a similar or superior bacteriologic eradication rate and clinical cure compared to that achievable with 10 days administration of oral penicillin V ***(12)***. Azithromycin may be administered for 5 days because this antibiotic persists in tonsillopharyngeal tissues for approximately 10 days after discontinuation of the drug (total of 15 days therapy). If bacteriologic eradication is the primary measure of effective GABHS treatment, as it is the only corollary for the prevention of acute rheumatic fever, then superior bacteriologic eradication with a compliance-enhancing short course of cephalosporin or azithromycin may prove a significant advance.

Explanations for Antibiotic Failure

Compliance

For optimal absorption, oral penicillin V should be administered one hour before or two hours after meals. A reduction in the number of times a day a patient must take any medication and the ability to take doses at meal time will improve patient compliance. Three-times-daily dosing typically is associated with 30–50% compliance whereas 1–2-times-daily dosing produces 70–90% compliance. Intramuscular benzathine penicillin injections obviates compliance issues.

A good taste of suspension formulation for oral antibiotics can be compliance-enhancing for children. On the contrary, a marginal or poor taste may lead to the child refusing, spitting, or vomiting the drug. Penicillin V suspension does not have a good taste whereas most children find the taste of amoxicillin quite pleasant.

Patients who have recurrent bouts of GABHS tonsillopharyngitis and/or in whom penicillin does not eradicate GABHS might be colonized with copathogens. Selecting an alternative antibiotic which is beta-lactamase stable and can be bactericidal to GABHS is advisable.

GAHBS Carriage

High rates of GABHS carriage may account for apparent penicillin failures. The presence of GABHS on throat culture or as detected through rapid diagnostic testing does not distinguish between children with an acute viral sore throat who happen to be a GABHS carrier from a bona fide infection. Asymptomatic GABHS carriage may persist despite intensive penicillin treatment. Eradication of the GABHS carrier state is achievable with clindamycin, rifampin plus penicillin, and cefprozil ***(13, 14)***.

Duration of Illness

The number of days the child is ill prior to treatment may also be an important factor in determining treatment success rate with penicillin. If the patient has been ill for 2 days or more, the likelihood of a treatment success exceeds 80%, but if the patient has been ill for less than 2 days before penicillin is started, the success rate approaches 60%. With longer illness there may be a greater inflammation of the tonsillopharynx and the higher penicillin levels in this inflamed tonsillopharyngeal tissue might explain the lower failure rate.

Age may influence penicillin treatment outcome. Treatment of children in the age group 2–5 years may be successful in only 60% of cases. Many of these young patients may have had previous courses of amoxicillin, so there may be copathogen co-colonization. In 6–12-year olds about 75% are cured and in teenagers and young adults about 85% are cured ***(15,16)***.

Guidelines

Recommendations for GABHS tonsillopharyngitis from the American Academy of Pediatrics, the Infectious Disease Society of America, and the American Heart Association are summarized in Table 2 ***(7,9)***. Antibiotics are only advised for patients with symptomatic pharyngitis and laboratory-proven GABHS (rapid antigen detection test or culture). Although penicillin is advocated as the treatment of choice, amoxicillin is acknowledged for children as a suitable alternative due to a better, compliance-enhancing taste in suspension formulation for younger children.

Conclusions

Optimal management of AOM, ABRS, and GAHBS tonsillopharyngitis is a clinical challenge. Accurate diagnosis is a critical first step. Once the diagnosis is accurately made, the clinician must consider the patient's prior history and predisposing factors in order to develop an appropriate treatment plan. Clinicians

Table 2 Recommendations for antimicrobial therapy for Group A streptococci pharyngitis

Route of administration, antimicrobial agent	Dosage	Duration[a]	Rating
Oral			
Penicillin V[b]	Children: 250 mg b.i.d or t.i.d	10 days	A-II
	Adolescents and adults: 250 mg t.i.d or q.i.d	10 days	A-II
Intramuscular			
Benzathine penicillin G	1.2×10^6 U	1 dose	A-II[c]
	6.0×10^5 U	1 dose[d]	A-II
Mixtures of benzathine and procaine penicillin G	Varies with formulation[e]	1 dose	B-II
Oral, for patients allergic to penicillin			
Erythromycin	Varies with formulation[f]	10 days	A-II
First-generation cephalosporins[g]	Varies with agent	10 days	A-II

[a] Although shorter courses of azithromycin and some cephalosporins have been reported to be effective for treating Group A streptococcal upper respiratory tract infections, evidence is not sufficient to recommend these shorter courses for routine therapy at this time
[b] Amoxicillin is often used in place of oral penicillin V for young children; efficacy appears to be equal. The choice is primarily related to acceptance of the taste of the suspension
[c] See the discussion of benzathine penicillin G therapy in Management of Group A Streptococcal Pharyngitis
[d] For patients who weigh <27 kg
[e] Dose should be determined on the basis of the benzathine component. For example, mixtures of 9×10^5 U of benzathine penicillin G and 3×10^5 U of procaine penicillin G contain less benzathine penicillin G than is recommended for treatment of adolescents or adults
[f] Available as stearate, ethyl succinate, estolate, or base. Cholestatic hepatitis may rarely occur in patients, primarily adults, receiving erythromycin estolate; the incidence is greater among pregnant women, who should not receive this formulation
[g] These agents should not be used to treat patients with immediate-type hypersensitivity to β-lactam antibiotics

selecting an antibiotic should consider compliance-influencing factors such as side effect profile, dosing frequency, duration of therapy, and taste/aftertaste. No single agent is ideal for all patients. The treatment strategy should be tailored to the patient's needs while appropriate attention to microbial resistance patterns is maintained.

With AOM and ABRS, the option of symptomatic treatment and watchful waiting might be considered in the child more than 3 years old, although careful follow-up must be available in the event of clinical deterioration or development of a complication (e.g., mastoiditis). If an antibiotic is used, then selection of appropriate therapy should take into account the major pathogens (*S. pneumoniae*, *H. influenzae*, and *M. catarrhalis*) and the occurrence of antibiotic resistance.

With GAHBS tonsillopharyngitis, the clinician must consider the patient's prior history and predisposing factors to penicillin treatment failure. Selection of appropriate therapy should take into account the changes in penicillin treatment success observed over time and the explanation for antibiotic failure - compliance, copathogens, alteration of microbial ecology, and carriage.

References

1. Pichichero, ME, Reiner, SA, Brook, I, Gooch III, WM, Yamauchi, TY, Jenkins, SG, Sher, L. Controversies in the medical management of persistent and recurrent acute otitis media. Recommendations of a Clinical Advisory Committee. *Annals of Otology, Rhinology&Laryngology* 2000; 109(Supplement 183):1–12.
2. Brook, I, Gooch III, WM, Jenkins, SG, Pichichero, ME, Reiner, SA, Sher, L, Yamauchi, T. Medical management of acute bacterial sinusitis. Recommendations of a Clinical Advisory Committee on Pediatric and Adult Sinusitis. *Annals of Otology, Rhinology&Laryngology* 2000; 109 (Supplement 182):1–20.
3. Dowell, SF, Butler, JC, Giebink, GS, Jacobs, MR, Jernigan, D, Musher, DM, Rakowsky, A, Schwartz, B, et al. Acute otitis media: management and surveillance in an era of pneumococcal resistance - A report from the Drug-Resistant Streptococcus pneumoniae Therapeutic Working Group. *Pediatric Infectious Disease Journal* 1999; 18:1–9.
4. American Academy of Pediatrics and American Academy of Family Physicians, Subcommittee on Management of Acute Otitis Media, Clinical Practice Guideline. Diagnosis and management of acute otitis media. *Pediatrics* 2004; 113:1451–1466.
5. American Academy of Pediatrics, Subcommittee on Management of Sinusitis and Committee on Quality Improvement. Clinical practice guideline: management of sinusitis. *Pediatrics* 2001; 108:798–808.
6. Sinus and allergy health partnership antimicrobial treatment guidelines for acute bacterial rhinosinusitis.

Otolaryngology - Head and Neck Surgery 2004; 130(Suppl.):1–45.

7. Practice guidelines for the diagnosis and management of Group A streptococcal pharyngitis. *Clinical Infectious Diseases* 2002; 35:113–125.
8. Pichichero, ME. Acute otitis media: part II. Treatment in an era of increasing antibiotic resistance. *American Family Physician* 2000; 61:2410–2415.
9. Bisno, AL. Acute pharyngitis. *New England Journal of Medicine* 2001; 344:205–212.
10. Casey, JR, Pichichero, ME. Higher dosages of azithromycin are more effective in Group A streptococcal tonsillopharyngitis treatment. *Clinical Infectious Diseases* 2005; 40:1748–1755.
11. Casey, JR, Pichichero, ME. Meta-analysis of cephalosporin versus penicillin treatment of Group A streptococcal tonsillopharygitis in children. *Pediatrics* 2004; 113:866–882.
12. Casey, JR, Pichichero, ME. Meta-analysis of the short course antibiotic treatment for Group A streptococcal tonsillopharyngitis. *Pediatric Infectious Disease Journal* 2005; 10:909–917.
13. Pichichero, ME, Casey, JR. Systematic review of factors contributing to penicillin treatment failure in Streptococcus pyogenes pharyngitis. *Otolaryngology - Head and Neck Surgery* 2007; 137:851–857.
14. Pichichero, ME, Hoeger, W, Marsocci, SM, Lynd Murphy, AM, Francis, AB, Dragalin, V. Variables influencing penicillin treatment outcome in streptococcal tonsillopharyngitis. *Archives of Pediatrics&Adolescent Medicine* 1999; 186:565–572.
15. Brook, I. Penicillin failure and copathogenicity in streptococcal pharyngotonsillitis. *The Journal of Family Practice* 1994; 38:175–179.
16. Brook, I, Gober, AE. Role of bacterial interference and β-lactimase-producing bacteria in the failure of penicillin to eradicate Group A streptococcal phayrngotonsillitis. *Archives of Otolaryngol Head & Neck Surgery* 1995; 121:1405–1409.

Pediatric Hearing Assessment

Stanton Jones

Key Points

- This chapter outlines the methods of hearing assessment that are appropriate for children from birth to adolescence.
- The importance of timely referral of children with suspected hearing loss for a full hearing assessment cannot be overemphasized. This can be accomplished in a screening and/or a diagnostic hearing assessment.
- The audiogram is the true measure of threshold sensitivity and is considered the "gold standard" for hearing assessment.
- Hearing in children can be assessed from an extremely young age. A reasonable assessment of hearing is now possible in children using physiologic assessment tools including otoacoustic emissions (OAEs), evoked potentials, and tympanometry.
- Behavioral audiologic assessment can include visual response audiometry, conditioned play audiometry, conventional audiometry, speech audiometry, speech reception thresholds, or speech discrimination testing.
- Test batteries consisting of a number of assessment tools are used to make a diagnosis of hearing loss and identify a probable site of lesion. No single tool can provide all of that information.
- Hearing thresholds can range from normal (air conduction better than 15 dB at all frequencies) to a profound loss (one or more thresholds at 80 dB or more) and can be conductive, sensorineural, or mixed.

S. Jones
Cochlear Implant Program, Department of Otolaryngology – Head and Neck Surgery, Saint Louis University School of Medicine, St. Louis, MO, USA
e-mail: sjones50@slu.edu

Keywords: Newborn hearing screening • Otoacoustic emissions • Auditory evoked potentials • Play audiometry • Visual response audiometry

Introduction

Hearing assessment is an integral part of evaluating a child with a speech or hearing problem. Hearing loss has the highest incidence rate for any pediatric disability and should be detected as early as possible. Parents may report signs and symptoms of reduced hearing, or the practitioner may identify the symptoms during a routine evaluation of the child. The importance of timely referral of children with suspected hearing loss for a full hearing assessment cannot be overemphasized. The use of informal methods of hearing assessment, such as the whisper test, can lead to late diagnosis of hearing loss and should be discouraged. With modern screening and diagnostic equipment, hearing can and should be quantified. This can be accomplished in a screening and/or a diagnostic hearing assessment.

Hearing thresholds and speech discrimination measurements as well as site-of-lesion detection, are routine practice in the field of audiology. The audiologist can assist in the diagnosis and the determination of the type and degree of hearing loss. With this information, the physician can assess the likely impact of hearing loss on the development of speech and language skills and whether reduced hearing is part of a syndrome. Rehabilitation and intervention measures can then be planned, including medical and surgical therapy, dispensing hearing aids, or evaluating the child for cochlear implants.

R.B. Mitchell and K.D. Pereira (eds.), *Pediatric Otolaryngology for the Clinician,*
DOI: 10.1007/978-1-60327-127-1_2, © Humana Press, a part of Springer Science + Business Media, LLC 2009

Symptoms of Hearing Loss

The symptoms of hearing loss depend on the degree and nature of the disability. If a child presents with one or more of the following symptoms, a hearing assessment should be considered:

- Delayed language development *(1)*
- Delayed speech development *(1)*
- Asking for repetition *(1)*
- Not waking up to loud sounds
- Not responding when called *(1)*
- Unable to locate a sound source *(1)*
- Places ear close to television or speaker or wants television or radio louder
- Speech and language development has slowed down or ceased *(1)*
- Speech production has become less clear *(1)*
- Not noticing loud sounds in the environment such as an airplane or dog barking

Risk Factors for Hearing Loss

The incidence of sensorineural hearing loss is 1–3 per 1,000 healthy births and 2–4 per 100 in high-risk children *(2)*. The following is a list of factors that may place children at risk of hearing loss, either congenital or acquired:

- Family history of hearing loss
- Genetic disorders or syndromes
- Problematic pregnancy
- Drugs or alcohol use during pregnancy
- Maternal infections during pregnancy such as rubella, sexually transmitted diseases, cytomegalovirus, and numerous others
- Trauma during pregnancy
- Trauma during birth
- Anoxia at birth
- Apgar scores below 5 at 1 min or less than 6 at 5 min
- Postnatal infections
- Hyperbilirubenemia
- Ototoxic medications including aminoglycosides alone or in combination with loop diuretics
- Patients undergoing chemotherapy or radiation for cancer treatment
- Craniofacial anomalies
- Recurrent otitis media with or without ventilation tubes
- Mumps, measles
- Noise exposure, particularly excessive use of personal listening devices

Methods of Hearing Assessment in Pediatrics

The audiogram is the true measure of threshold sensitivity and is considered the "gold standard" for hearing assessment *(3)*. Obtaining an audiogram is not always practical due to the age of the child, level of cognitive functioning, or other confounding factors. Nonetheless, every effort should be made to obtain an audiogram in a child with possible hearing loss.

Hearing in children can be assessed from an extremely young age. A reasonable assessment of hearing is now possible in newborns using otoacoustic emissions (OAEs), evoked potentials, and tympanometry. Testing leads to early intervention measures which ultimately aim to minimize developmental delays. Newborn hearing screening programs are currently mandated by the federal government. All children born in the United States have to undergo a hearing screen soon after birth. Children with congenital hearing loss are therefore identified and diagnosed very early and can be fitted with hearing aids as early as 2 months of age. Below is an outline of the tools and general hearing assessment methods used in different age groups.

Physiologic Assessment Tools

Otoacoustic emissions (OAE) are tests that determine cochlear status, specifically hair cell function. They are mostly used to screen hearing in neonates, infants, or individuals with developmental disabilities. OAEs were first described by Kemp in 1978 *(4)*, when he measured spontaneous and evoked emissions in the human ear. Spontaneous emissions are sounds emitted from the cochlea without an acoustic stimulus and have little or no clinical application. Evoked emissions are sounds emitted from the cochlea in response to acoustic stimuli and play an important role in screening or diagnosing hearing loss in neonates. A probe is placed in the ear canal of the child. The probe houses two receivers (speakers) and a microphone. The resulting sound from the cochlea that is picked up by the microphone is digitized and processed using signal averaging methodology. The type of stimulus presented into the ear determines the type of evoked emission. The following two Otoacoustic Emissions are the most common types utilized: (a) Distortion product otoacoustic emissions (DPOAEs) *(4)* are sounds emitted from the cochlea in response to two simultaneous tones of different frequencies. The response occurs only if there is a sufficient number of outer hair cells in the area of stimulation. (b) The second type, transient evoked otoacoustic emissions (TEOAEs) *(4)*, are sounds emitted from the cochlea in response to acoustic stimuli of very short duration, usually in the form of clicks, but can also be tone bursts. The stimulus is comprised of numerous frequencies and evokes responses from a large portion of the cochlea. OAEs measure only the peripheral auditory system, which includes the outer ear, middle ear, and cochlea. To obtain an OAE, one needs an unobstructed outer ear canal, absence of significant middle ear pathology, and functioning cochlear outer hair cells. Common reasons for not obtaining OAEs in a normal hearing ear include a lack of an optimal probe fit, cerumen impaction, or a middle ear effusion.

Auditory evoked potentials (AEP) (3), also referred to as auditory brainstem responses (ABRs), may be used to screen the hearing of newborns or as a diagnostic tool in a full hearing assessment. The auditory brainstem response is an early audiologic, electrophysiological response originating from the cochlea nerve and lower brainstem. Responses are elicited by a click stimulus presented at 25–30 dB in a screening or varied intensities in a diagnostic assessment. Click stimuli are used in screenings, and tone bursts stimuli are used in diagnostic assessments. Responses are recorded by placing electrodes at the vertex of the scalp and ear lobes. Earphones are placed in the ears to deliver the click stimulus into each ear. Several hundred responses are collected and averaged to reduce background recording noise and increase signal-to-noise ratio.

Tympanometry and acoustic reflexes (5). Tympanometry is used to assess numerous middle ear functions including: the ear canal volume (large canal volumes may indicate a perforation of the tympanic membrane) (Fig. 1, amount of sound admittance and sound impedance at varying pressure levels, ear drum movement, eustachian tube function, and acoustic reflex thresholds (ARTs) *(5)*. Reduced movement of the eardrum may be indicative of fluid in the middle ear or of ossicular dysfunction as seen in children with craniofacial abnormalities. Acoustic reflexes are involuntary contractions of the stapedius and tensor tympani muscles in response to loud noise *(6)*. Conductive or sensorineural hearing loss will cause elevation of these thresholds. These

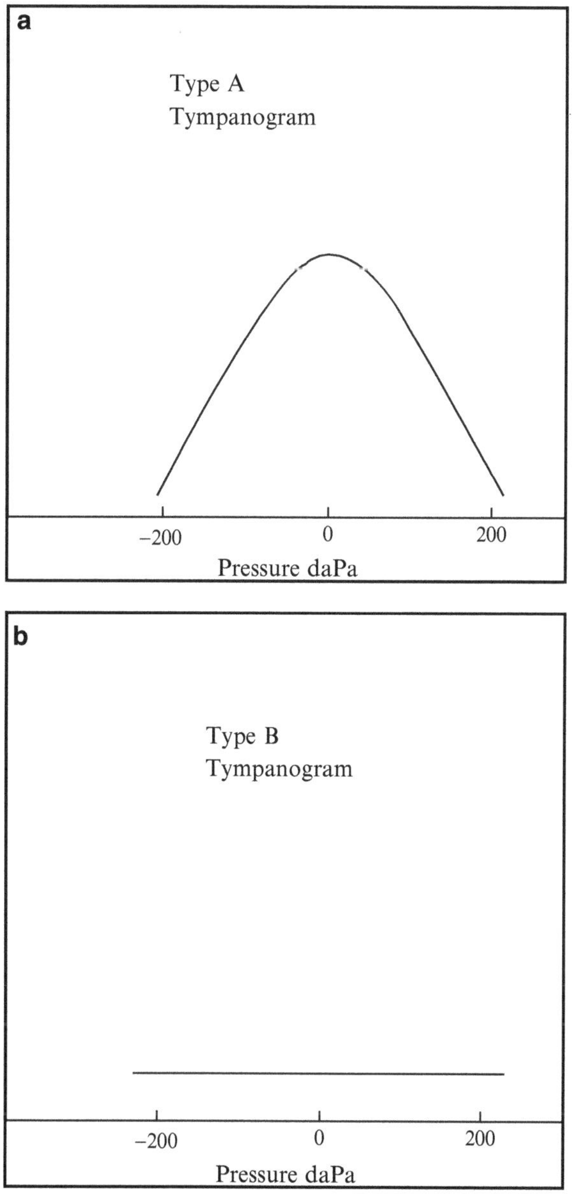

Fig. 1 Type A tympanograms indicate normal ear pressures. Type B tympanograms are seen with a tympanic membrane perforation, a patent tube (large ear canal volume), or with fluid in the middle ear cleft (small ear canal volume). Type C tympanograms are seen with eustachian tube dysfunction and a negative middle ear pressure

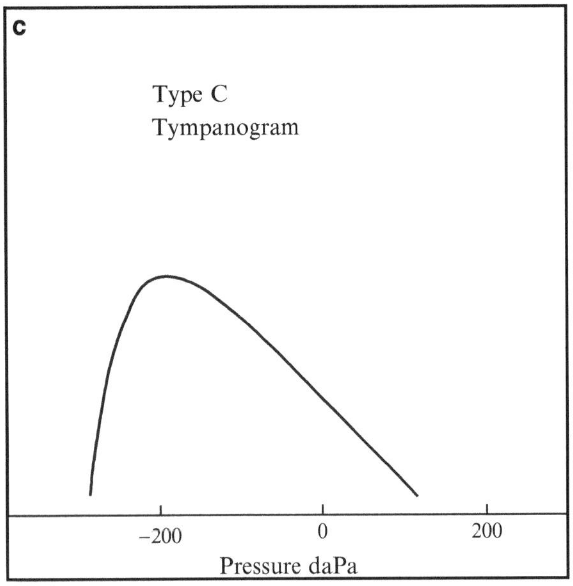

Fig. 1 (continued)

reflexes are usually absent if there is a moderate, severe, or profound hearing loss.

Air conduction and bone conduction testing. Stimuli may be presented to the test subject via circum-aural earphones, insert phones, or speakers. This method of stimulus delivery is known as air-conduction testing. The same stimuli may be presented through a bone vibrator usually placed on the mastoid of the test ear. This essentially directs the sound to the cochlea and bypasses the outer and middle ear systems by setting up vibrations in the skull, which are then transmitted into the fluids of the cochlea. Air and bone conduction testing establishes the presence of a conductive or sensorineural hearing loss.

Behavioral Audiologic Assessment

Visual response audiometry (VRA) (6) relies on the child's ability to localize to the side of the sound source. The child is placed in a sound booth, often seated on the caregiver's lap, with earphones placed in the ear canals. Speakers may be used in a sound field if the child would not tolerate earphones. The use of earphones provides ear-specific information. A stimulus, usually a pure tone, narrow band noise, or warble tone (at 500, 1,000, 2,000, 4,000, and 8,000 Hz), is presented to each ear individually at decreasing intensities, until a threshold is obtained. If the child localizes toward the sound, a visual reinforcer is given to maintain the child's responses. The reinforcement is given only if the child responds to the sound immediately following the sound stimulus *(6)*.

Conditioned play audiometry (CPA) (6) requires the child to be conditioned to the stimulus and to provide a motor response. The response is a play task such as placing a block in a box or a peg in a board, once the stimulus has been heard. Verbal praise is provided as reinforcement to encourage the child to continue the responses. The play activity should be age-appropriate so as to maintain the child's interest but not be too demanding so as to detract from the response. Frequencies that are measured range from 250 to 8,000 Hz at decreasing intensities until a threshold is established.

Conventional audiometry (7) measures require the child to raise a hand or press a button when the stimulus is heard. Frequencies between 250 Hz and 8,000 Hz are assessed at decreasing intensities until a threshold is established at each frequency.

Speech audiometry is used to assess the child's ability to hear speech accurately. Speech stimuli may be used in any of the above behavioral measures rather than tones to obtain a *speech awareness threshold (SAT)*.

Speech reception thresholds (SRT) are established using phonetically balanced words at decreasing intensities. This test requires the child to be able to repeat the words or identify them in pictures.

Speech discrimination testing (SD) assesses the child's ability to comprehend words at suprathreshold levels. This test may require the child to repeat the words. Pointing to pictures may be used if the child has impaired speech production.

Test Batteries

Test batteries consisting of a number of assessment tools are used to make a diagnosis of a hearing loss and identify a probable site of lesion. No single tool can provide all of that information. Table 1 serves as a guide to determine which assessment tools are used at different ages.

It is not unusual to adapt a test battery to the needs and capabilities of the child (Table 1). AEPs and OAEs

split and head in opposite directions within a single bed or it may cross into adjacent beds to form a composite joint.[28]

Evidence for self-correcting rupture is found when stress concentration points in bedded sedimentary rocks force an odd-shaped initial rupture.[30] Occasionally primary growth involves an initial growth spurt producing an elliptical shape followed by a decrease in ellipticity in the central portion of a bed. This happens because v_{tl} becomes faster in the direction of the short axis. The short axis catches up in length to the long axis, thereby returning the rupture to a circular shape (Fig. 13). In some instances the rupture continues to grow in what was the direction of the short axis. The higher velocity portion of the crack tip does not decelerate instantaneously so the former short axis continues propagating and becomes the long axis. The effect is that an elliptical rupture seems to turn at right angles to itself in the interior of a bed (Fig. 13). In these cases, the rupture evolves seamlessly from elliptical to circular and back to elliptical. While circular crack growth occurs during unstable rupture, self-correction does not because in the critical realm there is no correlation between v_{tl} and K_{Ic}. Self-correction requires that $v_{tl} = f(K_{Ic})$.

INCREMENTAL JOINT PROPAGATION BY THE THERMOELASTIC CONTRACTION AND FLUID-DRIVE MECHANISMS

Joint propagation is commonly periodic. In the Catskill Delta Complex this is periodicity is manifest by cycles of gradual roughening of joint surfaces before an abrupt hesitation or complete arrest (Fig. 14). During cooling of basalt that flows onto the Earth's surface, columnar jointing takes place in a series of cycles as a cooling front moves from the edge of the basalt flow to its interior (Fig. 15). Joints in granite can grow cycle by cycle in a series of increasingly larger radius fringe cracks (Figs. 11, 12).

A self-gravitating Earth generates large compressive stresses in its interior. Nevertheless, there are a number of mechanisms by which tensile stresses superimpose on gravitationally generated stress. Joint growth requires the superposition of large enough tensile stresses to create a net tension that is called a tensile effective stress in the geoscience literature.[64] Two of the most common mechanisms for producing a net tension are thermoelastic contraction and fluid pressure generation.[38] The former also produces an absolute tension.

Thermoelastic Contraction

Thermoelastic contraction is strongest following the emplacement of magma into plutons in the Earth's interior or flow lava onto the surface of the Earth. Cooling causes a contraction. Because rocks, including freshly intruded magma or extruded lava, are fixed to external boundaries, the surrounding Earth prevents such contraction and a thermoelastic tensile stress is generated instead. Basalt flows on the Earth's surface are famous for their columnar jointing which is a manifestation of thermoelastic contraction. Early microcracking is very common in

Table 1 Age-appropriate assessment tools

Age	Assessment tool	Table key
Birth (screening)	Neonatal screening using AEP or OAE or both	DPOAE: distortion product otoacoustic emissions TEOAE: transient evoked otoacoustic emissions
Birth to 4 months (diagnostic)	DPOAE/TEOAE	AEP: auditory evoked potential
	AEP	VRA: visual response audiometry
	Tympanometry	SAT: speech awareness threshold CPA: conditioned play audiometry
4 to 18 months	VRA (air and bone conduction) SAT Tympanometry Acoustic reflexes	SD: speech discrimination
18 months to 5 years	CPA (air and bone conduction) SAT/SD Tympanometry Acoustic reflexes	
5 years and over	Conventional audiometry (air and bone conduction) Tympanometry SRT/SD Acoustic reflexes	

are often carried out in children at any age if accurate and reliable information cannot be obtained from behavioral tests. AEPs may require sedating the child in the clinic or operating room in order to obtain the information quickly and accurately. Hearing can then be classified into one of the following categories *(8)*:

1. *Normal hearing*. Air conduction thresholds are better than 15 dB at all frequencies.
2. *Slight hearing loss*. Any one or more thresholds are between 15 and 25 dB at any frequency.
3. *Mild hearing loss*. Any one or more thresholds are between 25 and 40 dB at any frequency.
4. *Moderate hearing loss*. Any one or more thresholds are between 40 and 60 dB at any frequency.
5. *Severe hearing loss*. Any one or more thresholds are between 60 and 80 dB at any frequency.
6. *Profound hearing loss*. Any one or more thresholds are 80 dB or more.

Information from these tests can also help identify the possible cause of hearing loss. A *conductive* hearing loss

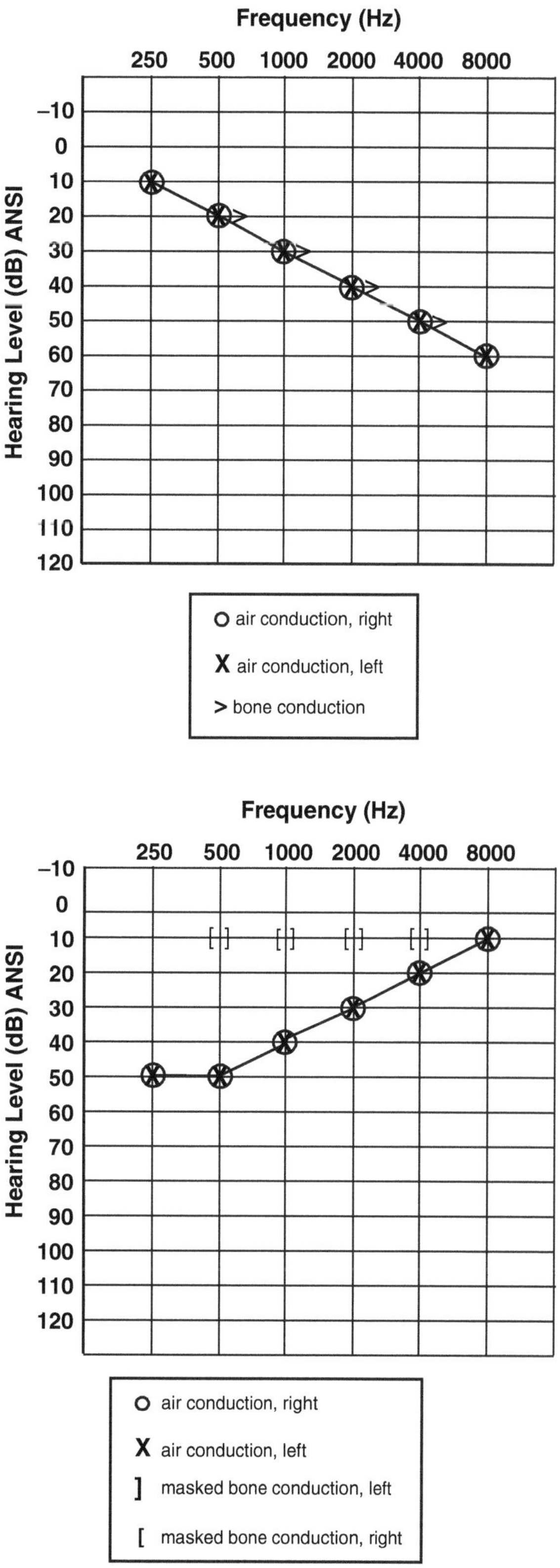

Fig. 2 (**a**) Conductive hearing loss; (**b**) sensorineural hearing loss

originates from the outer or middle ear. Atresia, cerumen impaction, otitis media, or ossicular discontinuity will result in a conductive hearing loss (Fig. 2). A *sensorineural* hearing loss originates from the cochlea or higher auditory pathways. Ototoxic medication or genetic-based hearing loss can give rise to a sensorineural hearing loss. A *mixed* hearing loss originates from the outer or middle ear and cochlea and may be seen in children with craniofacial anomalies that affect the embryologic development of the inner, middle, and outer ear.

References

1. Hear-It. Symptoms of hearing loss. © 2006 Internet webpage available at http://www.hear-it.org/page.dsp?page = 364
2. Cunningham M, Cox EO. Hearing assessment in infants and children: recommendations beyond neonatal screening. *Pediatrics* 2003; 111(2): 436–440.
3. Minnesota Department of Health. Minnesota Newborn Hearing Screening Program. © 2004 Internet webpage available at http://www.health.state.mn.us/divs/fh/mch/unhs/resources/riskinfant.html
4. Marilyn D, Glattke T, Earl R. Comparison of transient evoked otoacoustic emissions and distortion product otoacoustic emissions when screening hearing in preschool children in a community setting. *International Journal of Pediatric Otorhinolaryngology* 2007; 71: 1789–1795.
5. Grimes A. Acoustic immittance: tympanometry and acoustic reflexes. In: Lalwani AK and Grundfast KM (editors). Pediatric Otology and Neurotology, Lippencott-Raven, Philadelphia, 1996.
6. Kemper AR, Downs SM. Evaluation of hearing loss in infants and young children. *Pediatric Annals* 2004; 33(12): 811–821.
7. Gravel J. Behavioral audiologic assessment. In: Lalwani AK and Grundfast KM (editors). Pediatric Otology and Neurotology, Lippencott-Raven, Philadelphia, 1996.
8. American Speech and Hearing Association. Type, degree and configuration of hearing loss. © 2006 Internet webpage available at http://www.asha.org/public/hearing/disorders/types.htm

Speech, Voice, and Swallowing Assessment

Jean E. Ashland

Key Points

- The speech language pathologist (SLP) and otolaryngologist may collaborate effectively in the assessment and treatment of children with speech, resonance, and feeding/swallowing disorders.
- Assessment protocols may involve multidisciplinary efforts, such as a feeding or airway team.
- Knowledge of speech and feeding developmental milestones can help guide the practitioner in identification of problems and the referral process to a SLP.
- SLPs with specialty training in pediatric dysphagia and/or resonance disorders are optimal referral sources for children with issues in these areas. For school age children, the SLP specialist may collaborate with the school speech language pathologist to guide the treatment process or act as a resource when needed.
- The use of FEES to assess swallowing continues to increase in the pediatric population, but there are limits secondary to age and cooperation.
- Children with gagging problems and food refusal behaviors related to food textures likely have sensory-based feeding issues and not a swallowing problem. These children do not require instrumental assessment such as videoflouroscopic exam, but are better served with a feeding evaluation by a feeding specialist.

Abstract This chapter provides a summary of pediatric speech, resonance, and feeding/swallowing disorders. Information regarding normal development, assessment procedures, and referral guidelines are outlined in each of these topic areas. There is discussion of how the speech language pathologist and otolaryngologist may collaborate in such clinical cases. Differential diagnosis of speech disorders includes developmental, structural, and neurological causes. Both instrumental and noninstrumental assessment of resonance issues involving velopharyngeal dysfunction is discussed including nasopharyngoscopy, multiview videofluoroscopy, and nasometry. Feeding and swallowing disorders are differentiated to assist with the diagnosis and referral process. Sample parent interview questions are provided to assist the practitioner in discerning underlying problems in these three areas of speech, voice, and swallowing.

Keywords: Speech • Articulation • Resonance • Velopharyngeal dysfunction • Hypernasality • Dysphagia • Aspiration • Modified barium swallow • FEES • Feeding team

Speech, Voice, and Swallowing Assessment

Altered function of the upper aerodigestive tract can impact not only biological functions such as respiration and digestion, but also nonbiological functions such as speech and voice. The otolaryngologist and speech language pathologist (SLP) often collaborate with particular diagnoses such as speech, voice and resonance disorders, and dysphagia (*1–4*). This chapter will summarize normal and disordered pediatric speech, voice, and swallowing function as well as describe approaches to assessment and intervention.

J.E. Ashland
Department of Speech Language and Swallowing Disorders, Massachusetts General Hospital, Boston, MA, USA
e-mail: jashland@partners.org

R.B. Mitchell and K.D. Pereira (eds.), *Pediatric Otolaryngology for the Clinician*,
DOI: 10.1007/978-1-60327-127-1_3, © Humana Press, a part of Springer Science + Business Media, LLC 2009

Speech/Articulation

Normal Speech Development

Speech develops in relation to muscle maturation, from simple to complex muscle motions. From an anatomical point of view, the general order of sound development occurs from the front of the mouth and progresses posteriorly. For example, labial or lip sounds generally emerge first with /m, p, b/, such as "mama, papa, baby." Then tongue tip elevation (lingual alveolar) sounds emerge: /t, d, n/. For example: "no, hot, dada." Posterior tongue sounds follow: /k, g/, such as "car, go." Early emerging sounds tend to be plosive or stop sounds that require stopping and releasing the air. Sounds that require more control of the air stream, such as fricatives or sibilants: /s, z, sh, ch, f/ are generally acquired later and/or are produced with greater errors. Figure 1 provides a summary of sound development milestones and how sounds are classified by articulator placement.

Speech Disorders

Pediatric speech and/or articulation problems involve compromised speech intelligibility related to imprecise or inaccurate speech sound productions. In addition, rate of speech and degree of mouth opening can also impact intelligibility. Speech production problems may include sound substitution errors (e.g., tat/cat), omissions (e.g., _at/cat), or distortions, such as a frontal distortion (e.g., thuzy/Suzy). Less common speech disorders may be due to motor planning problems for placement of the articulators resulting in inconsistent speech errors and difficulty with oral and speech imitation acts. This problem may be referred to as developmental apraxia ***(5,6)***. Finally, stuttering or dysfluent speech can present as sound or word repetitions with more serious symptoms including speech prolongations, blocking, or secondary motor responses (e.g., eye blinking, facial grimacing). Young children can experience normal periods of nonfluency between 2 and 4 years of age when vocabulary is quickly expanding and they are "thinking faster than they can speak." Children's speech intelligibility progresses with age, so it is important to know what speech errors are expected based on age. Toddlers between 18 months and 2 years generally exhibit ~50% intelligible speech to a familiar listener. This increases to ~70% between 2 and 3 years of age and up to 80% by age 4. Parents can be excellent sources regarding their child's speech development (see Fig. 2).

Differential Diagnoses of Speech Disorders

Developmental delay is the most common etiology for speech difficulties in children. In addition, structural issues, neurological compromise, and acquired deficits are other differential diagnoses to consider. Developmental problems generally present as typical speech errors that might be seen in a younger child who has normal developing speech for his or her age.

Structural issues that impact speech production may include dental occlusion, restricted tongue mobility related to ankyloglossia, congenital anomaly of the jaw, or cleft palate (including submucous cleft). When forward tongue carriage is present during speech acts, it can also be helpful to rule out a tongue thrust pattern, or myofunctional disorder ***(7–9)***. Other structural complications, such as ankyloglossia or a short lingual

Milestones for speech development

- p, m, b, h, n, w, b (90% by age 3)
- k, g, d, t, ng, f, y (90% by age 4)
- r, l, s; sh, ch, z; j,v; th; dj, zh (6-8 yrs)
- Speech intelligibility: 70% age 2; 80% age 3; 90% age 4

Speech production classification by placement

- Labials (p, b, m)
- Labial and lingual-dental (f, v, th)
- Lingual Alveolars (t, d, n, l)
- Palatal (sh, zh, ch, dj)
- Velar (k, g, ng)
- Continuants (h)

Fig. 1 Speech milestones and sound classification

What to ask parents or caregivers at an office visit?

- Do you understand your child's speech half the time; most of the time?
- Does your child avoid talking with others or "give up" when others do not understand them?
- Does your child have temper tantrums in relation to their speech not being understood by others?
- Are you concerned with your child's speech?
- What words can your child say? (this can provide to clues in sound development).
  - expected sounds by age 2-3 years includes: /p, b, m, h, t, d/
  - Sounds at 4 years: /k, g, s, sh, ch, f/
  - Sounds at 5-7 years: /r, l/

Fig. 2 Parent questions about speech development and concerns

frenulum can restrict adequate tongue mobility for accurate articulation ***(10–12)***, especially for tongue tip sounds (e.g., /t, d, l, n, s/).

Neurological or motor speech disorders present as abnormal muscle tone or uncoordinated muscle function including stroke, cerebral palsy, progressive neurological disorder, seizures, or brain tumor. These children often present with feeding and/or swallowing difficulties as well.

Assessment approach: The SLP approaches speech assessment with formal and informal measures. Speech intelligibility is rated in single word productions, the sentence level, and during spontaneous conversation. The child may be asked to label pictures or objects as part of a formal testing tool. In addition, queries are made to the caregiver as to the degree that the speech patterns of the child are disrupting or affecting the child's ability to communicate with others. For example, is there frustration behavior or acts of avoiding talking with others because of speech not being understood? An inventory of speech errors is assembled and the errors are categorized as age appropriate (i.e., not yet acquired based on age) or disordered. An exam of the oral mechanism is also completed to determine if any structural or neuromuscular issues are contributing to the speech errors, such as dental occlusion, shape and movement of the articulators (tongue, palate, lips, jaw), or enlarged tonsils. Stimulability testing is also part of the assessment to determine if the child is able to achieve accurate production of the speech errors during sound and word imitation tasks. Children under 2 years of age generally do no warrant an evaluation of speech sound development as the focus at this age is typically language development. The exception would be extremely poor intelligibility, such as speech primarily characterized by use of vowels. Figure 3 summarizes general guidelines for when to refer children for a speech evaluation.

<u>When to refer for evaluation of speech</u>

Age 2-3
- Speech intelligibility less than 50%
- Omission of initial sounds in words
- Multiple sound errors for early developing sounds: /p, b, m, t, d, h, n, w/
- Frustrated behavior because speech is not understood

Age 4-5
- Speech intelligibility less than 70%
- Multiple sound errors for age appropriate sounds: /k, g, sh, f, ch, dj, y/
- Frustrated behavior because speech is not understood

Age 6-9
- Speech intelligibility is less than 90%
- Multiple sound errors for age appropriate sounds: /l, r, th/

Fig. 3 Speech referral guidelines by age

Voice and Resonance

Disordered Voice and Resonance

Etiologies may vary from hyperfunctional use of voice, a physical pathology, to a structural issue impacting production of voice. For example, etiologies may include deviant vocal cord movement, vocal nodules, or narrowing of the supra- or subglottic airway regions. The pediatric otolaryngologist may use the *Pediatric Voice-Related Quality-of-Life Survey* ***(13)***, a validated instrument to obtain the required information. Figure 4 outlines additional questions for families about their child's resonance.

Resonance disorders include deviant nasal balance characterized as excessive nasality or lack of nasality related nasal air leakage for non-nasal speech sounds or nasal air blockage for nasal speech sounds. These deviant nasal airflow patterns may present as hypernasality and hyponasality. Hypernasality related to soft palate dysfunction is referred to as velopharyngeal insufficiency (VPI) or velopharyngeal dysfunction (VPD) and is most often associated with the presence of a cleft palate or submucous cleft palate ***(14)***. Other etiologies for disrupting soft palate closure during speech may include low muscle tone, a congenitally short palate, or a motor planning difficulty that may be affiliated with apraxic speech. Sometimes enlarged tonsils can project into the velopharyngeal space and disrupt lateral pharyngeal wall closure. When children present with velopharyngeal dysfunction risk factors, the otolaryngologist may consider a speech and resonance evaluation prior to surgery and possibly a modified adenoidectomy, such as a superior-based adenoidectomy to preserve part of the adenoid pad for maintaining soft palate closure during speech.

Assessment of Resonance

Noninstrumental assessment: The SLP can conduct various objective measures of resonance including instrumental and noninstrumental assessment ***(15)***.

What to ask parents or caregivers at an office visit?
- Do you have concerns about your child's pronunciation?
- Do other people have difficulty understanding your child?
- Is your child receiving speech therapy services?
- Does your child speak with a nasal voice quality?
- Do you hear air coming from your child's nose or nasal snorting noises while your child is talking?
- Does your child have a history of a cleft palate?

Fig. 4 Parent questions about resonance

Noninstrumental or perceptual assessment may include intake of developmental articulation abilities for accuracy of articulator placement, nonspeech contributors to speech intelligibility (e.g., rate and loudness of speech, dental occlusion, degree of jaw opening, or intonation patterns), and rating scales of velopharyngeal (VP) function ***(16,17)***. These rating scales can provide guidance for those children that may achieve improvement with speech treatment alone (scores between 1 and 6) versus surgical intervention, such as a pharyngeal flap or oral prosthesis. If the etiology for nasal air leakage is structural, then a surgical option for correction can be explored. If the issue is functional or a learned speaking pattern, then speech intervention can be explored. There are continued efforts to establish a standardized assessment of nasality on a national and international basis to allow a more consistent objective description of resonance disorders, such as the nasality severity index ***(18)*** and cleft audit protocol for speech ***(19)***.

Instrumental assessment: Instrumental assessment may include nasometry or nasal aerodynamic instrumentation, multiview videofluoroscopy or nasopharyngoscopy ***(20,21)***. Typically, children are 4 years of age or older to participate in these exams. *Nasometry* measures nasal air flow during speech acts. For example, expected nasal air flow for target phrases: "pick up the puppy," or "take a tire" is ~10–12%. Other types of instrumental assessment to achieve a direct view of the VP mechanism during speech tasks include multiview videofluorscopy, lateral radiographs/cephalometrics and nasopharyngoscopy ***(22–25)***. Other innovative approaches for assessment of VP function include advanced technology, such as functional MRI ***(26)***. This is primarily in the clinical research field and has not yet translated to clinical use. Current findings reported include close correlation of functional MRI and videofluoroscopy outcomes with some additional information such as dynamics of levator palatine function, muscle alignment in occult submucous cleft palate, and pharyngeal wall movement ***(27–29)***.

Considerations for referral to a speech language pathologist

- Hypernasal voice quality with evidence of nasal air escape
- Cul de sac speech quality with observed bifid uvula
- Repaired cleft palate and residual speech errors and/or deviant nasal resonance

Fig. 5 Referral considerations to a speech language pathologist for resonance problems

Treatment Approaches for VPI

Nonsurgical: Speech intervention for mild to moderate VPI cases can be beneficial ***(15,22,23,30)***. It's optimal to have a SLP who has experience with resonance-based speech disorders. Sometimes, the school SLP will be providing the treatment with consultation from an SLP experienced with resonance disorders. Treatment approaches for resonance disorders focus on improving oral airflow for non-nasal sounds to achieve maximal resonance balance. Techniques such as slowed rate of speech, exaggerated mouth opening or lowered tongue positioning in the floor of the mouth, vowel prolongation, or a plosive sound leading into a sibilant sound (ttt-ssss oap: soap) can be helpful therapy techniques. Palatal obturator use can provide feedback for the child and some children have shown sustained improvement in VP closure after removal of a palatal obturator ***(31,32)***.

Surgical: Surgical approaches for moderate to severe VPI may include a palatal pharyngoplasty (pharyngeal flap) or sphincter pharyngoplasty or palate lengthening ***(33)***. Alternative approaches for minor midline gaps between the velum and pharynx include posterior pharyngeal wall enhancements ***(22,30,34–38)***. Pharyngeal flaps or sphincter palatoplasty approaches are typically used for moderate to severe central gaps between the soft palate and posterior pharyngeal wall. The airway status of the child is an important consideration and a pharyngeal flap is generally contra-indicated when it is compromised in conditions like sleep apnea or in laryngeal anomalies. Indications for referral to a speech pathologist for children with resonance disorders are summarized in Fig. 5.

Feeding and Swallowing

Developmental Nature of Feeding and Swallowing in Children

Children develop feeding abilities and swallowing coordination, much like they acquire other developmental milestones. Feeding milestones start with sucking and progress to cup drinking, spoon feeding, and chewable table foods over the first year of life. Feeding is differentiated from swallowing primarily by voluntary versus involuntary motor control. Feeding involves the process of taking food into the mouth and preparing the food to be swallowed in a coordinated fashion. This is also considered the oral preparatory stage of the swallow. Once food reaches the base of the tongue and begins to propel into the hypopharynx, the reflexive nature of swallowing comes into play. The swallow transports the food or liquid bolus through the pharynx, into the esophagus, and is completed when the bolus moves into the stomach. Coordinated swallowing requires sequencing breathing with swallowing in conjunction with controlled movement of the liquid or food from the mouth to the pharynx ***(39)***. In addition, there must be adequate sensation to detect the bolus as it moves through the mouth and pharynx to assist with triggering the swallowing and maintaining airway protection. A weak or uncoordinated tongue can result in early entry of a liquid or food bolus into the pharynx and an open airway. There must be a coordinated sequence of events to maintain airway protection and have sufficient pressure to drive the bolus through the pharynx into the esophagus. Also, when the sensory system is muted, such as when GERD is present, there can be a compromise of swallow coordination and an aspiration risk.

Disordered Feeding and Swallowing

Typical concerns with feeding and swallowing involve efficiency, coordination, and safety. Symptoms that generate concern may vary from prolonged meals, food refusal, poor weight gain or failure to thrive, weak or immature sucking for infants, weak or immature chewing for older infants and toddlers, gagging/coughing/choking behaviors, and aspiration. A feeding problem can be assessed through a multidisciplinary clinical evaluation ***(40,41)*** whereas a swallowing problem often requires instrumental assessment such as videofluoroscopy or nasoendoscopy ***(42,43)***.

Table 1 summarizes some key differences between feeding and swallowing problems.

Feeding Problems

Feeding problems are often categorized as developmental, motor-based, sensory-based, or behavioral. Because feeding is a complex process, it is not uncommon for multiple issues to be present, such as both motor and sensory-based feeding difficulties ***(44,45)***.

Developmental feeding problems: These may present as immature feeding behaviors expected of a younger child, such as slow acquisition of chewing skills in a child with general slow onset of motor milestones (sitting, crawling, walking). Parents may advance a child's diet based on chronological age and not consider the stage of actual development and readiness. This may result in gagging/choking behaviors with chewable solids if skills are too immature.

Sensory-based feeding issues: Sensory-based feeding issues may occur due to general heightened sensitivity to the environment (light, sound, touch), or with GERD from irritation of the upper airway. Typically, these children will gag on chewable foods, or sticky/mushy foods. The child may retain food in the mouth for long periods of time, spit food out after chewing, or swallow the smooth portion of the food and expel any "pieces" in the food. Reflux and food allergies often accompany sensory-based feeding difficulties as there may be irritation of the upper airway lining or increased mucous presence. Sometimes structural issues such as

Table 1 Symptoms and etiologies of feeding and swallowing problems

Feeding problem	Swallowing problem
Sensitive to textures	Uncoordinated swallow
Occurs prior to swallow	Reduced airway protection
Reduced oral control	Delayed laryngeal elevation/closure
Immature chewing skills	Occurs during the swallow
Response to taste or smell	Generally with liquids and not food
Gagging and enlarged tonsils	More common with neurological, cardiorespiratory, or upper airway structural anomalies
Occurs more with solid food than liquids	
Frequent history of reflux, constipation, delayed gastric emptying, food allergies	

enlarged tonsils can result in gagging behavior with chewable foods secondary to food pooling or being impeded by the tonsils. Parents have reported resolution of gagging issues after tonsillectomy in some cases.

Motor-based feeding issues: In comparison, motor-based feeding problems may present as prolonged chewing because of immature or weak motor function, loss of food from the mouth, or a weak or inefficient suck. As children experience gastrointestinal discomfort with feeding (e.g., reflux), unpleasant sensory responses to taste/texture, or sense parental stress with prolonged meals or insufficient calorie intake, *behavioral* issues can develop around the feeding process. Inevitably, forceful feeding by the parents is not successful to achieve more food intake as the child will generate greater resistance, with a snowball effect. In addition, children with delayed gastric emptying or constipation may show low hunger behavior and limited drive for eating.

Swallowing Problems

Swallowing disorders or dysphagia involve the pharyngeal stage and sometimes esophageal portion of the swallow. Children with neurological, respiratory, or structural airway anomalies are at a greatest risk for dysphagia *(46,47)*. Common *neurological* diagnoses associated with swallowing safety risks include: uncontrolled seizures, moderate to severe cerebral palsy, mitochondrial disease, progressive neurological diseases, and brain tumors impacting the cranial nerves or motor cortex. These children can present with multifaceted feeding and swallowing problems, compromised chewing, choking on liquids, difficulty clearing solid foods from the pharynx, and esophageal dysmotility in some cases. *Respiratory risk factors* for dysphagia may include history of prematurity and chronic lung disease, as well as laryngo or tracheomalacia. Coordinating breathing and swallowing can be disrupted causing risk for aspiration, especially with thin liquids. *Structural complications* can impact swallowing and can sometimes require tracheostomy. They include vocal cord paralysis, choanal atresia, laryngeal cleft, tracheoesophageal fistula, esophageal atresia, or subglottic or supraglottic stenosis.

Assessment of Feeding and Swallowing

Feeding: A feeding assessment is most commonly done by a "feeding specialist," typically a speech language pathologist or occupational therapist. There

Referral Considerations For Feeding and Swallow Problems.

Feeding Team:

- o Gagging or vomiting with chewable solid foods but tolerates liquids and smooth solids
- o Poor texture progression with foods
- o History of reflux
- o Poor weight gain, FTT, and/or Food Refusal
- o Multiple Medical Issues
- o Progression from tube feeding to oral feeding
- o Guidelines for feeding or swallow therapy

Modified Barium Swallow

- o Evaluation of swallow safety, rule out aspiration
- o Coughing and choking DURING or immediately following drinking
- o Wet, congested breath sounds immediately following drinking
- o History of URI, pneumonias
- o Neurological or developmental impairments

FEES

- o Evaluation of swallow safety, rule out aspiration
- o Concerns with upper airway physiology or anatomy contributing to dysphagia
- o Pooling pharyngeal secretions
- o Risk of non-compliance with toddler and preschool age children

Airway or Aerodigestive Team

- o Cardiopulmonary, neurological, and/or gastrointestinal disorders contributing to feeding or swallowing problems
- o Multidisciplinary assessment and management of dysphagia in the presence upper airway complications
- o Chronic cough

Fig. 6 Referral considerations for feeding and swallowing problems

may be a multidisciplinary team evaluation in complex cases that will include a feeding specialist, a dietitian, a physician or nurse, and sometimes a behavioral specialist or psychologist/psychiatrist ***(40,48)***. Recommendations are provided regarding diet, mealtime approaches, feeding therapy, or need to pursue other specialists such as a gastroenterologist or a behavioral specialist ***(48)***.

Swallowing: The gold standard of swallowing assessment is typically a videofluoroscopic swallow study (VFSS) or modified barium swallow (MBS). Fiberoptic endoscopic examination of swallowing (FEES) has been gaining popularity as an alternative procedure in older children and adults ***(49,50)***. Both exams offer dynamic assessment of swallow function. During the MBS or VFSS, the child or older infant is seated in a chair and presented with barium contrast in liquid, paste, and solid food with paste consistencies to assimilate typical meal consistencies, depending on their developmental level of function and current diet. The FEES offers the opportunity to examine the swallow, management or aspiration of secretions, upper airway anatomy, and vocal cord function ***(5,51,52)***. This can be helpful to identify any edema from GERD or anatomical issues impacting swallowing. In addition, a FEES exam may be more sensitive in displaying episodes of microaspiration when compared to MBS in milder cases like a subtle laryngeal cleft ***(53,54)***. However, young children in the toddler and preschool age group may not be compliant with FEES exams resulting in false positive dysphagia findings especially if they are distressed during the exam. Figure 6 provides summary of referral guidelines for feeding and swallowing problems, including instrumental and non-instrumental assessment.

References

1. Coie, JD, Watt, NF, West, SG, et al. The science of prevention: a conceptual framework and some directions for a national research program. *Am Psychol* 1993; 48(10): 1013–1022.
2. Hix-Small, H, Marks, K, Squires, J, Nickel, R. Impact of implementing developmental screening at 12 and 24 months in a pediatric practice. *Pediatrics* 2007; 120(2): 381–389.
3. Zachor, DA, Isaacs, J, Merrick, J. Alternative developmental evaluation paradigm in centers for developmental disabilities. *Res Dev Disabil* 2006; 27(4): 400–410.
4. Wilcox, J. Delivering communication-based services to infants, toddlers, and their families: approaches and models. *Top Lang Disord* 1989; 10(1): 68–79.
5. Shriberg, LD, Green, JR, Campbell, TF, McSweeny, JL, Scheer, AR. A diagnostic marker for childhood apraxia of speech: the coefficient of variation ratio. *Clin Linguist Phon* 2003; 17(7): 575–595.
6. Marquardt, JA, Davis, BL. Consonant and syllable structure patterns in childhood apraxia of speech: developmental change in three children. *J Commun Disord* 2006; 39(6): 424–441.
7. Gommerman, SL, Hodge, MM. Effects of oral myofunctional therapy on swallowing and sibilant production. *Int J Orofacial Myolology* 1995; 21: 9–22.
8. Garretto, AL. Orofacial myofunctional disorders related to malocclusion. *Int J Orofacial Myology* 2001; 27: 44–54.
9. Mason, RM. A retrospective and prospective view of orofacial mycology. *Int J Orofacial Myology* 2005; 31(5): 5–14.
10. Lalakea, ML, Messner, AH. Ankyloglossia: does it matter? *Pediatr Clin North Am* 2003; 50: 381–397.
11. Messner, AH, Lalakea, ML. The effect of ankyloglossia on speech in children. *Otolaryngol Head Neck Surg* 2002; 127(6): 539–545.
12. Dollberg, S, Botzer, E, Grunis, E, Francis, BM. Immediate nipple pain relief after frenotomy in breast-fed infants with ankyloglossia: a randomized, prospective study. *J Pediatr Surg* 2006; 41: 1598–1600.
13. Boseley, ME, Cunningham, MJ, Volk, MS, Hartnick, CJ. Validation of the pediatric voice-related quality-of-life survey. *Arch Otolaryngol Head Neck Surg* 2006; 132(7): 717–720.
14. Miller, CK, Kummer, AW. Velopharyngeal dysfunction (VPD) and resonance disorders. In: Kummer AW, ed. Cleft Palate and Craniofacial Anomalies: Effects on Speech and Resonance. San Diego: Singular Publishing, 2001: 145–176.
15. Kuehn, DP, Henne, LJ. Speech evaluation and treatment for patients with cleft palate. *Am J Speech Lang Pathol* 2003; 12: 103–109.
16. Bzoch, K. Perceptual assessment instrument. Communicative Disorders Related to Cleft Lip and Palate, 4th Edition, Austin, TX: Pro-Ed, 1997.
17. McWilliams, BJ, Phillips, BJ. Velopharyngeal Incompetence: Audio Seminars in Speech Pathology, Philadelphia: WB Saunders, 1978.
18. Van Lierde, KM, Wuyts, FL, Bonte, K, Van Cauwenberge, P. The nasality severity index: an objective measure of hypernasality based on a multiparameter approach. A pilot study. *Folia Phoniatr Logop* 2007; 59(1): 31–38.
19. John, A, Sell, D, Sweeney, T, Harding-Bell, A, Williams, A. The cleft audit protocol for speech-augmented: a validated and reliable measure for auditing cleft speech. *Cleft Palate Craniofac J* 2006; 43(3): 272–281.
20. Johns, DF, Rohrich, RJ, Awada, M. Velopharyngeal incompetence: a guide for clinical evaluation. *Plast Reconstr Surg* 2003; 112: 1890–1897.
21. MacKay, IRA, Kummer, AW. MacKay-Kummer SNAP (Simplified Nasometric Assessment Procedures) Test, Lincoln Park, NJ: Kay Elemetrics Corp., 1994.
22. Marsh, JL. Management of velopharyngeal dysfunction: differential diagnosis for differential management. *J Craniofac Surg* 2003; 13(3): 621–628.

23. Loskin, A, Williams, JK, Burstein, FD, Malick, DN, Riski, JE. Surgical correction of velopharyngeal insufficiency in children with velocardiofacial syndrome. *Plast Reconstr Surg* 2006; 117: 1493–1498.
24. Lam, DJ, Starr, JR, Perkins, JA, Lewis, CW, Eblen, LE, Dunlap, J, Sie, KC. A comparison of nasendoscopy and multiview videofluoroscopy in assessing velopharyngeal insufficiency. *Otolaryngol Head Neck Surg* 2006;134(4): 394–402.
25. Witt, PD, Marsh, JL, McFarland, EG, Riski, JE. The evolution of velopharyngeal imaging. *Ann Plast Surg* 2000; 45: 665–673.
26. Kane, AA, Butman, JA, Mullick, R, Skopec, M, Choyke, P. A new method for the study of velopharyngeal function using gated magnetic resonance imaging. *Plast Reconstr Surg* 2002; 109(2): 472–481.
27. Beer, AJ, Hellerhoff, P, Zimmerman, A, Mady, K, Sader, R, Rummeny, EJ, Hannig, C. Dynamic near-real-time magnetic resonance imaging for analyzing the velopharyngeal closure in comparison with videofluoroscopy. *J Magn Reson Imaging* 2004; 20(5): 791–797.
28. Ettema, SL, Kuehn, DP, Perlman, AL, Alperin, N. Magnetic resonance imaging of the levator veli palatini muscle during speech. *Cleft Palate Craniofac J* 2002; 39(2): 130–144.
29. Kuehn, DP, Ettema, SL, Goldwasser, MS, Barkmeier, JC, Wachtel, JM. Magnetic resonance imaging in the evaluation of occult submucous cleft palate. *Cleft Palate Craniofac J* 2001; 38(5): 421–431.
30. Witt, P, O'Daniel, T, Marsh, JL, Grames, LM, Muntz, HR, Pilgram, TK. Surgical management of velopharyngeal dysfunction: outcome analysis of autogenous posterior pharyngeal wall augmentation. *Plast Reconstr Surg* 1997; 99(5): 1287–1296.
31. Sell, D, Mars, M, Worrell, E. Process and outcomes of multidisciplinary prosthetic treatment for velopharyngeal dysfunction. *Int J Lang Commun Disord* 2006; 41(5): 495–511.
32. Tachimura, T, Nohara, K, Wada, T. Effect of placement of a speech appliance on lavator veli palatini muscle activity during speech. *Cleft Palate Craniofac J* 2000; 37(5): 478–482.
33. Sloan, GM. Posterior pharyngeal flap and sphincter pharyngoplasty: the state of the art. *Cleft Palate Craniofac J* 2000; 57(2): 112–122.
34. Mehendale, FV, Birch, MJ, Birkett, L, Sell, D, Sommerlad, BC. Surgical management of velopharyngeal incompetence in velocardiofacial syndrome. *Cleft Palate Craniofac J* 2004; 41(2): 124–135.
35. Sipp, JA, Ashland, J, Hartnick, CJ. Injection pharyngoplasty with calcium hydroxyl apatite (CHA) for treatment of velopalatal insufficiency. Arch Otolaryngol Head Neck Surg 2008 Mar; 134(3): 268–271.
36. Golding-Kushner, KJ, Argamaso, RV, Cotton, RT, et al. Standardization for the reporting of nasopharyngoscopy and mulitview videofluoroscopy: a report from an international working group. *Cleft Palate J* 1990; 27(4): 337–348.
37. Sie, KCY, Tampakopoulou, DA, de Serres, LM, Gruss, JS, Eblen, LE, Yonick, T. Sphincter pharyngoplasty: speech outcome and complications. *Laryngosope* 1998; 108: 1211–1217.
38. Willging, JP. Velopharyngeal insufficiency. *Curr Opin Otolaryngol Head Neck Surg* 2003; 11: 452–455.
39. Derkay, CS, Schecter, GL. Anatomy and physiology of pediatric swallowing disorders. *Otolaryngol Clin North Am* 1998; 31(3): 397–404.
40. Lefton-Greif, MA, Arvedson, JC. Pediatric feeding/swallowing teams. *Semin Speech Lang* 1997; 18(1): 5–11.
41. Pentuik, SP, Kane Miller, C, Kaul, A. Eosihophilic esophagitis in infants and toddlers. *Dysphagia* 2007; 22: 44–48.
42. Wu, CH, Hsiaso, TY, Chen, JC, Chang, YC, Lee, SY. Evaluation of swallowing safety with fiberoptic endoscope: comparison with videofluorscopic technique. *Laryngoscope* 1997; 107: 396–401.
43. Lowery, SD. Assessment and measuring tools used in the evaluation of swallowing. *Curr Opin Otolaryngol Head Neck Surg* 2001; 9: 134–138.
44. Manikam, R, Perman, JA. Pediatric feeding disorders. *J Clin Gastroenterol* 2000; 30(1): 34–46.
45. Burklow, KA, Phelps, AN, Schultz, JR, McConnell, K, Rudolph, C. Classifying complex pediatric feeding disorders. *J Pediatr Gastroenterol Nutr* 1998; 27(2): 143–147.
46. Kosko, JR, Moser, JD, Erhart, N, Tunkel, DE. Differential diagnosis of dysphagia in children. *Otolaryngol Clin North Am* 1998; 31(3): 435–451.
47. Newman, LA, Keckley, C, Petersen, MC, Hamner, A. Swallowing function and medical diagnoses in infants suspected of dysphagia. *Pediatrics* 2001; 108(6): 1–4.
48. Sheppard, JJ. Case management challenges in pediatric dysphagia. *Dysphagia* 2001; 17: 74.
49. Hiss, S, Postma, GN.Fiberoptic evaluation of swallowing. *Laryngoscope* 2003; 113(8): 1386–1393.
50. Langmore, S, Schatz, K, Olson, N. Fiberoptic endoscopic evaluation of swallowing safety: a new procedure. *Dysphagia* 1988; 2: 216–219.
51. Hartnick, CJ, Miller, C, Hartley, BEJ, Willging, JP. Pediatric fiberoptic endoscopic evaluation of swallowing. *Ann Otol Rhinol Laryngol* 2000; 109: 996–999.
52. Leder, SB, Karas, DE. Fiberoptic endoscopic examination of swallowing in the pediatric population. *Laryngoscope* 2000; 110: 1132–1136.
53. Chien, W, Ashland, J, Haver, K, Hardy, SC, Curren, P, Hartnick, CJ. Type I laryngeal cleft: establishing a functional diagnostic and management algorithm. *Int J Pedeiatr Otorhinolaryngol* 2006; 70(12): 2073–2079.
54. Boseley, ME, Ashland, J, Hartnick, CJ. The utility of the fiberoptic evaluation of swallowing (FEES) in diagnosing and treating children with Type I laryngeal clefts. *Int J Pediatr Otorhinolaryngol* 2006; 70(2): 339–343.

Methicillin-Resistant *Staphylococcus aureus* (MRSA) Infections of the Head and Neck in Children

Tulio A. Valdez and Alexander J. Osborn

Key Points

- MRSA infections have been on the rise over the last 5 years in the United States.
- The USA300 clone is responsible for most cases of community-acquired MRSA.
- Suppurative lymphadenitis is a common manifestation of MRSA infections.
- Lateral neck infections are more common than deep neck infections and are commonly seen in children less than 1 year.
- Clindamycin, Trimethoprim, and Sulfamethoxazole provide excellent coverage against MRSA.
- Incision and drainage is the treatment of choice for suppurative lymphadenitis.

Keywords: Methicillin-resistant *Staphylococcus aureus* (MRSA) • Neck infections • Head and neck • Children

Clinical Presentation

The last decade has seen a dramatic increase in the prevalence of community-acquired methicillin-resistant *Staphylococcus aureus* (CA-MRSA) infections in children. Multiple studies have shown that the proportion of head and neck abscesses caused by CA-MRSA have increased from 0–9% at the start of the millennium to 33–64% in its latter half ***(1–3)***. A recent study has even shown the proportion of CA-MRSA to be as high as 76% ***(4)***. The rate of nasal carriage of MRSA among healthy children appears to have increased from 1% to nearly 10% in just 3 years ***(5)***. Specific risk factors for the acquisition of CA-MRSA in children include underlying chronic illness, previous MRSA infection, contact with family members with MRSA infection, and situations that place the child in close contact with others who might be infected. Outbreaks have been associated with daycare attendance and participation in contact sports ***(6)***. Interestingly, health-related, demographic, and contact-associated risks do not appear to be different for MRSA and methicillin-sensitive *Staphylococcus aureus* (MSSA) infections ***(7)***.

The most common manifestation of CA-MRSA is skin and soft tissue infections such as cellulitis, furuncle, carbuncle, or abscess ***(6)***. In the head and neck, children can present with superficial facial or neck abscesses of the skin, lymphadenitis, or deep lymph node abscesses of the jugular chain, posterior triangle nodes, or submandibular region. Also possible are medial abscesses of the retropharyngeal, parapharyngeal, and peritonsillar regions ***(2,3)***. Presenting signs and symptoms include a mass or swelling, fever, pain, decreased neck mobility, sore throat, decreased oral intake, irritability, leukocytosis, and a preceding upper respiratory tract infection. There do not appear to be differences between MSSA and MRSA with respect to age, location, and presenting symptoms ***(3)***. Compared with nonstaphylococcal infections, however, MRSA and MSSA tend to affect younger individuals in general and have a much higher propensity to afflict specifically those less than 1 year of age ***(7)***. *S. aureus* is much more likely to cause lateral (anterior and posterior triangle nodes) as well as submandibular or submental abscesses, whereas the medial abscesses mentioned above are much more commonly caused by nonstaphylococcal organisms. The most

T.A. Valdez (✉)
Assistant Professor Pediatric Otolaryngology, Connecticut Children's Medical Center
e-mail: tvaldez@ccmckids.org

A.J. Osborn
Bobby Alford Department of Otolaryngology – Head and Neck Surgery, Baylor College of Medicine, Houston, TX, USA

R.B. Mitchell and K.D. Pereira (eds.), *Pediatric Otolaryngology for the Clinician*,
DOI: 10.1007/978-1-60327-127-1_4,

common non-*S. aureus* organisms to cause abscesses of the head and neck are Group A *Streptococcus*, namely, *Streptococcus milleri* and *Streptococcus epidermidis*. Up to 10% of neck infections will grow mixed flora and approximately 25% may yield no growth when cultured *(7)*. These factors should be taken into consideration when treatment options are considered.

Although most CA-MRSA infections are of the skin and soft tissue, this organism can cause severe, life-threatening sepsis and necrotizing pneumonia. In two small series focusing specifically on children, presenting signs and symptoms of systemic CA-MRSA infection included fever, localized joint pain, myalgia, diffuse rash, and leukocytosis or leucopenia *(8,9)*. Pulmonary involvement included complicated parapneumonic effusions, scattered septic emboli, and necrotizing pneumonia with resultant bronchopleural fistula. Clearly, CA-MRSA can potentially lead to much more serious and dangerous infections of which the practitioner must be aware.

Staphylococcus aureus: Mechanisms of Resistance, Evolution and Epidemiology, and Virulence

Penicillin, the original β-lactam antibiotic, was fortuitously discovered as a fungally produced inhibitor of *S. aureus* growth. These antibiotics inhibit enzymes that are essential for cell wall synthesis. Continued cell division in the absence of cell wall synthesis leads to cell death, and thus the β-lactam antibiotics are considered bacteriocidal, not bacteriostatic.

Two fundamental means of β-lactam resistance exist. The first means is the production of β-lactamase, an extracellular enzyme that binds to and enzymatically cleaves the β-lactam ring, rendering the antibiotic inactive. The semisynthetic β-lactamase-resistant penicillins, such as methicillin, were developed in response to the discovery of β-lactamase-conferred penicillin resistance. The second means of β-lactam resistance is the alteration of the peptidoglycan crosslinking enzymes *(10)*. This type of β-lactam resistance is effective against methicillin and other β-lactamase-resistant penicillins because it alters the final target of the antibiotic. In *S. aureus*, the emergence of the *gene mec* resulted in the alteration of the peptidoglycan crosslinking enzymes and was responsible for the appearance of MRSA within just a couple of years of the introduction of methicillin into clinical practice in the early 1960s.

The *mecA* gene appears to have originated from *Staphylococcus sciuri* a widespread relative of *S. aureus*. All strains of this near ubiquitous colonizer of humans and livestock possess a *mecA* homologue, which when upregulated confers methicillin resistance to otherwise susceptible strains of *S. sciuri* and *S. aureus*. The parallel evolution of *mecA* and its subsequent horizontal transfer to *S. aureus* would explain the emergence of MRSA so rapidly after the introduction of methicillin *(11)*.

These initial MRSA strains became prominent in the healthcare setting and gradually acquired, under the selective pressure of the environment, genetic determinants of resistance to a broader variety of antibiotics. Risk factors for contracting these hospital-acquired MRSA (HA-MRSA) infections include hospital and ICU admission, central venous catheter placement, endotracheal intubation, dialysis, and long-term care residency. Recently, however, CA-MRSA has emerged in individuals that do not possess these traditional healthcare-associated risk factors. CA-MRSA tends to be susceptible to more antibiotics than traditional HA-MRSA strains. The current evidence suggests that CA-MRSA arose as a separate evolutionary event within the community, rather than being seeded into the community from the healthcare setting.

A recent multicenter study of adult ER visits for skin and soft tissue infections demonstrated the presence of CA-MRSA in 59% of patients, whereas MSSA was present in 17% of patients and other bacteria or no organisms were isolated in 24% of patients *(12)*. The vast majority (97%) of these CA-MRSA isolates belonged to a single strain called USA300. Although the frequency of CA-MRSA varied among centers from 15 to 74%, in all but one center this pathogen was the most common cause of skin and soft tissue infections.

The USA300 strain of *S. aureus* is the most common CA-MRSA strain in the USA *(12)*. USA300 grows more rapidly, causes more severe infections, and spreads more widely geographically than other MRSA and MSSA strains *(13)*. Indeed the USA300 strain may even be outcompeting traditional hospital-acquired MRSA (HA-MRSA) strains in the healthcare setting *(14,15)*. Future research about the virulence mechanisms of MRSA might provide us with insights into novel adjunct therapies for MRSA infection.

Treatment

Prevention

The United States Centers for Disease Control and Prevention has published excellent evidence-based guidelines for the treatment and prevention of CA-MRSA infections. Prevention measures are listed below and are in addition to guidelines established for the healthcare setting to prevent the spread of HA-MRSA ***(16,17)***. Practitioners should be familiar with these guidelines so that they may properly counsel patients and attempt to minimize or prevent the spread of the pathogen:

1. Keep wounds that are draining covered with clean, dry, bandages.
2. Clean hands regularly with soap and water or alcohol-based hand gel (if hands are not visibly soiled). Always clean hands immediately after touching infected skin or any item that has come in direct contact with a draining wound.
3. Maintain good general hygiene with regular bathing.
4. Do not share items that may become contaminated with wound drainage, such as towels, clothing, bedding, bar soap, razors, and athletic equipment that touches the skin.
5. Launder clothing that has come in contact with wound drainage after each use and dry thoroughly.
6. If you are not able to keep your wound covered with a clean, dry bandage at all times, do not participate in activities where you have skin to skin contact with other persons (such as athletic activities) until your wound is healed.
7. Clean equipment and other environmental surfaces with which multiple individuals have bare skin contact with an over-the-counter detergent/disinfectant that specifies *S. aureus* on the product label and is suitable for the type of surface being cleaned.

Antibiotic Choice

Treatment of CA-MRSA cellulitis and superficially purulent skin infections is primarily by antibiotic therapy. CA-MRSA tends to be, but is not uniformly sensitive to clindamycin, rifampin, trimethoprim-sulfamethoxazole, and sometimes the tetracyclines. Rates of resistance to these agents tend to be less than 10% but this does vary by geographic area ***(18,19)***. CA-MRSA is by definition resistant to the penicillins, is clinically resistant to cephalosporins, and tends to have high rates of resistance to quinolones and macrolides. Typically, fewer than 10% of CA-MRSA isolates demonstrate erythromycin-induced clindamycin resistance, or so-called type B macrolide-lincosamide-streptogramin (MLS_B) resistance, but again variability depending on geographic region exists ***(20,21)***. It has been suggested that empiric therapy with clindamycin in areas with high rates of MLS_B resistance should be avoided. Of course it may be used for definitive therapy should the individual culture results indicate full susceptibility to the drug. Choices for intravenous antibiotics include vancomycin and gentamicin, both of which have excellent efficacy against CA-MRSA. Antibiograms are typically available from area hospitals or academic centers and can be valuable guides in determining the community physician's choice in empiric antibiotic therapy.

One pressing question concerning antibiotic therapy is whether or not consistent empiric use of an agent to which CA-MRSA is susceptible will lead to the development of resistance to that agent. This does not appear to be the case. In at least one academic center, the consistent empiric use of clindamycin as a first line therapy for CA-MRSA did not alter the proportion of clindamycin resistance over 2 years (98% vs. 97%) ***(22)***.

Surgical Management

Abscesses are traditionally treated with incision and drainage (I&D), with or without the concomitant use of antibiotics. Studies that included patients who were given placebo or ineffective antibiotics after incision and drainage demonstrate that high rates of cure are achieved regardless of effective antibiotic treatment ***(23,24)***. The only factor that seems to predict failure of I&D alone is abscess size greater than 5 cm. Demographic, comorbidities, and other abscess parameters are poor predictors of failure ***(23)***. The average hospital stay after I&D is 2–3 days ***(23)***.

Treatment Algorithm

With the above caveats in mind, the following treatment algorithm for CA-MRSA infections of the head and neck is proposed. Given the significant symptomatic overlap between staphylococcal and nonstaphylococcal infection lymphadenitis, initial empiric therapy should be directed at both types of infection. Clindamycin is an appropriate choice of therapy for this purpose. In addition, trimethoprim-sulfamethoxazole provides excellent coverage and may be useful in areas where clindamycin-resistant MRSA is prevalent. Children with neck lymphadenopathy and high fever with evidence of a phlegmon on imaging should be admitted for intravenous therapy. A failure to improve within 48 h warrants surgical treatment. Otolaryngologic consultation for airway evaluation and surgical intervention can be made earlier at the discretion of the admitting team. Contrast-enhanced CT may help differentiate abscess from lymphadenitis or phlegmon and is important for surgical planning in order to ensure that multiple loculations or occult abscesses are surgically drained (See Figs. 1 and 2). However, given the small but apparently real risk of malignancy associated with high-resolution CT of the head and neck *(25)*, the decision for CT may be reserved for those patients who may present with a possible deep space abscess and when the physical findings of erythema, pain, and fluctuance are not obvious. Ultrasound is a good alternative for patients that present with superficial or lateral neck lymphadenitis. Abscesses larger than 5 cm are likely to require both I&D and a longer course of antibiotic therapy. The treatment of systemic MRSA illness, pneumonia, or sepsis requires intravenous antibiotic therapy and intensive care unit support, a full discussion of which is beyond the scope of this chapter.

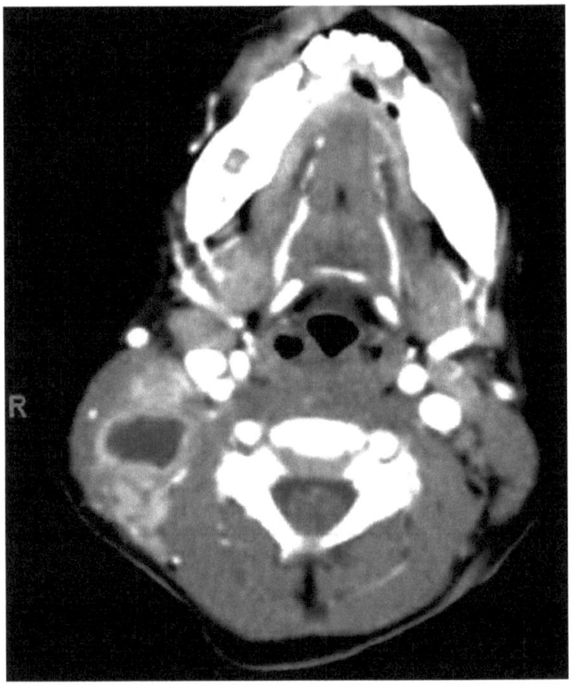

Fig. 1 Axial CT scan with contrast with posterior neck ring enhancing fluid collection secondary to MRSA infection

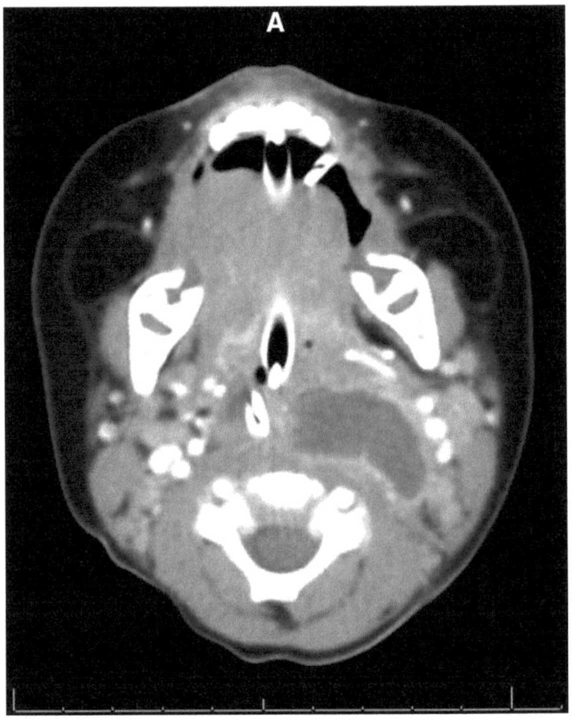

Fig. 2 Axial CT scan with contrast with showing a retropharyngeal abscess in a 10 month old that grew MRSA in cultures

Future Directions

Currently vancomycin is effective against virtually all MRSA strains. Thankfully reports of vancomycin-resistant *Staphylococcus aureus* (VRSA) are rare with only seven cases reported in the United States between 2002 and 2006 *(26)*. Nonetheless, the emergence of complete penicillin resistance, within a decade of its introduction into clinical practice, is a testament to the adaptive power of *S. aureus*. Consequently the threat of widespread vancomycin-resistant *S. aureus* is one that looms ever present in the collective conscious of the medical community. Accordingly, a number of new antibiotics have been developed and are in limited use against MRSA *(27)*. These antibiotics include quinopristin-dalfopristin (Synercid®), linezolid (Zyvox®), daptomycin (Cubicin®), and tigecycline (Tygacil®). With the exception of tigecycline, an advanced member of the tetracycline family, all these antibiotics possess unique mechanisms of action, which bodes well for their combined effectiveness over time as well as for the possibility of improvements with subsequent generations. Even more antibiotics effective against MRSA are in early clinical trials and new fascinating methods of drug discovery, including the mining of ancient medicinal texts *(28,29)*, are being employed in the discovery of new agents.

In addition to the development of new antimicrobial drugs, efforts have also been directed toward the development of antistaphylococcal vaccines. Two phase III trials, one of a staphylococcal capsular vaccine in hemodialysis patients *(30)* and one of antistaphylococcal immunoglobulin infusion in neonates *(31)*, have, however, failed to demonstrate a meaningful reduction in the rates of *S. aureus* infection. Further work including multiple doses and additional antigen combinations may yet yield more effective and substantial gains in the arena of vaccine development.

References

1. Guss J, Kazahaya K. Antibiotic-resistant Staphylococcus aureus in community-acquired pediatric neck abscesses. International Journal of Pediatric Otorhinolaryngology 2007;71(6):943–8.
2. Ossowski K, Chun RH, Suskind D, Baroody FM. Increased isolation of methicillin-resistant Staphylococcus aureus in pediatric head and neck abscesses. Archives of Otolaryngology-Head & Neck Surgery 2006;132(11):1176–81.
3. Thomason TS, Brenski A, McClay J, Ehmer D. The rising incidence of methicillin-resistant Staphylococcus aureus in pediatric neck abscesses. Otolaryngology and Head and Neck Surgery 2007;137(3):459–64.
4. Kaplan SL. Community-acquired methicillin-resistant Staphylococcus aureus infections in children. Seminars in Pediatric Infectious Diseases 2006;17(3):113–9.
5. Creech CB, 2nd, Kernodle DS, Alsentzer A, Wilson C, Edwards KM. Increasing rates of nasal carriage of methicillin-resistant Staphylococcus aureus in healthy children. The Pediatric Infectious Disease Journal 2005;24(7):617–21.
6. Daum RS. Clinical practice. Skin and soft-tissue infections caused by methicillin-resistant Staphylococcus aureus. The New England Journal of Medicine 2007;357(4):380–90.
7. Coticchia JM, Getnick GS, Yun RD, Arnold JE. Age-, site-, and time-specific differences in pediatric deep neck abscesses. Archives of Otolaryngology-Head & Neck Surgery 2004; 130(2):201–7.
8. Castaldo ET, Yang EY. Severe sepsis attributable to community-associated methicillin-resistant Staphylococcus aureus: an emerging fatal problem. The American Surgeon 2007;73(7):684–7; discussion 7–8.
9. Gonzalez BE, Martinez-Aguilar G, Hulten KG, et al. Severe Staphylococcal sepsis in adolescents in the era of community-acquired methicillin-resistant Staphylococcus aureus. Pediatrics 2005;115(3):642–8.
10. Malouin F, Bryan LE. Modification of penicillin-binding proteins as mechanisms of beta-lactam resistance. Antimicrobial Agents and Chemotherapy 1986;30(1):1–5.
11. de Lencastre H, Oliveira D, Tomasz A. Antibiotic resistant Staphylococcus aureus: a paradigm of adaptive power. Current Opinion in Microbiology 2007;10(5):428–35.
12. Moran GJ, Krishnadasan A, Gorwitz RJ, et al. Methicillin-resistant S. aureus infections among patients in the emergency department. The New England Journal of Medicine 2006;355(7):666–74.
13. Nygaard TK, DeLeo FR, Voyich JM. Community-associated methicillin-resistant Staphylococcus aureus skin infections: advances toward identifying the key virulence factors. Current Opinion in Infectious Diseases 2008;21(2):147–52.
14. Klevens RM, Morrison MA, Nadle J, et al. Invasive methicillin-resistant Staphylococcus aureus infections in the United States. JAMA 2007;298(15):1763–71.
15. Diep BA, Gill SR, Chang RF, Phan TH, Chen JH, Davidson MG, Lin F, Lin J, Carleton HA, Mongodin EF, Sensabaugh GF, Perdreau-Remington F. Complete genome sequence of USA300, an epidemic clone of community-acquired meticillin-resistant Staphylococcus aureus. Lancet 2006;367: 731–9.
16. Strategies for clinical management of MRSA in the community: Summary of an experts' meeting convened by the Centers for Disease Control and Prevention, 2006 (accessed at http://www.cdc.gov/ncidod/dhqp/ar_mrsa_ca.html).
17. Huskins WC. Interventions to prevent transmission of antimicrobial-resistant bacteria in the intensive care unit. Current Opinion in Critical Care 2007;13(5):572–7.
18. Le J, Lieberman JM. Management of community-associated methicillin-resistant Staphylococcus aureus infections in children. Pharmacotherapy 2006;26(12):1758–70.
19. Marcinak JF, Frank AL. Treatment of community-acquired methicillin-resistant Staphylococcus aureus in children. Current Opinion in Infectious Diseases 2003;16(3):265–9.
20. Buescher ES. Community-acquired methicillin-resistant Staphylococcus aureus in pediatrics. Current Opinion in Pediatrics 2005;17(1):67–70.
21. Siberry GK, Tekle T, Carroll K, Dick J. Failure of clindamycin treatment of methicillin-resistant Staphylococcus

aureus expressing inducible clindamycin resistance in vitro. Clinical Infectious Diseases 2003;37(9):1257–60.
22. Szczesiul JM, Shermock KM, Murtaza UI, Siberry GK. No decrease in clindamycin susceptibility despite increased use of clindamycin for pediatric community-associated methicillin-resistant Staphylococcus aureus skin infections. The Pediatric Infectious Disease Journal 2007;26(9):852–4.
23. Lee MC, Rios AM, Aten MF, et al. Management and outcome of children with skin and soft tissue abscesses caused by community-acquired methicillin-resistant Staphylococcus aureus. The Pediatric Infectious Disease Journal 2004;23(2):123–7.
24. Rajendran PM, Young D, Maurer T, et al. Randomized, double-blind, placebo-controlled trial of cephalexin for treatment of uncomplicated skin abscesses in a population at risk for community-acquired methicillin-resistant Staphylococcus aureus infection. Antimicrobial Agents and Chemotherapy 2007;51(11):4044–8.
25. Rice HE, Frush DP, Farmer D, Waldhausen JH. Review of radiation risks from computed tomography: essentials for the pediatric surgeon. Journal of Pediatric Surgery 2007;42(4):603–7.
26. Sievert DM, Rudrik JT, Patel JB, McDonald LC, Wilkins MJ, Hageman JC. Vancomycin-resistant Staphylococcus aureus in the United States, 2002–2006. Clinical Infectious Diseases 2008;46(5):668–74.
27. Lentino JR, Narita M, Yu VL. New antimicrobial agents as therapy for resistant gram-positive cocci. European Journal of Clinical & Microbiology Infectious Diseases 2008;27(1):3–15.
28. Buenz EJ, Bauer BA, Johnson HE, et al. Searching historical herbal texts for potential new drugs. British Medical Journal (Clinical Research ed.) 2006;333(7582):1314–15.
29. Buenz EJ, Bauer BA, Schnepple DJ, Wahner-Roedler DL, Vandell AG, Howe CL. A randomized Phase I study of Atuna racemosa: a potential new anti-MRSA natural product extract. Journal of Ethnopharmacology 2007;114(3):371–6.
30. Shinefield H, Black S, Fattom A, et al. Use of a Staphylococcus aureus conjugate vaccine in patients receiving hemodialysis. The New England Journal of Medicine 2002; 346(7):491–6.
31. Capparelli EV, Bloom BT, Kueser TJ, et al. Multicenter study to determine antibody concentrations and assess the safety of administration of INH-A21, a donor-selected human Staphylococcal immune globulin, in low-birth-weight infants. Antimicrobial Agents and Chemotherapy 2005; 49(10):4121–7.

Polysomnography in Children

Cindy Jon

Key Points

- Polysomnography is the gold standard test for the diagnosis of sleep-disordered breathing (SDB) in children.
- Pediatric polysomnography should be performed in a sleep laboratory equipped for children and staffed by qualified personnel following the American Thoracic Society (ATS) standards for testing.
- In 2007, the American Academy of Sleep Medicine (AASM) standardized scoring of sleep stages and definitions for sleep-disordered breathing events in children.
- Controversy remains regarding preoperative screening for SDB in normal children undergoing adenotonsillectomy (T&A).
- All children with risk factors for respiratory complications postoperatively should have a baseline polysomnogram before T&A.
- Children requiring positive airway pressure therapy must have a baseline and a titration polysomnogram to evaluate therapeutic effect.
- Alternative types of sleep studies with variable channels have not been fully validated in children.

Keywords: Polysomnography • Children • Sleep stage scoring • Sleep-disordered breathing • Adenotonsillectomy • Continuous positive airway pressure • Portable monitoring • Decannulation

C. Jon
Division of Pediatric Pulmonary and Critical Care Medicine, Department of Pediatrics, University of Texas Health Science Center at Houston, Houston, TX, USA
e-mail: Cindy.Jon@uth.tmc.edu

Introduction to Polysomnography

Sleep-disordered breathing (SDB) has been associated with significant cardiovascular, neurologic, and metabolic abnormalities in adults. The impact of recurrent sleep fragmentation and hypoxemia from SDB may be more deleterious in a developing child. In children, obstructive sleep apnea (OSA) has been associated with pulmonary hypertension, failure to thrive, and possibly systemic hypertension. Recent literature has linked OSA with decreased intellectual function and worsening behavioral problems, such as hyperactivity and aggressive behaviors *(1,2)*.

Polysomnography identifies and quantifies the type and severity of SDB. Various physiologic measurements are obtained during polysomnography that provide an objective measure of sleep disturbance. Polysomnography is the "gold standard" for the diagnosis of a sleep disturbance due to respiratory abnormalities and sleep-related movement disorders.

Indications for Polysomnography in Children

SDB usually manifests as restless sleep, snoring, mouth breathing, gasping during sleep, and frequent awakenings. Clinical history may not be able to differentiate between primary benign snoring and OSA. The American Academy of Pediatrics (AAP) published a clinical practice guideline which recommended screening all children for snoring *(3,4)*. Snoring alone is not associated with hypoxemia, hypercapnia, sleep disruption, or daytime symptoms. However, OSA may lead to significant, nocturnal hemodynamic changes

R.B. Mitchell and K.D. Pereira (eds.), *Pediatric Otolaryngology for the Clinician,*
DOI: 10.1007/978-1-60327-127-1_5, © Humana Press, a part of Springer Science + Business Media, LLC 2009

and potentially harmful neurocognitive outcomes. Polysomnography can differentiate between benign and pathologic SDB *(5)*.

Indications to perform a polysomnogram on children are listed below *(1)*:

- To differentiate primary snoring from other SDB that may require intervention
- To ascertain if SDB is contributing to a disturbed sleep pattern, excessive hypersomnia, pulmonary hypertension, failure to thrive, or polycythemia
- To determine if surgical intervention is warranted (i.e., T&A) and to determine the required intensity of postoperative monitoring
- To determine the etiology of persistent snoring or symptoms of SDB after T&A
- To recognize SDB in children who have laryngomalacia, pulmonary hypertension, failure to thrive, or worse symptoms at night
- To titrate positive airway pressure therapy to alleviate SDB
- To evaluate children with sickle cell disease who have SDB symptoms or frequent veno-occlusive crises
- To determine the effectiveness of weight loss on the severity of SDB

In addition, polysomnography identifies non-SDB-related sources of restless sleep or excessive daytime somnolence. Children who are considered high risk for SDB include patients with adenotonsillar hypertrophy, neuromuscular disease, obesity, genetic syndromes, and craniofacial abnormalities. Other children may require prolonged cardiopulmonary monitoring, such as patients with bronchopulmonary dysplasia with recent adjustment in oxygen therapy or progressive daytime hypoxemia in cystic fibrosis. Polysomnography may be deferred in children with obvious airway obstruction during sleep that is witnessed by the medical staff or evident on audiovisual recording to allow for immediate intervention *(1)*.

Polysomnography

During overnight polysomnography, every effort should be made to approximate the child's usual sleep pattern. The testing facility should be child friendly and provide appropriate accommodations for the accompanying parent. The medical staff should be skilled in working with children and certified in Basic Life Support and Pediatric Advanced Life Support. The use of sedatives or sleep deprivation prior to testing is discouraged since it may artificially worsen SDB *(1)*.

The American Thoracic Society (ATS) published standards for cardiopulmonary sleep studies in children in 1996 *(1)*. The consensus statement recommends simultaneous measurement of various physiologic Parameters in a sleep laboratory to include (Fig. 1):

- respiratory movement and effort by plethysmography (RIP), piezo crystal belts, or esophageal manometry
- airflow by nasal pressure, oral and nasal thermistor, or less commonly pneumotachograph
- ventilation by end tidal or transcutaneous CO_2 monitoring
- oxygenation by pulse oximetry
- cardiac rhythm by EKG
- sleep staging by EEG monitoring
- motor activity of the limbs, eyes, and jaw by noninvasive EMG monitoring
- audiovisual recording by video and microphone

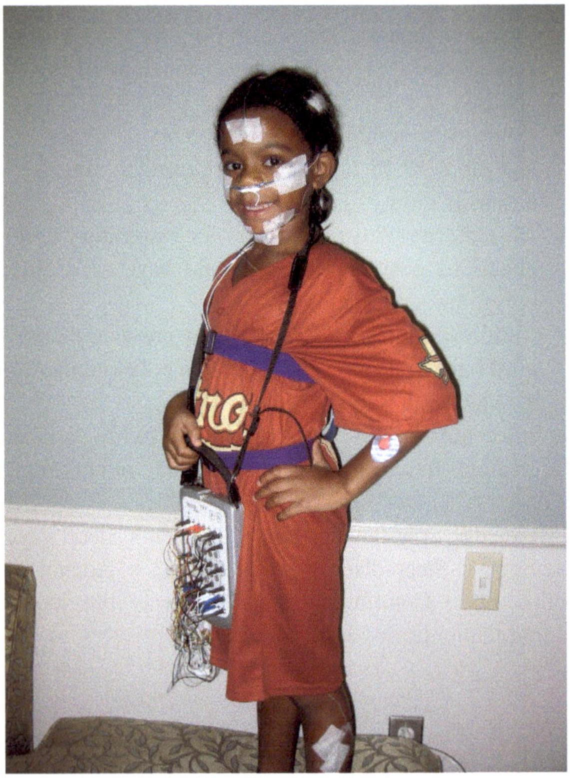

Fig. 1 A child undergoing a polysomnogram with multiple channels, including electroencephalogram, electro-oculogram, nasal and oral airflow detectors, respiratory effort belts, pulse oximetry probe, chin and anterior tibialis electromyograms, and snoring microphone

Respiratory movements are detected by sensor belts which are wrapped around the chest and abdomen. The most common types of belts are the respiratory inductive plethysmography (RIP) or piezo crystal belts *(6)*. RIP belts may detect paradoxical chest and abdomen movements which are suggestive of upper airway obstruction. The most sensitive method to detect respiratory effort is by esophageal manometry, which measures increasing negative esophageal and thus intrathoracic pressures with increasing airway obstruction. Most sleep laboratories do not offer esophageal manometry *(7)*.

Airflow may be measured by nasal pressure transduction and/or oral and nasal thermistor temperature probes. Although the reference standard for measuring airflow is pneumotachograph, the tight-fitting facemask may be too uncomfortable for the patient and it may disrupt sleep. Instead, nasal pressure prongs are well tolerated and have been validated in providing semiquantitative data regarding the degree of airflow limitation *(8,9)*. Oral and nasal thermistor provides a qualitative detection of both nose and mouth air movement based on temperature changes.

Ventilation assessment is especially important in children. Most children with SDB do not have discrete episodic cessation in breathing. Instead, they typically have prolonged partial upper airway obstruction resulting in hypercapnia. Marcus et al. measured the critical closing pressure in the upper airway of normal children and adults. The adult pharyngeal airway closed at a discrete subatmospheric pressure resulting in cessation of airflow. However, children were able to maintain upper airway patency despite increasing negative pressures, which suggests age-dependent differences in neuromotor upper airway tone *(10)*.

Most sleep laboratories detect hypoventilation with end tidal CO_2 ($ETCO_2$) monitoring which may be combined with the nasal pressure detectors. Although $ETCO_2$ detection is convenient and well tolerated, it may not be reliable if the signal does not display an adequate plateau to establish a true end exhalation CO_2 sample. In addition, concomitant use of oxygen by nasal cannula or positive airway pressure may interfere with adequate $ETCO_2$ detection *(7)*. The recorded $ETCO_2$ may underestimate arterial CO_2 ($PaCO_2$) by as much as 10–15 mmHg when a patient is asleep and breathing room air.

Trancutaneous CO_2 ($TcCO_2$) monitors detect CO_2 on the skin surface. The heating unit of the $TcCO_2$ probe increases the local skin temperature to enhance CO_2 diffusion from vasculature in the upper dermis. The probe should be placed over an area where there is high capillary density and decreased skin thickness, such as the forearm or chest. Thermal injury may occur if the $TcCO_2$-heated probe is used for a prolonged period of time. Conventionally, $TcCO_2$ monitoring should be transitioned between different sites every 2–4 h. In general, $TcCO_2$ overestimates $PaCO_2$ which may be partly due to the increased local skin metabolism from the heating unit. Although $TcCO_2$ measurements are simultaneously obtained with other physiologic readings, there is a 1–2-min delay in recording hemodynamic changes from onset of the event. This may be due to the delay in blood flow to the skin from the time of the event and specific type of probe used *(11,12)*.

Oxygenation saturation (SaO_2) is measured by pulse oximetry. Optimal placement of the SaO_2 probe is necessary to obtain an adequate signal and waveform and to decrease artifact, such as motion and low perfusion *(12)*. The recommended signal averaging time is 3 s or less *(9)*. Electrocardiogram (EKG) measures heart rate and rhythm. In children dysrhythmias are less prevalent than in adults. Bradycardia, usually due to hypoxemia, may be seen *(12–14)*.

Electroencephalogram (EEG) is included to determine sleep stages. The recommended recording montage is C3 and C4 referenced to an auricular lead. Occipital leads may be added. This configuration optimizes detection of sleep stage-specific EEG changes. This derivation does not replace conventional EEG for diagnosis of neurologic diseases *(1,12)*.

Electromyogram (EMG) detects motor activity. Noninvasive EMG leads are placed on the chin to assist in sleep stage identification and over the anterior tibialis to detect leg movement. Sleep-related movement disorders, such as periodic limb movement disorder, bruxism, and rhythmic movement disorder, may be identified during polysomnography *(13)*.

Electro-oculogram (EOG) measures eye movement necessary to determine rapid eye movement (REM) sleep. One lead is placed lateral to the outer canthus of each eye to detect movement *(1)*.

Audiovisual recording during polysomnography allows the medical staff to correlate recorded data with visual or auditory events. It is particularly helpful in distinguishing wakefulness from sleep and sleep-related movement disorders. Home audiovisual recordings for screening SDB may be helpful if obvious

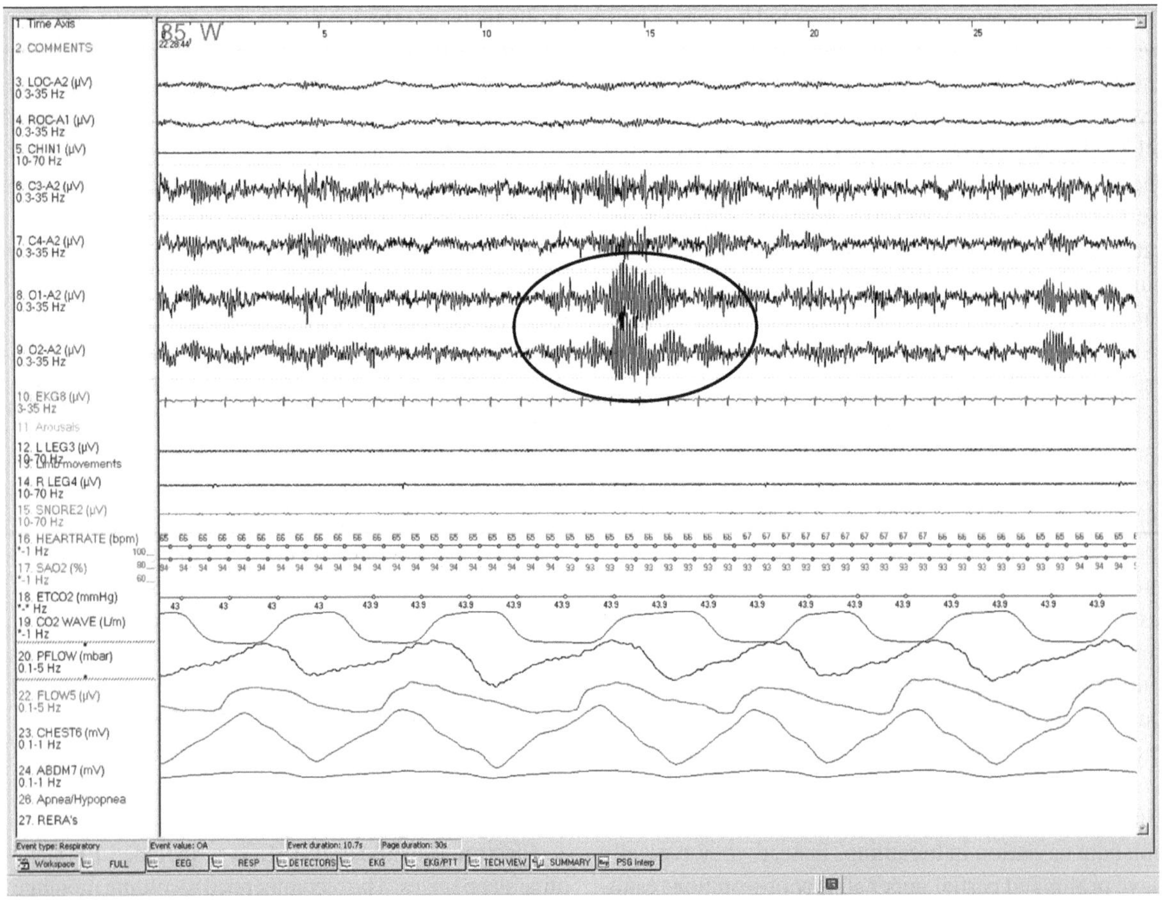

Fig. 2 Wakefulness with eyes closed. Dominant posterior or alpha rhythm (*oval*) is predominantly seen on the occipital EEG leads (O1-A2 and O2-A1)

events occur, especially apneas or periods when the child is struggling to breathe. However, it has poor predictive value, if it is negative *(4)*.

Scoring a Polysomnogram

All polysomnograms performed on children should be scored using pediatric scoring criteria. Applying adult parameters may underestimate the presence and severity of SDB. Depending on independent sleep laboratory standards, polysomnogram performed in children between 13 and 18 years of age may be scored using adult criteria *(9)*.

In 2007, the American Academy of Sleep Medicine (AASM) published a new manual to score sleep stages and events for patients who are 2 months postterm or older. This revised the previous parameters set by Rechtschaffen and Kales and standardized the scoring for respiratory events that were previously poorly defined in children *(15)*. This section summarizes the general features of each sleep stage and respiratory events. The specific details may be found in The AASM Manual for the Scoring of Sleep and Associated Events *(9)*.

Polysomnograms are scored by epochs which are usually 30 s in length. Sleep stage is identified when greater than 50% of the epoch has the characteristic EEG changes.

Sleep Stage Scoring (9)

- W = Wakefulness is characterized by increased chin EMG tone, fast moving and blinking eyes, and alpha or dominant posterior rhythm EEG activity (Fig. 2).
- N1 = The first stage of sleep represents the transition of wakefulness to sleep. Low-amplitude and mixed-frequency EEG activity is noted. Slow rolling eye movements may be seen (Fig. 3).

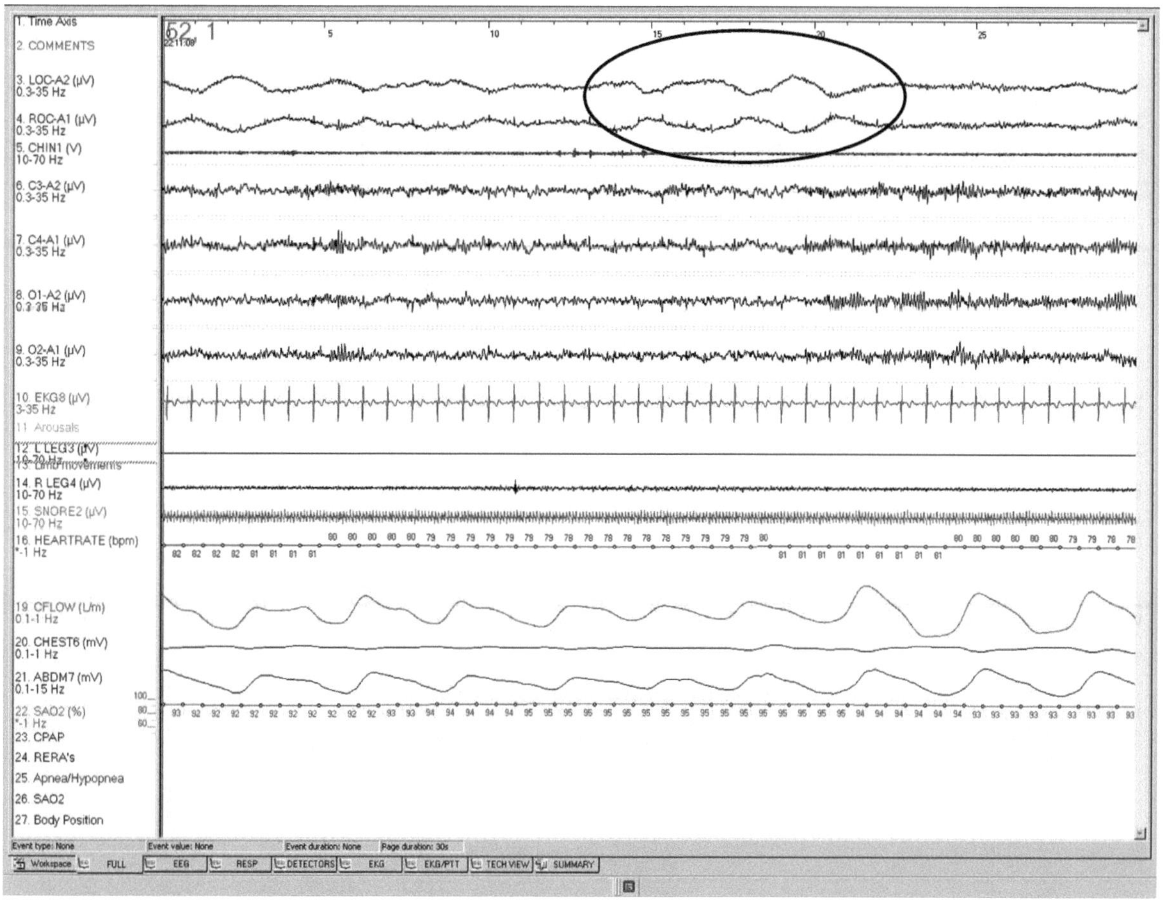

Fig. 3 Sleep stage N1. Mixed-frequency low-amplitude EEG. Slow rolling eye (*oval*) movements may be seen on LOC-A2 and ROC-A1 channels

- N2 = The second stage of sleep is characterized by K complexes and sleep spindles. K complexes are bipolar sharp waves that last for at least 0.5 s. Sleep spindles are distinct episodic high-frequency (11–16 Hz) waveforms. Most patients spend approximately half the total sleep time in this stage, especially older children and adults (Fig. 4).
- N3 = The third sleep stage represents slow wave sleep. It is identified when there are low-frequency (0.5–2 Hz) and high-amplitude (>75 mV) waveforms for greater than 20% of the epoch. This stage combines sleep stages 3 and 4 previously described by Rechtschaffen and Kales (Fig. 5).
- N = This stage represents non-REM sleep in infants who do not have identifiable EEG characteristics to distinguish between N1, N2, or N3.
- R = REM sleep is characterized by low voltage and mixed-frequency EEG pattern with rapid eye movements on EOG leads and low chin EMG tone. In general, the percent of stage R sleep decreases with advancing age in children without SDB (Fig. 6).

Respiratory Events (9)

- Obstructive apnea (OA) = An OA is scored if its duration is at least two respiratory cycles, the airflow signal is decreased by greater than 90% from baseline, and there is persistent or increased respiratory effort. The apnea event is measured from the end of the last normal breath to the start of first breath that is comparable to baseline. In children, oxygen desaturation is not required to score this event (Fig. 7).

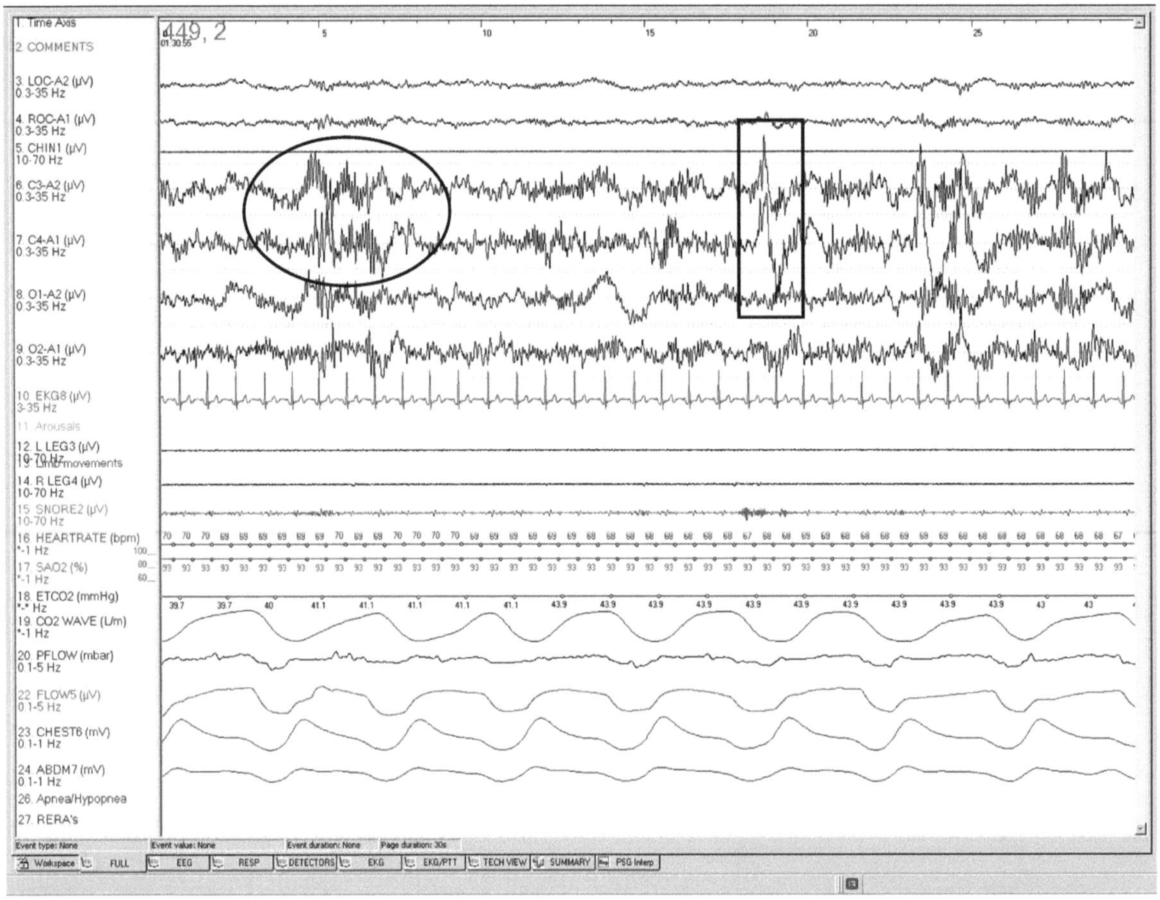

Fig. 4 Sleep stage N2. Low-amplitude high-frequency EEG with sleep spindles (*oval*) and intermittent K complexes (*box*) are characteristic of N2 sleep stage

- Mixed apnea (MA) = Scoring an MA has similar criteria to OA, except that there is absent respiratory effort at the beginning of the event followed by increasing respiratory movements by the end of the event.
- Hypopnea (H) = A hypopnea occurs when there is decreased but not absent airflow with persistent respiratory effort. A hypopnea event occurs when there is at least 50% decrease in nasal pressure amplitude which lasts at least 90% of the designated event. Hypopneas last for two respiratory cycles or longer and are associated with an arousal, awakening, or a desaturation of 3% or greater. All of the criteria must be met for scoring a hypopnea in children. Hypopnea may be diagnosed as obstructive, central, or mixed only if there is accompanying esophageal manometry or calibrated RIP (Fig. 8).
- Central apnea (CA) = A CA is scored if there is absent airflow and respiratory effort for at least 20 s or at least two respiratory cycles associated with an arousal, awakening, or desaturation of 3% or greater. If a CA event occurs after a snore, arousal, sigh, or respiratory event, it is not scored unless the CA leads to an arousal, awakening, or desaturation (Fig. 9).
- Respiratory effort-related arousal (RERA) = RERA was first described using esophageal manometry ***(16)***. However, due to the invasiveness of the esophageal manometer, its use has not been universally adopted by majority of the sleep laboratories. Nasal pressure probes may be used as an alternative for detecting RERA events since it provides semiquantitative measurement. When using esophageal manometry, a RERA event may be scored if there is progressively increased respiratory effort. When

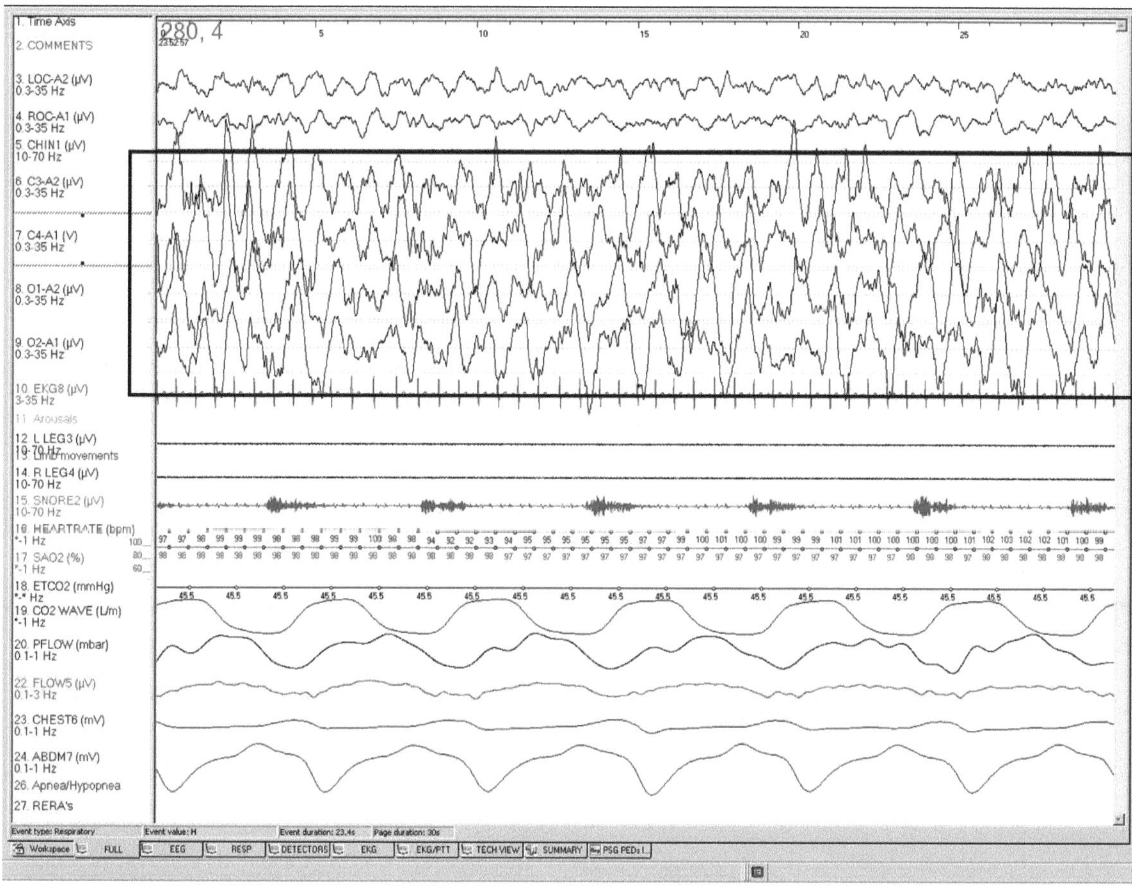

Fig. 5 Sleep stage N3. High-amplitude low-frequency EEG waveforms for at least 20% of the epoch

nasal pressure monitoring is used, a RERA event may be scored if there is a 50% or greater fall in amplitude of a flattened nasal pressure waveform when compared to baseline. In both cases, the respiratory event must last for at least two respiratory cycles and be associated with snoring, noisy breathing, increased $ETCO_2$, or visual evidence of increased respiratory effort.

- Periodic breathing (PB) = PB is primarily seen in premature infants. It is scored if there are more than three central apnea episodes separated by 20 s or less of normal breathing. Each central apnea event lasts more than 3 s in duration.
- Arousal (A) = An arousal is a distinct EEG change from baseline for at least 3 s which is preceded by at least 10 s of sleep at any stage. During REM sleep, these EEG changes must be accompanied by increased chin EMG tone for at least 1 s.

Sleep-Disordered Breathing

The culmination of the events results in designation of certain respiratory indices. The apnea index (AI) describes the number of apneas per hour of sleep. The apnea hypopnea index (AHI) indicates the number of apneas and hypopneas per hour of sleep. Respiratory disturbance index (RDI) describes all respiratory events per hour of sleep.

Based on normative data regarding respiratory events, healthy children do not have significant respiratory events during sleep. Based on a study of 50 normal children, the obstructive apnea index was 0.1 obstructive apnea per hour of sleep *(17)*. Due to the low incidence of obstructive sleep apnea, an obstructive apnea index of 1 or greater has been chosen to designate abnormality. However, the clinical

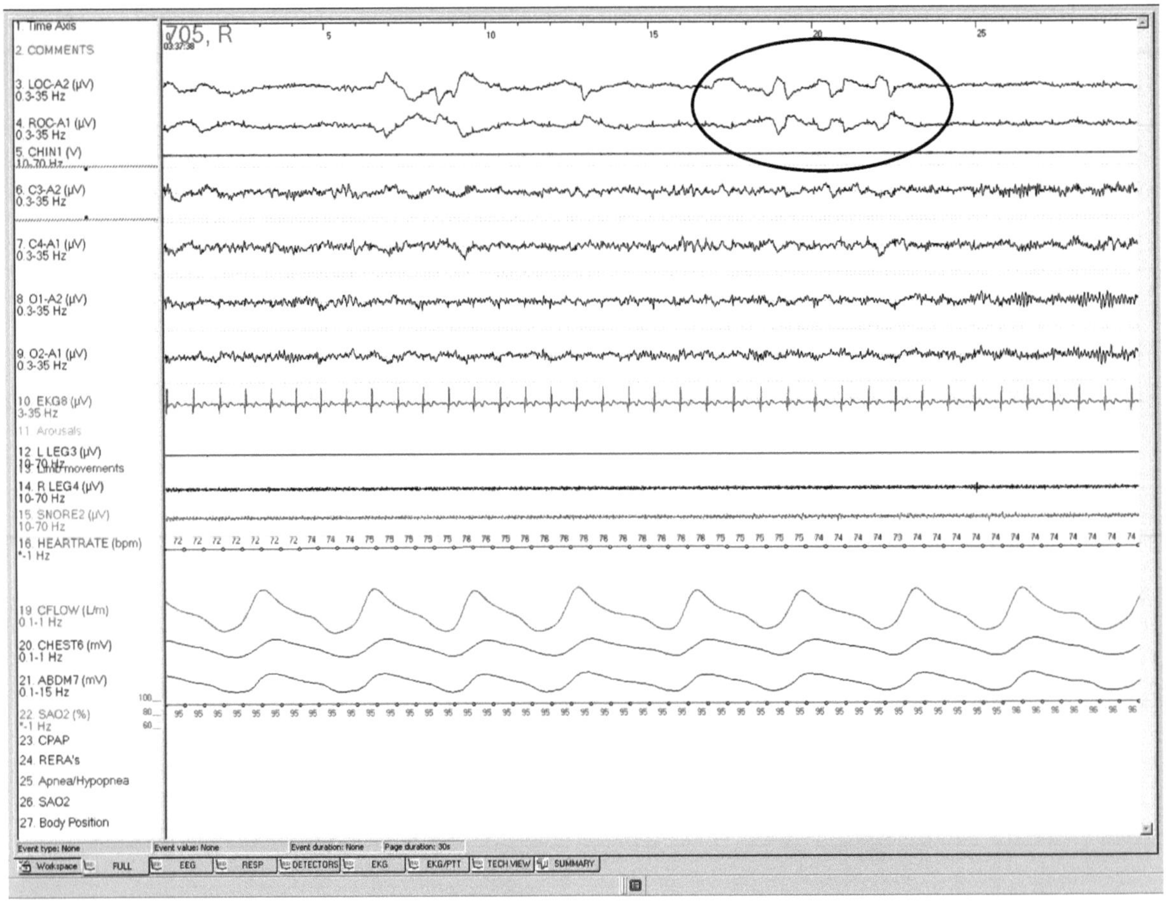

Fig. 6 Sleep stage R. High-frequency low-amplitude EEG waveform with occasional sawtooth configuration. Rapid eye movements (*oval*)

significance of this parameter has not been determined ***(18,19)***.

The following definitions for SDB disorders are based on current literature (Fig. 10).

Obstructive sleep apnea in children is diagnosed when all criteria from the International Classification of Sleep Disorders' definition are met ***(20)***.

(1) Snoring, labored breathing, and/or obstructed breathing is reported by the caregiver
(2) The caregiver reports one of the following: paradoxical inward chest movement upon inspiration, movement arousals, diaphoresis, neck hyperextension during sleep, behavioral changes (excessive daytime somnolence, hyperactivity, or aggressive behavior), slow growth rate, morning headaches, or secondary enuresis
(3) Polysomnogram records at least one respiratory event per hour of apneas and hypopneas
(4) Polysomnogram reveals one of the following:
    (a) Frequent arousals associated with increased respiratory effort, oxygen desaturation associated with apnea events, hypercapnia during sleep, or markedly negative esophageal pressure changes
    (b) Periods of hypercapnia and/or desaturation during sleep associated with snoring, Paradoxical inward chest movement during inspiration, and frequent arousal or markedly negative esophageal pressure swings
(5) No other disorder can explain these findings

Obstructive hypoventilation in children is diagnosed when $ETCO_2$ or $TcCO_2$ is elevated above 50 mmHg for greater than 25% of total sleep time ***(9)***.

Upper airway resistance syndrome (UARS) was initially identified in patients who had episodic

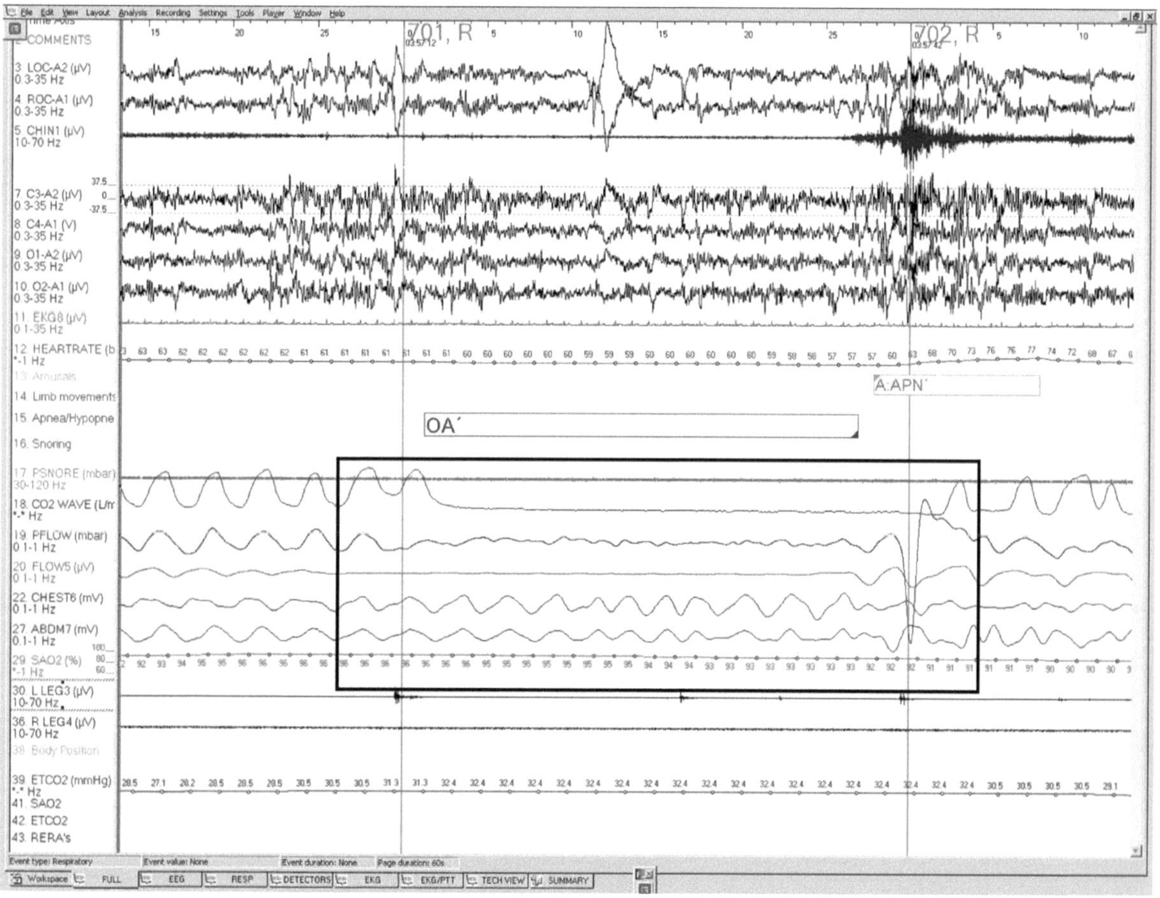

Fig. 7 Obstructive apnea resulting in no airflow in PFLOW and FLOW 5 channels with persistence of respiratory effort noted in CHEST6 and ABDM7 leads. Oxygen desaturation is noted but is not required for scoring an OA in children

increased negative esophageal pressures triggering an arousal from sleep. The hypersomnia due to sleep fragmentation from increased number of arousals resolved with positive airway pressure therapy. UARS in children is not clearly delineated *(16,21)*.

Primary snoring is defined as snoring that is not associated with oxygen desaturation, arousal, cardiac disturbance, insomnia, or hypersomnia *(5)*.

Central sleep apnea in children is defined as three or more events per hour of sleep *(1)*.

Positive Airway Pressure Therapy

Continuous positive airway pressure (CPAP) therapy is an option for children who are not surgical candidates or who have persistent symptoms despite T&A. If CPAP therapy is anticipated, a polysomnogram must be performed to ascertain the presence and degree of SDB. Unlike adults who have set parameters to determine the initiation of CPAP, there are no such standards in children. CPAP initiation is based on clinical judgment.

When the decision for CPAP therapy has been made, the patient should have a repeat polysomnogram for positive airway pressure titration. The goal of the titration study is to eliminate all or most SDB and restore adequate oxygenation and ventilation. The baseline study may be used to gauge the effectiveness the CPAP therapy. Transition to bilevel positive airway pressure (BiPAP) therapy may be done to improve patient comfort or hypoventilation disorders *(22)*.

The effectiveness of CPAP therapy in children has been established. Once CPAP has been initiated, close clinical monitoring is recommended to improve compliance and evaluate for persistent symptoms. A CPAP re-titration should be considered if there is significant weight change, worsening or development of new

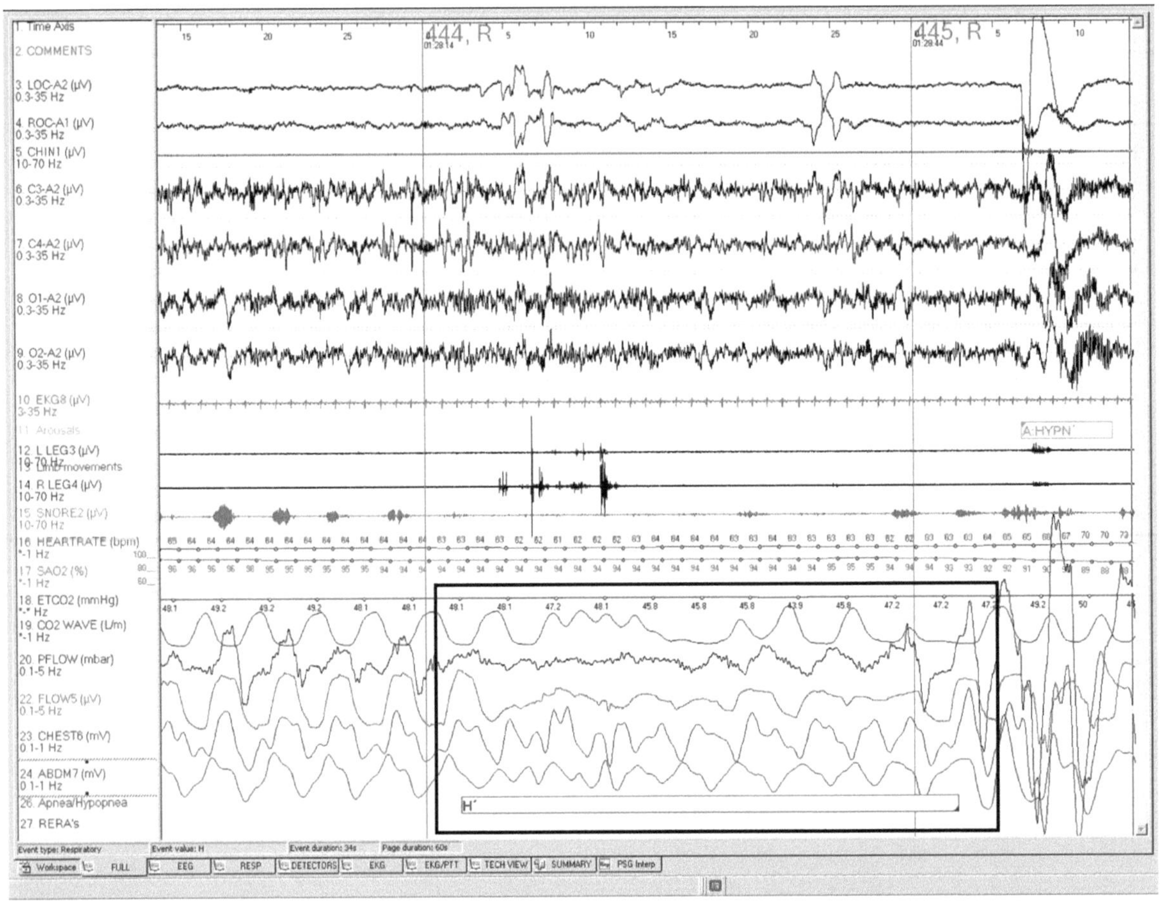

Fig. 8 Hyopnea is characterized by decreased airflow in channels PFLOW and FLOW5 from baseline with persistence of respiratory effort in the CHEST6 and ABDM7 leads that is associated with an arousal, awakening, and/or oxygen desaturation

symptoms, or significant growth. The periodicity of re-titration studies is individualized *(4)*.

As with any intervention, adverse effects may occur with prolonged CPAP use. Some of the potential complications include nasal dryness, epistaxis, skin ulceration, conjunctivitis, ear pain, sleep disruption, and midface hypoplasia. Careful fitting and addition of heated humidification may decrease the development of these effects and improve compliance with therapy *(23)*.

Until recently, positive airway pressure (PAP) therapy was not FDA approved to be used in children. Since there has been no equipment indicated for pediatric use, clinicians have fitted children with available small adult masks. In 2006, a specially designed mask and PAP machine system was FDA approved for children who are older than 7 years of age or more than 40 pounds with a diagnosis of OSA *(24)*.

Other Types of Sleep Studies

Abbreviated daytime polysomnography (ADP) or nap studies have been proposed as an alternative method of detecting SDB. A positive ADP study for SDB correlated well with overnight polysomnogram. However, if ADP did not identify SDB, the negative predictive value was as low at 17%. Therefore, ADP may be a useful screening tool if SDB is detected, but overnight polysomnography is required to confirm a negative ADP result. In addition, studies evaluating nap studies used chloral hydrate to induce naps during the daytime which may also affect upper airway tone. Circadian rhythm variations and possible lack of REM sleep detection during ADP may lead to poor correlation of results to overnight polysomnography and its tendency to underestimate SDB severity *(4,25,26)*.

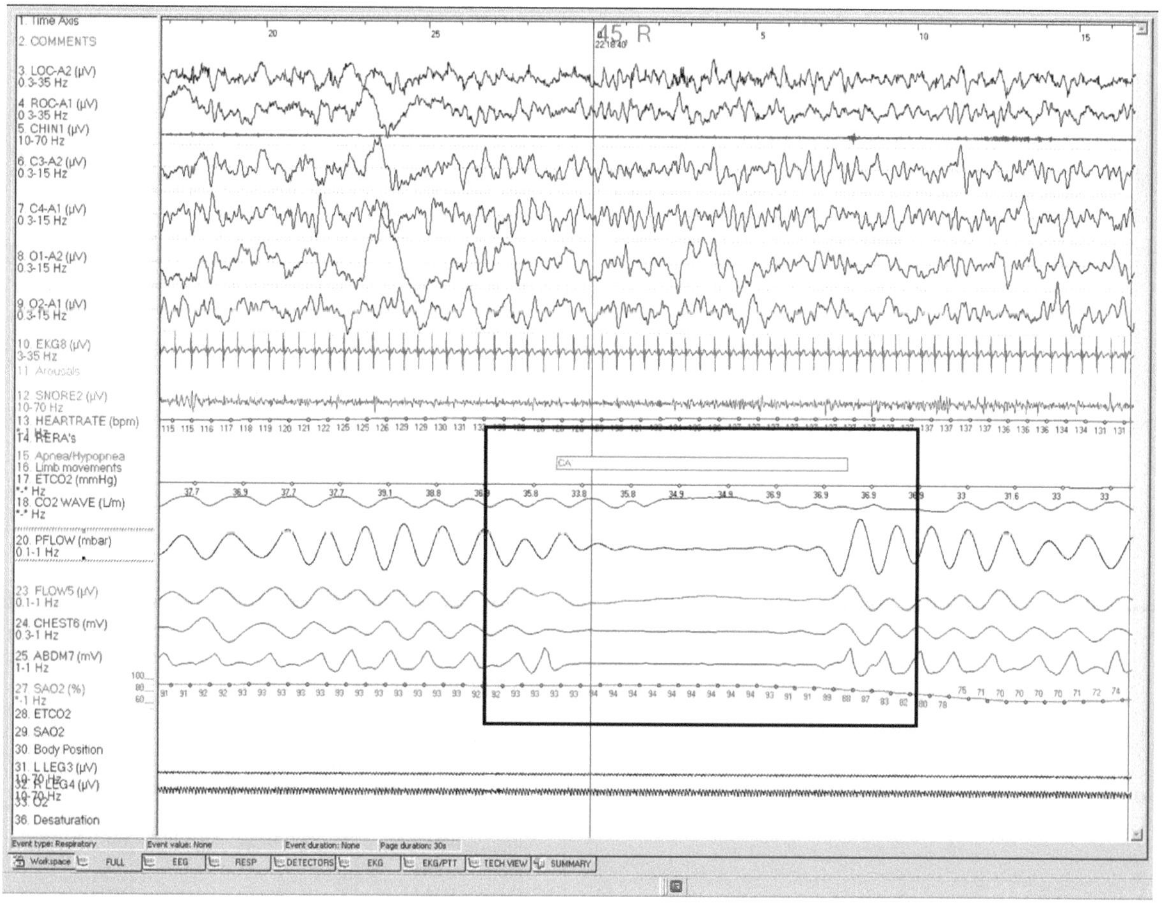

Fig. 9 Central apnea with absent airflow by PFLOW, FLOW5, and ETCO2 detection and absent effort by CHEST6, and ABDM7 belts

Practice parameters were published to standardize the types of portable sleep studies available. Four types of sleep studies have been distinguished. Type 1 polysomnography is an in-laboratory comprehensive study requiring at least seven channels and attendance of a qualified personnel. Type 2 studies are unattended polysomnograms that monitor at least seven channels. Type 3 portable monitoring usually requires four to seven channels. Type 4 analysis only has one to two channels which usually includes pulse oximetry *(27,28)*.

In children, few studies have compared the efficacy and accuracy of portable monitoring with in-laboratory polysomnography. Home studies had similar AHI, RDI, and desaturation indices, and equal or improved sleep efficiency and total sleep time when compared to polysomnography. None of the portable monitoring studies evaluated CO_2 monitoring which is important in identifying obstructive hypoventilation *(29–31)*.

Although portable monitoring may be a potential alternative method of evaluating SDB, the AAP recommends further testing to confirm the accuracy of portable monitoring with overnight polysomnogram *(32)*.

Limited data exist to compare overnight pulse oximetry with in-laboratory polysomnography in children. The positive predictive value can be as high as 97% for detection of OSA by pulse oximetry. However, a recent study revealed poor correlation between AHI by polysomnography and desaturation index by pulse oximetry. The disparity may be due in part to movement and poor detection of pulse waveform which resulted in data that were difficult to distinguish from true events. In addition, not all children have significant oxygen desaturation with SDB, such as UARS, obstructive hypoventilation, and less severe OSA *(32–34)*.

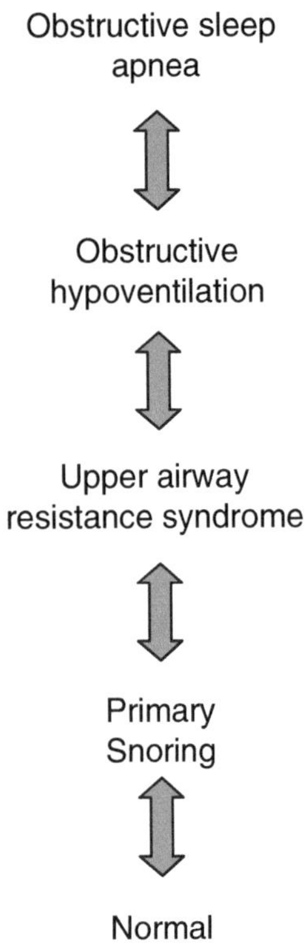

Fig. 10 Continuum of airway obstruction in sleep-disordered breathing

Role of Polysomnography in Tracheostomy Tube Decannulation

The decision for tracheostomy tube decannulation is primarily based on the clinical judgment of the child's general health, resolution of initial indication for tube placement, and endoscopic findings. Recently, tracheostomy tubes have been placed more for dynamic airway abnormalities, such as OSA and significant ventilatory control disorders. Conventional assessment of upper airway patency and tolerance of decannulation may not take into account the neuromotor changes that occur during sleep. Two studies evaluated the effectiveness of polysomnography in assessing readiness for decannulation and both confirmed that polysomnography provided additional data to facilitate the decision-making process *(35,36)*. Pre-decannulation polysomnography has therefore been increasingly used in the management of children with a tracheostomy.

References

1. American Thoracic Society, Official Statement. Standards and indications for cardiopulmonary sleep studies in children. Am J Respir Crit Care Med 1996;153:866–878.
2. Gozal D. Sleep-disordered breathing and school performance in children. Pediatrics 1998;101:616–620.
3. Carroll JL, McColley SA, Marcus CL, Curtis S, Loughlin GM. Inability of clinical history to distinguish primary snoring from obstructive sleep apnea syndrome in children. Chest 1995;108:610–618.
4. American Academy of Pediatrics, Section on Pediatric Pulmonology, Subcommittee on Obstructive Sleep Apnea Syndrome. Clinical practice guideline: diagnosis and management of childhood obstructive sleep apnea syndrome. Pediatrics 2002;109:704–712.
5. American Academy of Sleep Medicine. The International Classification of Sleep Disorders, Revised. Diagnostic and Coding Manual. Chicago, IL: American Academy of Sleep Medicine, 2001.
6. Adams JA, Zabaleta IA, Stroh D, Johnson P, Sackner MA. Tidal volume measurements in newborns using respiratory inductive plethysmography. Am Rev Respir Dis 1993;148(3):585–588.
7. American Academy of Sleep Medicine Task Force Report. Sleep-related breathing disorders in adults: recommendations for syndrome definition and measurement techniques in clinical research. Sleep 1999;22(5):667–689.
8. Heitman SJ, Atkar RS, Hajduk EA, Wanner RA, Flemons WW. Validation of nasal pressure for the identification of apneas/hypopneas during sleep. Am J Respir Crit Care Med 2002;166:386–391.
9. The AASM Manual for the Scoring of Sleep and Associated Events, Rules, Terminology and Technical Specifications, 2007.
10. Marcus CL, Lutz J, Hamer A, Smith PL, Schwartz A. Developmental changes in response to subatmospheric pressure loading of the upper airway. J Appl Physiol 1999;87:626–633.
11. Sanders MH, Kern NB, Costantino JP, Stiller RA, Strollo PJ, Studnicki KA, Coates JA, Richards TJ. Accuracy of end-tidal and transcutaneous PCO_2 monitoring during sleep. Chest 1994;106:472–483.
12. Principles and Practice of Sleep Medicine, 4th edition. In: Kryger MH, Roth T, Dement WC. Philadelphia: Elsevier, 2005.
13. Principles and Practice of Pediatric Sleep Medicine. In: Sheldon SH, Ferber R, Kryger MH. Philadelphia: Elsevier, 2005.
14. D'Andrea LA, Rosen CL, Haddad GG. Severe hypoxemia in children with upper airway obstruction during sleep does not lead to significant changes in heart rate. Pediatr Pulmonol 1993;16:362–369.
15. Rechtschaffen A, Kales A. A manual of standardized terminology, techniques and scoring system for sleep stages of human subjects. Washington, DC: National Institutes of Health, 1968.
16. Guilleminault C, Stoohs R, Clerk A, Cetel M, Maistros P. A cause of excessive daytime sleepiness: the upper airway resistance syndrome. Chest 1993;104:781–787.

17. Marcus CL, Omlin KJ, Basinki DJ, Bailey SL, Rachal AB, Von Pechmann WS, Keens TG, Ward SL. Normal polysomnographic values for children and adolescents. Am Rev Respir Dis 1992;146:1235–1239.
18. American Thoracic Society, Workshop Summary. Cardiorespiratory sleep studies in children: establishment of normative data and polysomnographic predictors of morbidity. Am J Respir Crit Care Med 1999;160:1381–1387.
19. Uliel S, Tauman R, Greenfeld M, Sivan Y. Normal polysomnographic respiratory value in children and adolescents. Chest 2004;125:872–878.
20. American Academy of Sleep Medicine. Obstructive sleep apnea syndromes, adult and pediatrics. In: Sateia MJ, ed. The International Classification of Sleep Disorders: Diagnostic & Coding Manual, 2nd edition, 2005:51–59.
21. Guilleminault C, Kim YD, Chowdhuri S, Horita M, Ohayon M, Kushida C. Sleep and daytime sleepiness in upper airway resistance syndrome compared to obstructive sleep apnoea syndrome. Eur Respir J 2001;17:838–847.
22. Kushida CA, Littner MR, Hirshkowitz M, Morgenthaler T, Alessi CA, Bailey D, Boehlecke B, Brown TM, Coleman J Jr, Friedman L, Kapen S, Kapur VK, Kramer M, Lee-Chiong TL, Owens J, Pancer JP, Swick TJ, Wise MS. Practice parameters for the use of continuous and bilevel positive airway pressure devices to treat adult patients with sleep-related breathing disorders. Sleep 2006;29(3):375–380.
23. Sleep breathing in children: a developmental approach. In: Loughlin GM, Carroll JL, Marcus CL, eds. Lung Biology in Health and Disease. Lenfant C. Exec. Ed. New York: Marcel Dekker, 2000; Vol. 147.
24. US Department of Health and Human Services, Public Health Service, Food and Drug Administration. Pre-Market Approval Letter, April 7, 2006. Available at: www.fda.gov/cdrh/pdf6/K060105.pdf Accessed September 12, 2006.
25. Marcus CL, Keens TG, Ward SL. Comparison of nap and overnight polysomnography in children. Pediatr Pulmonol 1992;13:16–21.
26. Saeed MM, Keens TG, Stabile MW, Bolokowicz J, Ward SL. Should children with suspected obstructive sleep apnea syndrome and normal nap sleep studies have overnight sleep studies? Chest 2000;118:360–365.
27. Collop NA, Anderson WM, Boehlecke B, Claman D, Goldberg R, Gottlieb DJ, Hudgel D, Sateia M, Schwab R – Task Force Members. Clinical guidelines for the use of unattended portable monitors in the diagnosis of obstructive sleep apnea in adult patients. J Clin Sleep Med 2007;3(7):737–747.
28. American Sleep Disorders Association and Sleep Research Society, ASDA Standards of Practice Committee. Practice parameters for the use of portable recording in the assessment of obstructive sleep apnea. Sleep 1993;17(4):372–377.
29. Jacob SV, Morielli A, Mograss MA, Ducharme FM, Schloss MD, Brouillette RT. Home testing for pediatric obstructive sleep apnea syndrome secondary to adenotonsillar hypertrophy. Pediatr Pulmonol 1995;20:241–252.
30. Goodwin JL, Enright PL, Kaemingk KL, Rosen GM, Morgan WJ, Fregosi RF, Quan SF. Feasibility of using unattended polysomnography in children for research - report of the Tucson Children's Assessment of Sleep Apnea Study (TuCASA). Sleep 2001;24(8):937–944.
31. Brouillette RT, Jacob SV, Morielli A, Mograss M, Lafontaine V, Ducharme F, Schloss M. There's no place like home: evaluation of obstructive sleep apnea in the child's home. Pediatr Pulmonol Suppl 1995;11:86–88.
32. American Academy of Pediatrics, Schecter MS, and the Section on Pediatric Pulmonology, Subcommittee on Obstructive Sleep Apnea Syndrome. Technical report: diagnosis and management of childhood obstructive sleep apnea syndrome. Pediatrics 2002;109(4):1–20.
33. Brouillette RT, Morielli A, Leimanis A, Waters KA, Luciano R, Ducharme FM. Nocturnal pulse oximetry as an abbreviated testing modality for pediatric obstructive sleep apnea. Pediatrics 2000;105(2):405–412.
34. Kirk VG, Bohn SG, Flemons WW, Remmers JE. Comparison of home oximetry monitoring with laboratory polysomnography in children. Chest 2003;124:1702–1708.
35. Tunkel DE, McColley SA, Baroody FM, Marcus CL, Carroll JL, Loughlin GM. Polysomnography in the evaluation of readiness for decannulation in children. Arch Otolaryngol Head Neck Surg 1996;122:721–724.
36. Mukherjee B, Bais AS, Bajaj Y. Role of polysomnography in tracheostomy decannulation in the paediatric patient. J Laryngol Otol 1999;113:442–445.

Otology

External Otitis

Marc C. Thorne and Ralph F. Wetmore

Key Points

- A careful history and physical examination are typically sufficient to accurately diagnose the cause of external otitis.
- Topical therapy is the first line for uncomplicated acute otitis externa.
- Topical agents with a potential for ototoxicity should be avoided in the setting of a known or suspected nonintact tympanic membrane.
- Fungal otitis externa presents with pruritis as the predominant complaint, and is more common in tropical climates and after topical antibiotic therapy.
- Malignant otitis externa should be suspected in children with diabetes or other immune dysfunction.
- Aggressive antimicrobial therapy aimed at *Pseudomonas* is necessary to prevent morbidity and mortality in malignant otitis externa.

Keywords: Ear • External • Otitis externa • Furunculosis • Atopic dermatiti • Contact dermatitis • Child

External otitis represents a group of disorders that share the condition of inflammation of the external ear canal. Acute external otitis is one of the most common infectious conditions for which patients seek medical care. Other diagnostic considerations include furunculosis (localized external otitis), fungal external otitis (otomycosis), chronic dermatitis, and malignant external otitis. Accurate diagnosis can typically be achieved through a careful history and physical examination. Treatment is tailored to the underlying cause, with topical therapy generally preferred over systemic therapy for uncomplicated cases.

Acute Otitis Externa

Acute otitis externa (AOE) is characterized by diffuse inflammation of the external ear canal, with symptoms typically appearing within 1–2 days of onset of inflammation. With an annual period prevalence of 1.2% ***(1)***, AOE is one of the more common infectious conditions for which patients seek medical care.

The lining of the external ear canal is composed of keratinizing stratified squamous epithelium. The squamous epithelium of the lateral cartilaginous external ear canal also contains sebaceous and ceruminous glands. Cerumen (wax) is a mixture of secretions from the sebaceous and ceruminous glands along with desquamated keratin debris. Cerumen serves to protect the ear canal from moisture and maceration due to its high lipid content. In addition, the acidic pH of cerumen helps to inhibit microbial growth. Water contamination and localized trauma may allow pathogenic bacteria to bypass these natural host defenses. Trauma to the external ear canal may be affected by means of instrumentation (such as with cotton-tipped applicators) or digital manipulation. The most common pathogenic organisms are *Pseudomonas aeruginosa* (60–70%) and *Staphylococcus aureus* (20–30%), with other Gram-negative organisms isolated much less frequently ***(2,3)***.

M.C. Thorne
Division of Pediatric Otolaryngology, Department of Otolaryngology – Head and Neck Surgery, University of Michigan, Ann Arbor, MI, USA

R.F. Wetmore (✉)
Division of Pediatric Otolaryngology, The Children's Hospital of Philadelphia, Philadelphia PA, USA
e-mail: wetmare@email.chap.edu

R.B. Mitchell and K.D. Pereira (eds.), *Pediatric Otolaryngology for the Clinician*,
DOI: 10.1007/978-1-60327-127-1_6, © Humana Press, a part of Springer Science + Business Media, LLC 2009

Diagnosis

Diagnosis of AOE can typically be achieved through a careful history and physical examination. Predisposing factors, such as water contamination and instrumentation or manipulation of the ear canal should be sought. Patients with AOE will typically complain of acute onset (<48 h) of unilateral ear pain, itching, and a sense of aural fullness. The pain of AOE is exacerbated by manipulation of the tragus, pinna, or ear canal, and by opening and closing of the jaw, findings that help to differentiate AOE from acute otitis media, in which case there is no change in the level of discomfort. A history of diabetes or other immunocompromised states should be sought, as children with these conditions are predisposed to malignant external otitis (discussed in more detail later). A history of tympanic membrane perforation or tympanostomy tube placement should also be sought, as this will impact the choice of therapy.

Physical examination will reveal erythema and edema of the canal, which may progress to complete occlusion of the canal and a resulting conductive hearing loss. In more severe cases, the infection may spread to the surrounding skin and regional lymphatics and present with cellulitis and regional lymphadenitis. Otoscopic evaluation will reveal moist ceruminous and exudative debris in the canal. Frequently, the discharge is associated with a pungent odor characteristic of *Pseudomonas* infection. Purulent discharge may be seen with acute otitis media with perforation or chronic otitis media. Therefore, inspection of the tympanic membrane is desirable, but may be precluded by patient discomfort or the degree of canal edema. Routine culture of the discharge from the ear is typically unnecessary and is not recommended.

Treatment

Strategies to prevent AOE are directed toward preventing excess water contamination and avoiding trauma to the external canal. The use of alcohol drops or a hair dryer on a cool setting after water exposure are advocated by some experts as a means of drying the external ear canal. Otic drops containing acetic acid may be used either before or after water exposure to maintain the acidic pH of the ear canal. Direct comparisons of the efficacy of different preventative measures have not been performed.

Recent clinical practice guidelines for the treatment of AOE emphasize the need for adequate assessment of pain and appropriate analgesic therapy *(4)*. It is not uncommon for the pain of AOE to be so severe as to require narcotic analgesic therapy. In uncomplicated cases of AOE, treatment with ototopical drops for a 7–10-day course should be administered. Systemic therapy should be reserved for patients with diabetes, other immunosuppression, or extension of infection beyond the external ear canal *(4)*.

In order for ototopical therapy to be effective, aural toilet may be required to remove obstructing debris and allow access of the drops to the infected tissue. Wick placement should be performed if the canal edema is severe enough to prevent entry of the drops. Adequate delivery is enhanced by having someone other than the patient apply the drops *(5)*. Specific instructions should be provided to caregivers regarding application of drops, including having the patient lie with the affected ear up during and for a period of 3 min following application, and for manipulation of the tragus to "pump" the drops into the more medial ear canal.

Available ototopical medications for treatment of AOE share similar efficacy; therefore, choice of agent may be determined by clinician experience and patient preference. Table 1 provides a list of commonly used topical antimicrobial preparations in the treatment of otitis externa. Topical therapy in the setting of known or suspected tympanic membrane perforation or tympanostomy tube presence warrants additional consideration. Due to concerns over potential ototoxicity, topical therapy in this setting should be limited to

Table 1 Common topical antimicrobial preparations

Active medication	Trade name
Acidifying agents	
Acetic acid, Aluminum acetate	Domeboro otic
Acetic acid, Hydrocortisone	VoSol HC
Antibiotics	
Ciprofloxacin	Ciloxan ophthalmic
Ciprofloxacin, Hydrocortisone	Cipro HC
Ciprofloxacin, Dexamethasone	Ciprodex
Neomycin, Polymyxin B, Hydrocortisone	Cortisporin otic
Ofloxacin	Floxin otic
Tobramycin	Tobrex ophthalmic
Tobramycin, Dexamethasone	Tobradex
Antifungals	
Clotrimazole	Lotrimin
Ketoconazole	Generic ointment
General antiseptics	
Gentian violet 2%	Generic
m-Cresyl acetate 25%	Cresylate

drops without ototoxic potential. Currently, this limits therapy in the setting of a nonintact tympanic membrane to a topical fluoroquinolone.

Clinical response to therapy is expected within 2–3 days. Failure of improvement over this time course should prompt medical reevaluation. Attention should be paid to factors which may be preventing adequate delivery of the medication, and to confirm the initial diagnostic impression. Contact sensitivity of the external ear canal should also be considered, a problem most commonly seen in ototopical preparations containing neomycin. During therapy, care should be taken to avoid water exposure, manipulation of the ear canal, or its occlusion (e.g., with headphones or hearing aids).

Furunculosis (Localized Otitis Externa)

A furuncle is a localized abscess that results from infection of an obstructed apocrine or sebaceous gland. These lesions are commonly seen in the lateral external ear canal, where these glands are numerous. The offending organism in furunculosis is typically *Staphylococcus aureus*. The clinical presentation may mimic acute external otitis, especially if the furuncle is large. However, careful history will typically reveal localized otalgia, in contrast to the more diffuse otalgia experienced with AOE. A history of drainage from the ear is uncommon with furunculosis. On examination, erythema and edema of the canal is found localized to the site of the abscess. Treatment with an oral antistaphylococcal antibiotic is typically effective. Lesions that fail to respond to antibiotic therapy may require incision and drainage.

Fungal Otitis Externa (Otomycosis)

Fungal otitis externa represents an infection of the external ear canal with a yeast or fungal organism. This condition is observed more frequently in tropical climates and following long-term topical antimicrobial therapy of the ear canal. *Aspergillus* species and *Candida* species are the most commonly identified causative organisms.

Fungal otitis externa presents with complaints of pruritis with or without associated otorrhea and aural fullness. Symptoms are typically more chronic than the presenting symptoms of AOE, and pain is not a prominent feature. On examination, *Aspergillus* typically appears as a white base spotted with gray-black debris. *Candidal* infections appear as white debris, with sprouting hyphae often visible under microscopic examination.

Treatment of fungal otitis externa requires thorough cleaning of the ear canal to remove the fungal debris. Mechanical debridement is followed by topical therapy. Several options for topical therapy are effective, including acidification of the canal with acetic acid or other solutions, topical antifungals (clotrimazole, nystatin, others), and general antiseptics (Gentian violet, *m*-Cresyl acetate).

Chronic Dermatitis

The squamous epithelium lining the external auditory canal is susceptible to a similar variety of dermatologic conditions that affect the skin throughout the rest of the body. Atopic dermatitis and contact dermatitis are two of the more commonly seen chronic dermatitis which may result in chronic otitis externa, both of which present with a chief complaint of pruritis. Patients with atopic dermatitis affecting the external ear will often report a history of asthma and hay fever, as well as atopic dermatitis affecting other skin sites. Examination reveals thickened, scaly skin with areas of weeping and crusting. The itching associated with atopic dermatitis will frequently result in local trauma and a predisposition to episodes of AOE. Management consists of topical antibacterial therapy for episodes of AOE with application of topical steroids to control the underlying dermatologic condition.

Contact dermatitis is a local inflammatory response triggered by exposure to a specific offending agent. Metal sensitivity is the most common form of chronic dermatitis involving the external ear, with nickel being the most common causative metal. Nickel may be released from stainless steel and other alloys in earrings, even after gold or silver plating. As previously noted, contact dermatitis resulting from exposure to antibiotic drops containing neomycin is especially problematic, with a hypersensitivity reaction occurring in up to 30% of patients treated for chronic otitis externa ***(6)***. Treatment involves removal of the offending agent and topical steroid therapy to decrease the inflammation.

Malignant Otitis Externa

Malignant otitis externa (MOE), also termed skull base osteomyelitis, is a serious progressive infection most commonly seen in older diabetic patients and others with immune dysfunction. However, MOE has been described in children with immune dysfunction from a variety of causes, including primary immunodeficiency, malnutrition, malignancy, and new-onset Type 1 diabetes mellitus. *Pseudomonas aeruginosa* is the predominant pathogen identified in MOE.

Diagnosis of MOE requires the clinician to maintain a high index of suspicion when evaluating complaints of otalgia. Predisposing factors, other than immune dysfunction, are similar to those for AOE. The onset of otalgia is typically acute, and the pain may be characterized as severe and unrelenting. On examination, granulation tissue at the bone-cartilage junction of the ear canal is a frequent finding. Necrosis of the tympanic membrane and involvement of the facial nerve are seen more frequently and earlier in the disease course than in adults. Laboratory evaluation will typically reveal elevation of the erythrocyte sedimentation rate *(7)*. Several imaging modalities offer complementary information in the evaluation of MOE. Computed tomography provides information regarding bony breakdown, while magnetic resonance imaging provides superior definition of soft-tissue involvement. Radionuclide imaging, such as single-photon emission computed tomography (SPECT), may also be helpful in establishing the diagnosis and following response to therapy *(8)*.

Treatment begins with biopsy of the granulation tissue in order to rule out the possibility of neoplastic disease and to provide tissue for culture. Surgical therapy plays a limited role, consisting mainly of cleaning the ear of debris and necrotic tissue. Medical therapy includes supportive care as well as antibiotic therapy directed against *Pseudomonas*. Recurrence of disease is typically less common in children than in adults, therefore a 2–3-week course of therapy may be sufficient if an appropriate clinical response is seen *(7)*. The mortality rate for children with MOE appears to be lower than their adult counterparts.

Conclusions

External otitis represents a group of disorders that share the condition of inflammation of the ear canal. Accurate diagnosis can typically be achieved through a careful history and physical examination. Acute otitis externa (AOE) is one of the most common infectious conditions for which patients seek medical care. First-line treatment for uncomplicated AOE consists of topical therapy. Potentially ototoxic medications should be avoided in the setting of a known or suspected nonintact tympanic membrane. Furunculosis is a condition of localized abscess formation caused by obstruction of sebaceous and ceruminous glands, and may be seen in the lateral ear canal. Treatment with oral antibiotics directed against the most commonly identified organism, *Staphylococcus aureus*, is typically effective. Fungal otitis externa is more common in tropical climates and following topical antimicrobial therapy with pruritis as the predominant complaint. Dermatologic conditions such as atopic and contact dermatitis may affect the skin of the ear canal. Malignant otitis externa is a severe infection seen most commonly in adults, but may present in children with Type 1 diabetes or other immune dysfunction. Aggressive antibiotic therapy directed against *Pseudomonas aeruginosa* is necessary to prevent morbidity and mortality.

References

1. Rowlands S, Devalia H, Smith C, Hubbard R, Dean A. Otitis externa in UK general practice: a survey using the UK General Practice Research Database. *Br J Gen Pract*. 2001;51(468):533–538.
2. Jones RN, Milazzo J, Seidlin M. Ofloxacin otic solution for treatment of otitis externa in children and adults. *Arch Otolaryngol Head Neck Surg*. 1997;123(11):1193–1200.
3. Manolidis S, Friedman R, Hannley M, et al. Comparative efficacy of aminoglycoside versus fluoroquinolone topical antibiotic drops. *Otolaryngol Head Neck Surg*. 2004;130(3 Suppl):S83–S88.
4. Rosenfeld RM, Brown L, Cannon CR, et al. Clinical practice guideline: acute otitis externa. *Otolaryngol Head Neck Surg*. 2006;134(4 Suppl):S4–S23.
5. Agius AM, Reid AP, Hamilton C. Patient compliance with short-term topical aural antibiotic therapy. *Clin Otolaryngol Allied Sci*. 1994;19(2):138–141.
6. Smith IM, Keay DG, Buxton PK. Contact hypersensitivity in patients with chronic otitis externa. *Clin Otolaryngol Allied Sci*. 1990;15(2):155–158.
7. Rubin J, Yu VL, Stool SE. Malignant external otitis in children. *J Pediatr*. 1988;113(6):965–970.
8. Okpala NC, Siraj QH, Nilssen E, Pringle M. Radiological and radionuclide investigation of malignant otitis externa. *J Laryngol Otol*. 2005;119(1):71–75.

Diagnosis and Management of Otitis Media

Margaretha L. Casselbrant and Ellen M. Mandel

Key Points

- The presence or absence of signs and symptoms is the basis for proper diagnosis of the different types of otitis media.
- The pneumatic otoscope is the most important tool for assessment of middle ear status.
- The highest incidence of otitis media occurs between 6 and 11 months of age and decreases with age. Risk factors include both host and environmental factors.
- Prevention of disease through reducing risk factors and use of vaccines is desirable.
- Antihistamines and steroids are ineffective for the treatment of otitis media.
- For children 2 years or older with nonsevere acute otitis media, published guidelines have given the option of observing rather than treating with antibiotics immediately.
- Tympanostomy tube insertion is effective in reducing recurrent episodes of otitis media and persistent middle ear effusion.
- Adenoidectomy is recommended for children in whom a repeat surgical procedure is needed.

Keywords: Otitis media • Acute otitis media • Otitis media with effusion • Middle ear effusion

M.L. Casselbrant (✉) and E.M. Mandel
Division of Pediatric Otolaryngology Children's Hospital of Pittsburgh of UPMC, University of Pittsburgh School of Medicine, Pittsburgh, PA, USA
e-mail: Margaretha.Casselbrant@chp.edu

Abstract

Otitis media is, next to the common cold, the most commonly diagnosed disorder in children. Although considered to be a continuum, otitis media can be subclassified into acute otitis media (AOM) and otitis media with effusion (OME) based on signs and symptoms. AOM is usually treated with antibiotics but, because of the high spontaneous resolution rate, selected children may be observed rather than treated immediately. Presently, antibiotic treatment is not routinely recommended for OME. Surgical treatment consisting of tympanostomy tube insertion as a primary procedure, followed by adenoidectomy if further surgical treatment is needed, is reserved for those children with recurrent AOM or persistent effusion. The preferred management is prevention, through modifying risk factors and use of vaccines.

Definitions

Otitis media (OM) is thought of as a continuum of middle ear disease. However, disease types are defined by the presence or absence of specific symptoms and signs, and treatment varies with disease type.

Acute otitis media (AOM): Rapid onset of signs (bulging or fullness, erythema or perforation of the tympanic membrane with otorrhea) and symptoms (otalgia, irritability, or fever) accompanied by middle ear effusion.

Otitis media with effusion (OME): Middle ear effusion without symptoms of inflammation.

Middle ear effusion (MEE): Episodes of AOM, OME, or both.

R.B. Mitchell and K.D. Pereira (eds.), *Pediatric Otolaryngology for the Clinician*,
DOI: 10.1007/978-1-60327-127-1_7, © Humana Press, a part of Springer Science + Business Media, LLC 2009

Diagnosis

Pneumatic otoscopy is the primary diagnostic tool used to assess the status in an intact middle ear as it allows for evaluation of tympanic membrane mobility. Reduced or no mobility in an intact tympanic membrane indicates fluid in the middle ear or increased stiffness due to scarring or thickness of the tympanic membrane. The position of the tympanic membrane can also be assessed (retracted or bulging). Other features, such as fluid levels or bubbles, may be more easily discerned with movement of the tympanic membrane. Use of an *operating microscope* enhances the assessment of middle ear status as well as detection of scarring and atrophy of the tympanic membrane.

Immittence testing (tympanometry) is an excellent adjunct to the assessment of middle ear status, especially when the otoscopic evaluation is uncertain or difficult to perform. This test can also be used to document changes in middle ear status over time. A flat pattern with a small ear canal volume indicates MEE, while a large ear canal volume suggests a perforation or a patent tympanostomy tube.

Spectral gradient acoustic reflectometry has also been used to measure middle ear effusion probability but has been found to have limitations, although it may be useful for screening.

Audiometry

The assessment of hearing is essential to management, as hearing impairment can predispose to delay in speech and language development, and may eventually affect school performance. Audiometry should be used to determine management of the child, with more aggressive management considered if there is significant hearing impairment.

Behavioral audiometry requires cooperation of the child with the examination. The test is adapted to the age of the child. Hearing thresholds in the sound field or ear-specific are determined from 0.25, 0.5, 1, 2, 4, and up to 8 kHz depending on the age of the child.

Auditory brainstem audiometry (ABR)/Transitory otoacoustic emission (TOAE) are excellent methods for testing children who do not cooperate with a hearing evaluation because of very young age or developmental delay. In an infant an ABR can be performed without sedation or general anesthesia. The TOAE is usually very quick at any age, but testing is limited by MEE or if the child is noisy or crying.

Epidemiology

Prevalence

Otitis media is, next to the common cold, the most diagnosed disorder in infants and children. In the Third National Health and Nutrition Examination Survey (NHANES III), which conducted household interviews from 1988 to 1994, 68.2% of parents with children less than 6 years of age reported their child had one or more episodes of OM *(1)*. A recent report from a nationally representative longitudinal study of U.S. births in 2001 showed that the prevalence of medically diagnosed ear infections was 39.1% at age 9 months and 62.3% at age 2 years *(2)*.

Risk Factors

Risk factors can be host related or environmental *(3)*.

Host Related

Age – The highest incidence of AOM occurs between 6 and 11 months of age; the risk of persistent MEE after an episode of AOM is inversely correlated with age.

Gender – Some studies have found a higher incidence of AOM and persistent MEE in males; most studies find no difference between the sexes in the incidence of OME or time with MEE.

Race – Recent studies have shown no difference between Caucasian and African-American children. The incidence is higher in Hispanic children but the highest incidence is found in American Indians, Eskimos, and Aborigine children.

Allergy/immunodeficiency – Atopic disease and allergic rhinitis may increase the risk of persistent MEE but the role of allergy in OM is uncertain. Defective or immature immunologic responses in children may contribute to the development of OM.

Cleft palate/craniofacial malformation – OM is universal in nearly all children less than 2 years of age with unrepaired palate. Repair of the palate reduces the incidence of OM, but many children require multiple tube insertions.

Genetics – Twin studies have demonstrated a strong genetic susceptibility to OM. Genome-wide linkage analysis has suggested that regions on chromosome 19q and 10q contain genes contributing to the susceptibility to chronic OME/recurrent AOM *(4)*.

Environmental

Upper respiratory infection/season – The incidence of OM parallels that of URI and is highest in the fall and winter and lowest in spring and summer.

Siblings – First-born children have less AOM/OME in the first 2 years of life compared to children with older siblings.

Daycare/homecare – Children in daycare have an increased incidence of AOM and tympanostomy tube insertion compared to children cared for at home.

Passive smoking – Many studies have reported an association between passive smoking and risk of recurrent OM, but a conclusive relationship has not yet been determined.

Breast/bottle feeding – Breastfeeding for at least 6 months is considered to have a protective effect against middle ear disease.

Socioeconomic status – It has generally been thought that OM is more common in lower socioeconomic strata due to poorer sanitary conditions and crowding.

Pacifier – Pacifier use has been associated with an increased risk of OM.

Treatment

Prevention of disease through vaccines and elimination of risk factors is thought to be key to management. The treatment of otitis media is focused on medical and surgical therapies.

Prevention of Disease

Prevention of disease is desirable, as the three most common bacteria isolated from middle ear effusion (*Streptococcus pneumoniae* 25–50% [15–50% nonsusceptible to penicillin: 50% highly resistant and 50% intermediate], *Haemophilus influenzae* 20–30% [50% beta-lactamase producing], and *Moraxella catarrhalis* 3–20% [100% beta-lactamase producing]) have developed increased resistance to the commonly used antibiotics, which has raised serious concerns about overuse of antibiotics. Prevention/modification of risk factors and vaccine development are two recommended strategies.

Management of Environmental Risk Factors

Promotion of breast feeding in the first 6 months of life, avoidance of supine bottle feeding and pacifier use, and elimination of passive tobacco smoke may be helpful in reducing the risk of development of OM. Alteration of child care arrangements where the child is exposed to fewer children may also be beneficial.

Vaccines

Bacterial vaccines – The *S. pneumoniae* vaccines (Pneumovax, Prevnar) are presently the only bacterial vaccines available for otitis media. Pneumovax is a 23-valent polysaccharide vaccine, which is not efficacious in children 2 years or younger. On the other hand, Prevnar, a 7-valent (serotypes 4, 6B, 9V, 14, 18C, 19F, 23F) conjugate vaccine is recommended for universal use in children 23 months or younger in the US. It has been proven effective in reducing the number of episodes of AOM and tube insertion in children with recurrent AOM *(5)*. Infants immunized with pneumococcal vaccine are unlikely to elicit protective serum antibody concentration during the first 4–6 months of life when recurrent AOM begins. Maternal immunization with pneumococcal vaccine is another approach currently being studied. The development of nontypable *H. influenzae and M. catarrhalis* vaccines is in progress.

Viral vaccines – Respiratory viruses, such as respiratory syncytial (RSV), influenza, adenovirus, parainfluenza, and rhinoviruses, have been isolated in MEE using polymerase chain reaction (PCR) tests *(6)*. Presently, influenza vaccine is the only available viral vaccine and it is recommended by the American Academy of Pediatrics for all healthy children 6 months to 18 years of age *(7)*. There is strong evidence that viruses have an important role in the development of AOM *(8)*. Bacterial vaccines only prevent the bacterial complication of a viral infection, while viral vaccines act at an earlier stage in the pathogenesis of AOM. Thus viral vaccines have the potential to prevent viral upper respiratory infections, thereby preventing the development of AOM as a complication of bacteria in the nasopharynx.

Treatment of Disease

Guidelines

Guidelines for management of AOM *(9)* and OME *(10)* have been published. Both guidelines were evidence-based and the quality of the evidence was assessed. The AOM guidelines were aimed at otherwise healthy children aged 2 months to 12 years "without signs and symptoms of systemic illness unrelated to the middle ear." The guidelines for management of OME were aimed at children aged 2 months to 12 years with and without developmental disabilities or underlying conditions that predispose to OM. The recommendations reflected the quality of the evidence and the balance between benefit and harm that is anticipated when the recommendations are followed.

Acute Otitis Media

Medical Treatment

Observation – In an effort to reduce antibiotic use and stem the increasing resistance of microbes, observation without use of antibiotics is an option for selected children with AOM, based on diagnostic certainty, age of the child, illness severity, and access to medical care *(9)*. Severe disease is defined as moderate to severe otalgia, fever > 39°C (102°F) orally or 39.5°C rectally, or a toxic-appearing child. Children less than 6 months of age should be treated with antibiotics regardless; children 6–23 months, if nonsevere, could be observed if the diagnosis was uncertain, but if AOM is certain or severe, the child should be treated with antibiotics; children 24 months or older could be watched if the diagnosis is uncertain or disease is nonsevere but treated if AOM is severe.

Antibiotics – Many antibiotics are available, but amoxicillin (now recommended at 90 mg/kg/day in two divided doses) is still the first line antibiotic for nonsevere episodes of AOM. For severe episodes of AOM amoxicillin/clavulanic acid (amoxicillin 90 mg/kg/day and clavulanic acid 6.4 mg/kg/day in two divided doses) is recommended. Cephalosporins should only be considered as accepted first-line treatment for patients with penicillin allergy. Macrolides should be prescribed for patients with penicillin and cephalosporin allergies. The child is considered a treatment failure if symptoms and signs persist/recur 48–72 h after initial treatment assignment. The diagnosis should then be reassessed, antibiotics started if not given previously, or changed to a more broad spectrum agent if antibiotics were previously prescribed (amoxicillin/clavulanic acid if amoxicillin failed and ceftriaxone (3 days) if amoxicillin/clavulanic acid failed). Tympanocentesis (insertion of a needle through the tympanic membrane and aspiration of fluid from the middle ear space) should always be considered if the child does not respond to antibiotic treatment in order to identify the bacteria in the middle ear effusion and select an appropriate antibiotic.

Decongestants/Antihistamines – In a recent trial for AOM, antihistamine administered with an antibiotic did not result in improved clinical outcome and prolonged the duration of effusion *(11)*.

Steroids – In the same trial as above, corticosteroid (2 mg/kg given for 5 days) administered with an antibiotic did not provide any improvement in clinical outcome *(11)*.

Surgical Treatment

Myringotomy – Myringotomy is helpful for acute pain relief and obtaining MEE samples for targeted antibiotic selection but provides no advantage in duration of effusion or recurrence of AOM *(12)*.

Tympanostomy tubes – For children with recurrent episodes of AOM (three or more episodes AOM in 6 months or four or more episodes in 12 months with one episode of AOM in the past 6 months) tympanostomy tube insertion is an option. It prevents the recurrent episodes of systemic illness but episodes of otorrhea, usually without fever or otalgia, occur *(13)*.

Adenoidectomy with and without tonsillectomy – Adenoidectomy may provide modest improvement in children with recurrent AOM but is not recommended as a first procedure unless it is being done for airway obstruction. Tonsillectomy, in conjunction with adenoidectomy, provides no significant advantage compared to adenoidectomy alone ***(14)***.

Otitis Media with Effusion

Medical

Observation – For children at no risk for speech, language, or learning disabilities "watchful waiting" should be considered. Hearing tests should be done if MEE persists for 3 months or longer or at any time that language delay, learning difficulties, or significant hearing loss is suspected. If hearing is <20 dB watchful waiting is suggested, but if it is >40 dB in the better ear surgery is recommended. For children with hearing levels 21–39 dB in the better ear, management is based on the duration of effusion and severity of symptoms. For children at no risk, examination at 3- to 6-month intervals, until the fluid has resolved, hearing loss, language or learning delays are identified, or there are suspected structural abnormalities of the ear drum, is recommended ***(10)***.

Antibiotics – Despite short-term efficacy ***(15,16)***, antibiotics are not recommended for routine treatment of OME, due to lack of long-term efficacy, the high spontaneous cure rate, and concern about overuse of antibiotics.

Decongestant/antihistamine – These systemic medications have not been shown to have any efficacy in resolving OME and are not recommended ***(17)***.

Steroids – Steroids have demonstrated a slight advantage in resolving MEE compared to placebo, but due to the high recurrence rate, are not recommended ***(18)***.

Autoinflation – Studies using a number of devices have failed to show consistent efficacy and so it is not recommended for routine use at this time.

Surgical

Myringotomy – Myringotomy alone is ineffective for long-term management and is not recommended for chronic OME ***(19,20)***.

Tympanostomy tubes – Tympanostomy tube insertion is the initial surgical procedure recommended for children with OME at risk for speech, language, and learning disabilities and/or hearing loss and in whom a need for intervention has been identified.

Adenoidectomy with and without tonsillectomy – As an initial procedure, adenoidectomy should be reserved for those with signs/symptoms of nasal obstructions, recurrent rhinorrhea, and/or chronic adenoiditis. For repeat surgical procedures, tympanostomy tube insertion with adenoidectomy is recommended as there is some evidence that future need for repeat surgical treatment may be decreased ***(21)***. For children 4 years and older, adenoidectomy with myringotomy alone may be effective, but tube insertion is advised for younger children ***(19)***. Tonsillectomy is not recommended as treatment for OM because of lack of demonstrable efficacy and increased risk.

References

1. Auinger P, Lanphear BP, Kalkwarf HJ, Mansour ME. Trends in otitis media among children in the United States. Pediatrics 2003;112(3):514–520.
2. Hoffman HJ, Park J, Losonczy KG, Chiu MS. Risk factors, treatments, and other conditions associated with frequent ear infections in US children through 2 years of age: the early childhood longitudinal study – birth cohort (ECLS-B). Presented at 9th International Symposium on Recent Advances in Otitis Media (June 3–7, 2007, St. Pete Beach, FL).
3. Casselbrant ML, Mandel EM. Epidemiology. In: Rosenfeld RM, Bluestone CD, eds. Evidence-Based Otitis Media, 2nd edn. Hamilton, ON: BC Decker, 2003:147–162.
4. Daly KA, Brown WM, Segade F, Bowden DW, Keats BJ, Lindgren BR, et al. Chronic and recurrent otitis media: a genome scan for susceptibility loci. Am J Hum Genet 2004;75:988–997.
5. Fireman B, Black SB, Shinefield HR, Lee J, Lewis E, Ray P. Impact of the pneumococcal conjugate vaccine on otitis media. Pediatr Infect Dis J 2003;22:10–16.
6. Pitkäranta A, Virolainen A, Jero J, Arruda E, Hayden FG. Detection of rhinovirus, respiratory syncytial virus, and corona virus infections in acute otitis media by reverse transcriptase polymerase chain reaction. Pediatrics 1998;102(2):291–295.
7. Committee on Infectious Diseases, American Academy of Pediatrics. Prevention of influenza: recommendations for influenza immunization of children, 2008–2009. Pediatrics 2008;112:1135–1141.
8. Heikkinen T, Chonmaitree T. Importance of respiratory viruses in acute otitis media. Clin Microbiol Rev 2003;16(2):230–241.
9. Subcommittee on Management of AOM, American Academy of Pediatrics and American Academy of Family Physicians. Diagnosis and management of acute otitis media. Pediatrics 2004;113(5):1451–1465.

10. Subcommittee on Otitis Media with Effusion, American Academy of Family Physicians. American Academy of Otolaryngology–Head and Neck Surgery, American Academy of Pediatrics. Otitis media with effusion. Pediatrics 2004;113(5):1412–1429.
11. Chonmaitree T, Saeed K, Uchida T, Heikkinen T, Baldwin CD, Freeman DH Jr, et al. A randomized, placebo-controlled trial of the effect of antihistamine or corticosteroid treatment in acute otitis media. J Pediatr 2003;143: 377–385.
12. Kaleida PH, Casselbrant ML, Rockette HE, Paradise JL, Bluestone CD, Blatter MM, et al. Amoxicillin or myringotomy or both for acute otitis media: results of a randomized clinical trial. Pediatrics 1991;87(4):466–474.
13. Casselbrant ML, Kaleida PH, Rockette HE, Paradise JL, Bluestone CD, Kurs-Lasky M, et al. Efficacy of antimicrobial prophylaxis and of tympanostomy tube insertion for prevention of recurrent acute otitis media: Results of a randomized clinical trial. Pediatr Infect Dis J 1992;11:278–286.
14. Paradise JL, Bluestone CD, Colborn DK, Bernard BS, Smith CG, Rockette HE, et al. Adenoidectomy and adenotonsillectomy for recurrent acute otitis media. JAMA 1999;282(10):945–953.
15. Williams RL, Chalmers TC, Stange KC, Chalmers FT, Bowlin SJ. Use of antibiotics in preventing recurrent acute otitis media and in treating otitis media with effusion. JAMA 1993;270(11);1344–1351.
16. Rosenfeld RM, Post JC. Meta-analysis of antibiotics for the treatment of otitis media with effusion. Otolaryngol Head Neck Surg 1992;106(4):378–386.
17. Cantekin EI, Mandel EM, Bluestone CD, Rockette HE, Paradise JL, Stool SE, et al. Lack of efficacy of a decongestant-antihistamine combination for otitis media with effusion ("secretory" otitis media) in children. N Engl J Med 1983;308:297–301.
18. Mandel EM, Casselbrant ML, Rockette HE, Fireman P, Kurs-Lasky M, Bluestone CD. Systemic steroid for chronic otitis media with effusion in children. Pediatrics 2002;110(6):1071–1080.
19. Gates GA, Avery CA, Cooper JC, Prihoda TJ. Chronic secretory otitis media: effects of surgical management. Ann Otol Rhinol Laryngol (suppl) 1989;138:2–32.
20. Mandel EM, Rockette HE, Bluestone CD, Paradise JL, Nozza RJ. Efficacy of myringotomy with and without tympanostomy tubes for chronic otitis media with effusion. Pediatr Infect Dis J 1992;11:270–277.
21. Coyte PC, Croxford R, McIsaac W, Feldman W, Friedberg J. The role of adjuvant adenoidectomy and tonsillectomy in the outcome of the insertion of tympanostomy tubes. N Engl J Med 2001;344(16):1188–1195.

Tympanostomy Tubes and Otorrhea

Peter S. Roland and Tyler W. Scoresby

Key Points

- Otitis media represents failure of eustachian tube function.
- Patent tubes effectively address eustachian tube dysfunction.
- Most common indications are recurrent acute otitis media and chronic otitis media with effusion.
- Common complications are otorrhea, tympanic membrane perforation, and foreign body reaction.

Keywords: Tympanostomy tubes • Eustachian tube • Acute otitis media • Chronic otitis media with effusion

Introduction

Myringotomy with grommet insertion is the most common procedure performed in children, with around one million performed each year. The frequency with which this surgery is performed underscores the necessity for the otolaryngologist and pediatrician to be well versed in the indications and complications of the procedure.

Indications

A thorough discussion of otitis media is found elsewhere in this textbook; however, a brief review of the pathophysiology of this disease is relevant to any discussion of tympanostomy tubes. The universal theme among the indications for surgical tube placement is poor performance of one or more of the following functions of the eustachian tube:

- middle ear protection
- middle ear clearance
- ventilation/pressure regulation

Bacterial entry into the middle ear space from the nasopharynx through the eustachian tube leads to acute otitis media, a failure of middle ear protection. Otitis media with effusion in young children most often represents a persistent stage of acute otitis media, lasting greater than 30 days in 40% of children and greater than 90 days in 10% of children after an episode of acute otitis media (AOM) *(1)*. The eustachian tube in these children fails to clear bacteria and inflammatory mediators from the middle ear. A failure in ventilation and pressure regulation often results in significant, negative middle ear pressure, which can itself lead to middle ear effusion but may also lead to severe retraction of the tympanic membrane. Chronic retractions can lead to ossicular erosion or create pockets that may eventually form cholesteatoma.

Tympanostomy tubes can effectively address the shortcomings of a poorly functioning eustachian tube. The indications for tympanostomy tubes are found in Table 1 and are described in more detail below.

Chronic otitis media with effusion. This is the most common diagnosis code used for the placement of tympanostomy tubes. In some studies, children with longer duration of otitis media with effusion (OME) have shown lower IQ scores and significant language delay when compared with those with shorter duration of OME *(2)*. However, recently a large prospective study showed no difference in developmental outcomes at ages 9 and 11 in children with persistent OME regardless of whether tubes were inserted *(3)*.

T.W. Scoresby and P.S. Roland (✉)
Department of Otolaryngology-Head and Neck Surgery, University of Texas Southwestern Medical Center at Dallas, Dallas, TX, USA
e-mail: Peter.Roland@UTSouthwestern.edu

R.B. Mitchell and K.D. Pereira (eds.), *Pediatric Otolaryngology for the Clinician*,
DOI: 10.1007/978-1-60327-127-1_8, © Humana Press, a part of Springer Science + Business Media, LLC 2009

Table 1 Indications for tympanostomy tubes

Chronic otitis media with effusion
Recurrent acute otitis media
Complications of acute otitis media
Tympanic membrane abnormalities (e.g., atelectasis or retraction)
Medical conditions predisposing to eustachian tube dysfunction
Down syndrome
Cleft palate
Hyperbaric oxygen

Despite this data, most clinicians continue to recommend tube placement if an effusion has been present for more than 3 months, especially if hearing loss is greater than 15–20 dB.

Recurrent acute otitis media. The potential complications of AOM include tympanosclerosis, cholesteatoma, sensorineural hearing loss, facial nerve paralysis, meningitis, mastoiditis, labrynthitis, and brain abscess. Tympanostomy tube placement significantly reduces the frequency of acute otitis media *(4)* and mitigates its effect when it does occur. AOM in a ear with a functioning tympanostomy tube is rarely painful. Systemic symptoms, including fever, are also rarely present. AOM in a ear with a tube generally presents as painless otorrhea. Current guidelines from the American Academy of Otolaryngology-Head and Neck surgery indicate that tubes should be considered in children who have four episodes of AOM in a 6-month window or six episodes within 1 year *(5)*.

Atelectasis and retraction pockets. Placement of tubes help in replacing the role of a poorly functioning eustachian tube and equalizing the pressure on either side of the drum, allowing release of the retraction pocket and prevention of cholesteatoma.

Surgical Considerations

Except possibly when tubes are placed emergently for AOM, audiometry should be performed before placement of tubes. Uncomplicated effusions will occasionally have no hearing loss, suggesting a course of watchful waiting rather than tube placement. A few children will also have a sensorineural component which should be assessed prior to any operative intervention.

Most children will require a general anesthetic for placement of tubes; however, this is nearly always attained with oral sedation and mask inhalational agents. In adults and older children, local anesthesia using phenol or topical tetracaine may be used.

After adequate anesthesia is obtained, a myringotomy is made under binocular microscopy, usually in a radial direction and usually in the anterior inferior quadrant. The posterior inferior quadrant can be used as well if the ear canal is unfavorable for anterior placement. The posterior superior quadrant should be avoided because of the close proximity of the chorda tympani and the ossicles. The myringotomy should be large enough to easily place the selected tube but small enough to hold the tube in place.

The choice of tube is widely variable and no study has shown a clear winner. There are two basic types of tubes: grommets and t-tubes. Grommets come in varying lengths, materials, stiffness, diameter, and flange size. Most typically remain in the tympanic membrane about 6–12 months before being extruded. The advantage of t-tubes is that they last much longer and are therefore frequently placed in children who have required multiple sets of tubes, or in those with known chronic eustachian tube dysfunction, such as those who suffer from cleft palate or Down syndrome. The advantage of increased dwell time comes at the cost of higher perforation rates as noted below. T-tubes with shorter flanges are an option to reduce this risk but it remains higher than with grommets. Both grommets and t-tubes come in silver oxide-coated varieties, which have shown significantly decreased rates of otorrhea in one study *(6)*.

Postoperative Management

Most clinicians recommend the use of ototopical antibiotic drops in the immediate postoperative period since they have been shown to reduce the incidence of postoperative otorrhea *(7)*. Given the small but significant risk of ototoxicity with aminoglycoside-containing medications in the middle ear *(8)*, a consensus panel of the American Academy of Otolaryngology-Head and Neck Surgery recommends that drops containing aminoglycosides be avoided. A steroid-containing drop has a greater likelihood of eliminating significant granulation tissue if encountered. Many would argue that the inflammatory nature of chronically infected middle ear mucosa indicates the use of a steroid-containing drop for all postoperative tubes.

A follow-up audiogram is recommended to assess closure of the air-bone gap. Tympanograms demonstrating large volumes can assist in confirming the patency of the tubes. While the tubes are in place, they should be evaluated by an otolaryngologist every 6 months or more frequently if complications occur.

Consensus does not exist on the question of swimming and bathing with tubes. Most studies have shown no difference in frequency of otorrhea or otitis media between children who did or did not swim and those who used or did not use plugs *(9)*.

Complications

While tympanostomy tubes are extremely common and safe when compared to most surgical procedures, there are potential complications and these should be discussed clearly with parents prior to surgery (see Table 2).

Otorrhea. Drainage from the ear after tympanostomy tubes is very common. At least one episode of otorrhea can be expected in around half of patients with tubes *(10)*. When drainage develops in a ear with a tympanostomy tube, initial treatment is empiric. Treatment should begin with topical antibiotic drops. As mentioned above, aminoglycoside drops should be avoided because of ototoxicity. Quinolone-containing drops are the treatment of choice. Steroid-containing quinolone drops have been shown to result in resolution of otorrhea sooner than drops that do not contain a steroid *(11,12)*.

Commercial otic drops generally contain 0.3% antibiotic, giving a concentration of 3,000 μg/ml. These concentrations are higher than any recorded MIC for any relevant organism and usually exceed the MIC by a factor of 10 or more. Consequently, otic drops will eliminate infection if they can reach the middle ear space. They are fully effective even for organisms labeled "resistant" to floraquinolones by clinical laboratories. Clinical laboratories generally consider organisms with an MIC of 4 μg or higher resistant to fluoroquinolones since blood and tissue levels can often not exceed these levels after *systemic* administration. The high concentration of antibiotic in topical drops (3,000 mg/ml) will easily eliminate organisms with even relatively high MICs (i.e., 128–256). Since the concentration of antibiotic is so high in topical drops, all failures of therapy are failures of delivery, i.e., the medicine is simply not getting to the infected area.

Table 2 Complications of tympanostomy tubes

- Tympanic membrane perforation
- Otorrhea
- Myringosclerosis
- Granulation tissue
- Tube obstruction
- Prolonged retention of tube
- Early extrusion
- Tympanic membrane atrophy

Systemic antibiotics are generally not helpful in the treatment of otorrhea and probably should not be used as first-line therapy, especially in children where systemic fluoroquinolones are not approved for use. Pseudomonas and *Staphylococcus aureus* are grown from a very high percentage of children with posttympanostomy tube otorrhea. The microbiology of posttympanostomy tube otorrhea is therefore quite different from that of acute otitis media with an intact tympanic membrane. The beta lactam and macrolide antibiotics generally used for acute otitis media with an intact drum are therefore frequently of little or no use in treating posttympanostomy tube otorrhea.

When topical therapy is being utilized, sensitivity results from cultures, as noted above, are of little help. In a study by Dohar et al., resolution of otorrhea occurred much more rapidly and cure rates were significantly higher in children who received ototopic drops compared with children who received high-dose amoxicillin with clavulanic acid *(13)*.

If, however, topical therapy fails and a trial of systemic antibiotics is considered, then systemic therapy should be culture directed. If antibiotic therapy fails to resolve the infection, then the child should be carefully evaluated for persistent rhinitis, adenoid disease, an immune deficiency, and for the presence of a middle ear foreign body/cholesteatoma. If such a work-up fails to identify a cause for the persistent otorrhea, the tympanostomy tube is best removed.

Tympanic membrane perforation. Studies place the risk of long-term perforation after tube extrusion at around 1–2% for grommets *(14)* and around 15–30% for t-tubes *(15)*. Softer t-tubes with shorter flanges may have significantly lower perforation rates. Perforations caused by tubes are usually small and can often be managed with paper patch or fat graft myringoplasty. However, a small perforation can perform the function of a tympanostomy tube. For this reason, formal tympanoplasty should probably not be attempted until the child has developed more mature eustachian tube function.

Myringosclerosis. Scarring of the tympanic membrane is a very common finding after tube extrusion. This problem is almost entirely cosmetic with no significant adverse sequellae ***(16)***.

Granulation tissue. Inflammatory tissue can form around the tympanostomy tube as chronic infection or a foreign body reaction. It can produce significant otorrhea and can block the opening, resulting in a nonfunctioning tube. Steroid-containing drops can be used for prolonged periods in an attempt to reduce the inflammation causing the granulation tissue but fungal superinfection can become a problem ***(17)***. Failing this, the tube should be removed.

Tube obstruction. Wax, dry mucous, dry blood, or granulation tissue can block the tube's opening. In a tolerant child or adult, wax, mucous, or blood can sometimes be removed with a pick or Rosen needle in the clinic. Alternatively, hydrogen peroxide can be used. Severe pain with hydrogen peroxide indicates the obstruction has been removed and the solution is irritating the middle ear mucosa.

Prolonged retention of tube. Occasionally a tube will last much longer than predicted. If it is not causing a foreign body reaction or other complication, there is no clear indication to remove it; however, many clinicians would do so after 2–3 years.

Early extrusion. This complication may be caused by voluminous mucous flow through the tympanostomy before the tube can become integrated into the drum.

Tympanic membrane atrophy. Repeated sets of tubes can produce focal areas of atrophy in the ear drum. These areas are usually not associated with adverse outcomes but occasionally can form retraction pockets with their attendant risks of ossicular chain erosion and cholesteatoma. If significant retractions do occur, the affected areas of the drum should be excised and repaired with a graft.

Conclusion

Placement of tympanostomy tubes is an extremely common procedure. The indications for tubes, typically for recurrent acute otitis media and persistent otitis media with effusion, represent failure of effective eustachian tube function. Tubes effectively address the shortcomings of a poorly functioning eustachian tube. Tympanostomy tubes are common and effective for recurrent acute otitis media and chronic otitis media with effusion.

References

1. Teele DW, Klein JO, Rosner B: The Greater Boston Otitis Media Study Group. Epidemiology of otitis media during the first seven years of life in children in Greater Boston: a prospective cohort study. *J Infect Dis* 1989;160:83–94.
2. Klein JO, et al.: Otitis media and the development of speech, language, and cognitive abilities at seven years of age. In: Lim DJ, ed. Recent Advances in Otitis Media, Philadelphia: BC Decker, 1988:396–397.
3. Paradise JL, et al.: Tympanostomy tubes and developmental outcomes at 9 to 11 years of age. *N Engl J Med* 2007;356(3):248–261.
4. Le CT, Freeman DW, Fireman BH: Evaluation of ventilating tubes and myringotomy in the treatment of recurrent or persistent otitis media. *Pediatr Infect Dis J* 1991;10:2–11.
5. American Academy of Otolaryngology-Head and Neck Surgery: 1995 Clinical Indicators Compendium: Guidelines for Tonsillectomy, Adenoidectomy, Adenotonsillectomy, Alexandria, VA: American Academy of Otolaryngology-Head and Neck Surgery, 1995.
6. Chole RA, Hubbell RN: Antimicrobial activity of silastic tympanostomy tubes impregnated with silver oxide. A randomized double-blind trial. *Arch Otolaryngol Head Neck Surg* 1995;121:562–565.
7. Garcia P, Gates GA, Schechtman KB: Does topical antibiotic prophylaxis reduce post-tympanostomy tube otorrhea? *Ann Otol Rhinol Laryngol* 1994;103:54–58.
8. Podoshin L, Fradis M, Ben DJ: Ototoxicity of ear drops in patients suffering from chronic otitis media. *J Laryngol Otol* 1989;103:46.
9. Parker GS, et al.: The effect of water exposure after tympanostomy tube insertion. *Am J Otolaryngol* 1994;15:193–196.
10. Mandel EM, Casselbrant ML, Kurs-Lasky M: Acute otorrhea: bacteriology of a common complication of tympanostomy tubes. *Ann Otol Rhinol Laryngol* 1994;103:713–718.
11. Roland PS, Anon JB, Moe RD, et al.: Topical Ciprofloxacin/Dexamethasosne is superior to ciprofloxacin alone in pediatric patients with acute otitis media and otorrhea through tympanostomy tubes. *Laryngoscope* 2003;113:2116–2122.
12. Roland PS, Kreisler LS, Reese B, et al.: Topical ciprofloxacin/dexamethasone otic suspension is superior to ofloxacin otic solution in the treatment of children with acute otitis media with otorrhea through tympanostomy tubes. *Pediatrics* (online edition) January 2004;113:e40–e46.
13. Dohar J, Giles W, Roland P, Bikhazi N, Carroll S, et al.: Topical ciprofloxacin/dexamethasone is superior to oral amoxicillin/clavulanic acid in acute otitis media with otorrhea through tympanostomy tubes. *Pediatrics* 2006;118(3):e561–e569. Epub 2006 Jul 31.
14. Matt BH, et al.: Incidence of perforation with Goode T-tube. *Int J Pediatr Otorhinolaryngol* 1991;21:1–6.

15. Hawthorne MR, Parker AJ: Perforations of the tympanic membrane following the use of Goode-Type 'long term' tympanostomy tubes. *J Laryngol Otol* 1988;102:997–999.
16. Tos M, Stangerup SE: Hearing loss in tympanosclerosis caused by grommets. *Arch Otolaryngol Head Neck Surg* 1989;115:931–935.
17. Roland PS, Dohar JE, Lanier BJ, Hekkenburg R, Lane EM, Conroy PJ, Wall GM, Dupre SJ, Potts S: Topical ciprofloxacin/dexamethasone otic suspension is superior to ofloxacin otic solution in the treatment of granulation tissue in children with acute otitis media with otorrhea through tympanostomy tubes. *Otolaryngol Head Neck Surg* 2004; 130(6):736–741.Tyler W. Scoresby and Peter S. RolandP.S. Roland (✉)and T.W. ScoresbyDepartment of Otolaryngology-Head and Neck Surgery, University of Texas Southwestern Medical Center at Dallas, 5323 Harry Hines Blvd, Dallas, TX, 75390-9035, USAe-mail: Peter.Roland@UTSouthwestern.edu

Chronic Disorders of the Middle Ear and Mastoid (Tympanic Membrane Perforations and Cholesteatoma)

C.Y. Joseph Chang

Key Points

- Chronic disorders of the middle ear and mastoid include chronic tympanic membrane (TM) perforations with or without infection, chronic otitis media (COM) or the synonymous chronic suppurative otitis media (CSOM), and cholesteatomas.
- These conditions occur infrequently in the developed world but are more prevalent in areas with limited medical care.
- The typical symptoms include hearing loss and recurrent or persistent otorrhea usually without pain.
- Diagnosis can usually be made based on the history and examination of the ear.
- Work-up typically includes testing such as audiometry or auditory brainstem response (ABR) and in some cases computed tomography (CT) of the temporal bone.
- Medical treatments such as ototopical antibiotics are used to suppress infection but are typically not curative.
- Surgery such as tympanoplasty with or without mastoidectomy is needed for cure.
- Long-term follow-up after treatment is essential due to a significant rate of disease recurrence.

Keywords: Chronic otitis media • Chronic suppurative otitis media • Cholesteatoma

C.Y.J. Chang
Texas Ear Center and Department of Otolaryngology – Head and Neck Surgery, University of Texas – Houston Medical School, Houston, TX, USA
e-mail: drchang@texasent.com

Introduction

Chronic disorders that affect the middle ear and mastoid include a number of conditions that are typically associated with a previous history of recurrent acute otitis media (AOM). It is unclear why some children with recurrent AOM develop chronic ear disease, but the prevalence of chronic ear disease is higher in areas that have fewer resources to provide early medical intervention for AOM. Poor eustachian tube function is also considered an important factor in pathogenesis. It is important to diagnose this condition early since recurrent infections can lead to sequelae such as ossicular chain destruction that can result in conductive hearing loss or more serious life-threatening complications.

Definitions

A tympanic membrane (TM) perforation is any defect in the tympanic membrane resulting in exposure of the middle ear. TM perforations occur as a result of acute otitis media with TM rupture, trauma, or surgical interventions such as placement of a pressure equalization tube (PET). The large majority of perforations heal spontaneously but some do not for reasons that are not known. A TM with a PET that is retained for over 1 year is at a significant risk for developing a chronic perforation. Most agree that a TM perforation that shows no sign of healing at 3 months is unlikely to close spontaneously and can at that point be considered a chronic perforation, making surgical repair an appropriate step.

Chronic otitis media (COM) and chronic suppurative otitis media (CSOM) is the presence of a chronic TM

R.B. Mitchell and K.D. Pereira (eds.), *Pediatric Otolaryngology for the Clinician*,
DOI: 10.1007/978-1-60327-127-1_9, © Humana Press, a part of Springer Science + Business Media, LLC 2009

perforation with recurrent or persistent purulent otorrhea. COM and CSOM are synonymous. The degree and duration of otorrhea necessary to be considered CSOM rather than a TM perforation with occasional otorrhea is not strictly defined. Most cases of CSOM are associated with chronically thickened middle ear mucosa (Fig. 1).

Cholesteatoma is the presence of keratinizing squamous epithelium (surface layer of skin) in the middle ear or mastoid. The usual origin of the skin is the TM. Interestingly, when skin is present in the middle ear space, its behavior is altered in such a way that it can grow without inhibition and cause progressive bone erosion. If the cholesteatoma is exposed to the external environment, the bacterial contamination usually results in chronic infection and otorrhea. Cholesteatomas are categorized based on etiology into congenital, primary acquired, and secondary acquired lesions.

Congenital cholesteatoma is the presence of a middle ear or mastoid cholesteatoma with no previous history of TM perforation or ear surgery and intact TM. These cholesteatomas are typically difficult to diagnose, especially if the TM is opaque. Congenital cholesteatomas were thought to arise from failure of involution of an embryonic rest of epithelial cells near the eustachian tube. However, a more recent theory advocates the presence of microretractions of the TM squamous epithelium that pinch off from the TM and form cholesteatoma pearls in the middle ear.

Primary acquired cholesteatoma arise as a retraction of the TM with migration of the skin into the middle ear and are the most common form of cholesteatoma seen. These retractions can form in the pars tensa, which is the conical portion of the TM, or the small area in the superior part of the TM above the malleus long process, pars flaccida. Since these cholesteatomas are open to the ear canal and are contaminated by bacteria, there is a high incidence of otorrhea. These primary acquired cholesteatomas can be visualized directly on examination of the ear (Fig. 2a,b).

Secondary acquired cholesteatoma form as a result of inadvertent skin implantation during ear surgery such as TM perforation repair or pressure equalization tube (PET) placement. They can also form from migration of skin from the edges of a healing TM perforation. The TM can be intact at the time of presentation, with no otorrhea, making the diagnosis difficult by examination alone.

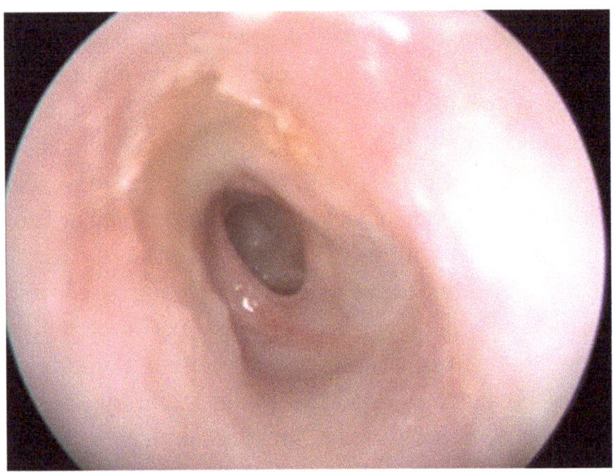

Fig. 1 Chronic otitis media (COM/CSOM) with tympanic membrane perforation, right ear

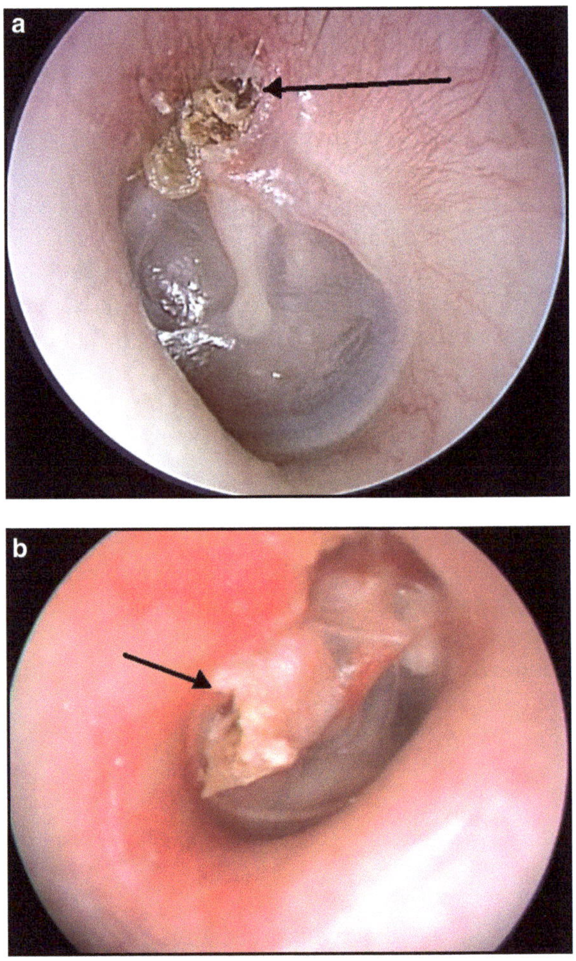

Fig. 2 Cholesteatoma arising from the tympanic membrane: (**a**) pars flaccida (***arrow***), left ear; (**b**) pars tensa (*arrow*), right ear

Prevalence

The prevalence of chronic ear disease in the developed world is thought to be around 0.3%, whereas in the less developed world, the figure may be as high as 15% *(1,2)*. The prevalence of cholesteatoma in the developed world may be in the order of 0.07%. The relative rarity of chronic ear disease in the developed world makes diagnosis and treatment of this condition difficult. The primary care physician, who sees the bulk of common acute otitis media, chronic otitis media with effusion (COME), and otitis externa, needs to have a high index of suspicion when evaluating patients with ear disease, especially if there are unusual symptoms in the presentation such as persistent otorrhea despite standard medical treatment.

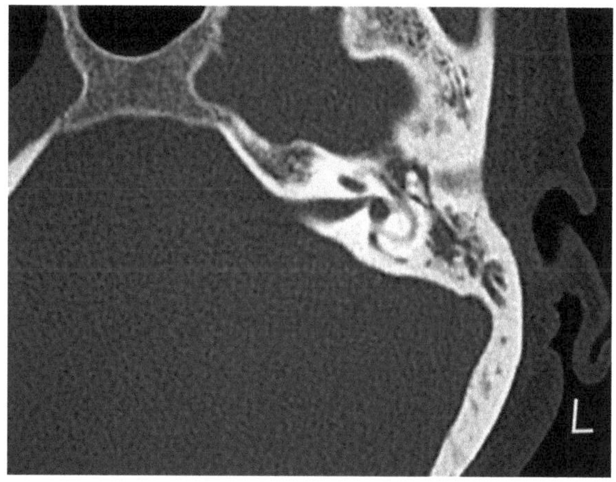

Fig. 3 CT showing left mastoid opacification without bone erosion. These findings can be consistent with AOM, COME, or COM/CSOM

Diagnosis

Clinical evaluation – Diagnosis is based on a history of recurrent acute otitis media or otorrhea, including hearing loss that persists even after the infection is controlled medically. The diagnosis is straightforward in cases where the TM perforation or cholesteatoma is readily visible. Occasionally, the otorrhea and debris in the external auditory canal (EAC) can obscure the view and make diagnosis difficult. This makes cleaning the EAC essential. In some children general anesthesia may be needed for an adequate evaluation. In cases of secondary acquired and congenital cholesteatoma, the lesion may be visible through the TM, but the TM may also appear completely normal. The only indication of a middle ear problem in these cases is the presence of a conductive hearing loss that is otherwise unexplained.

Hearing testing – It is important to establish the hearing level in patients with chronic ear disease. Bilateral hearing loss can lead to speech delay and deficits in learning, hence hearing restoration treatment will need to be considered urgently. Most children older than 2 years can be evaluated with behavioral audiometry. Younger or less cooperative patients may require auditory brainstem response (ABR) to record hearing thresholds.

Imaging – Computed tomography (CT) is the modality of choice when imaging of the temporal bone is needed to diagnose chronic ear disease. CT is vastly superior to plain films of the temporal bone. The CT scan is typically obtained in the axial and coronal planes using slice thicknesses of 0.6–1.5 mm and bone windows. It provides excellent delineation of the bony structure of the temporal bone, specifically areas of bone erosion, as well as any abnormal soft tissue or fluid that may be present in the middle ear or mastoid. It is important to note that the presence of soft tissue or fluid in the mastoid or middle ear does not necessarily indicate the presence of chronic ear disease, as acute otitis media can result in similar findings (Fig. 3). The CT abnormalities that are more specific to chronic ear disease include erosion of bone and ossicles. Bony changes are more commonly seen in cases of cholesteatoma than CSOM (Fig. 4a,b). MRI is not very useful for the delineation of middle ear and mastoid disease but can be useful in the evaluation of complications such as intracranial abscess and sigmoid sinus thrombosis.

Bacteriology – The organisms that are associated with chronic ear disease are typically very different from those that are found in acute otitis media. The typical bacteria found in chronic ear disease are more similar to those found in acute otitis externa such as *Pseudomonas aeruginosa*, Staphylococcus species, Proteus species, and occasionally anaerobes. Therefore, treatment of chronic ear disease with agents that are used typically for AOM is not usually effective. The most effective antibiotic classes for chronic ear disease include flouroquinolones and aminoglycosides. Fortunately, these antibiotics can usually be administered topically, avoiding the side effects and complications associated with systemic use.

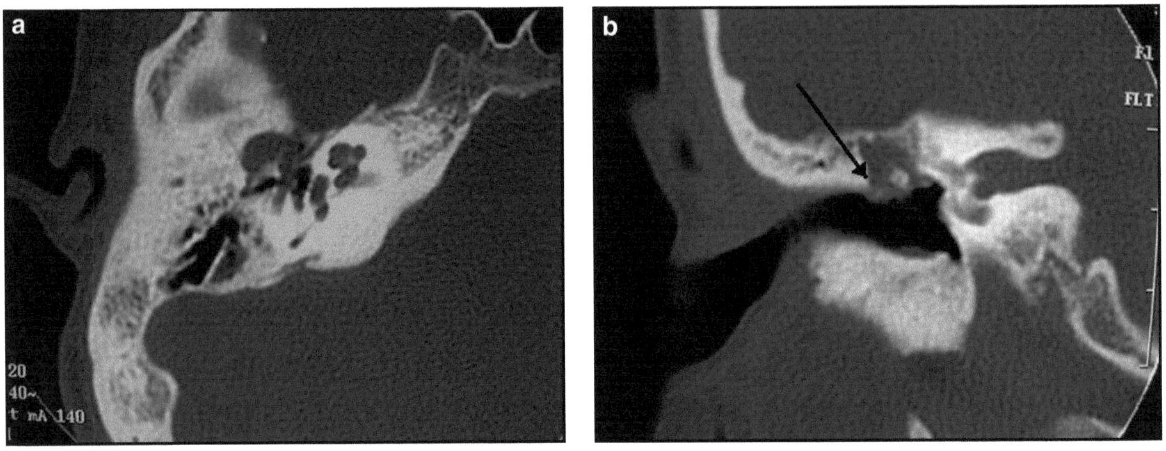

Fig. 4 CT showing mastoid opacification with bone erosion of the scutum (*arrow*) and mass in the middle ear and attic. These findings can be consistent with cholesteatoma. (**a**) Axial CT, right ear. (**b**) Coronal CT, right ear

Flouroquinolones are the drugs of choice as even topical use of aminoglycosides in chronic ear disease when there is a TM perforation can result in ototoxicity.

Complications of Chronic Ear Disease

Hearing loss – Conductive hearing loss (CHL) due to a mass effect of infected tissue and ossicular damage is common. Sensorineural hearing loss (SNHL) is also possible but less common. It may occur as a result of an induced inner ear inflammation from the adjacent purulent infection in the middle ear space. SNHL has also been implicated in a few cases of ototoxicity resulting from prolonged application of topical aminoglycosides.

Vestibular dysfunction – It is rare to have acute vertigo as a result of chronic ear disease. A labrynthine fistula with cholesteatoma can lead to vertigo but is not commonly encountered. Children rarely complain about disequilibrium unless the condition is severe. The mechanism may also be an induced inner ear inflammation from the adjacent purulent infection in the middle ear space.

Facial nerve injury – Facial nerve dysfunction rarely occurs in chronic ear disease. In cases of purulent otorrhea, there may be direct injury to the nerve by surrounding inflammation, especially in areas of dehiscence of the fallopian canal. In cases of cholesteatoma, there is the added possibility of mechanical compression caused by a growing cholesteatoma. Most cases of facial nerve dysfunction resolve after adequate treatment of the underlying chronic ear disease.

Acute mastoiditis – This condition is diagnosed by the presence of acute bone-erosive disease from purulent infection and extension of the inflammatory process to the surrounding tissues such as the postauricular skin. The presence of pus in the mastoid is technically considered "mastoiditis" but this condition occurs with all cases of acute otitis media and is not treated any differently. The term "acute mastoiditis" is reserved for cases in which the inflammation or infection extends to the postauricular skin, resulting in erythema, tenderness, and anterior displacement of the pinna, or where there is coalescence or bone erosion of the septae in the mastoid air cells, typically visible on a CT scan. In some cases, the purulent infection extends from the mastoid tip into the neck, forming a neck abscess (Bezold's abscess). Acute mastoiditis is typically treated with intravenous (IV) antibiotics and PET placement, although more aggressive treatments, including mastoidectomy, may be needed in certain cases such as coalescent mastoiditis. Any abscess also requires surgical drainage. Acute mastoiditis is not a common condition. Other complications of chronic ear disease, such as sigmoid sinus thrombosis and intracranial infection, are even less common but can be devastating.

Sigmoid sinus thrombosis – The extension of suppuration that results from acute mastoiditis can involve the sigmoid sinus, which is located posteriorly in the mastoid.

Inflammation results in thrombus formation in the sigmoid sinus, which can, in some cases, throw off septic emboli into the lungs causing picket-fence fevers. Otherwise, the symptoms of this condition are similar to acute mastoiditis. There is a higher incidence of intracranial complications associated with coalescent mastoiditis and sigmoid sinus thrombosis *(3)*, so it is typically treated aggressively, with IV antibiotics and surgical drainage with mastoidectomy.

Intracranial infections - This group of complications can be truly life-threatening if diagnosis and treatment are delayed. Possible problems include bacterial meningitis, epidural or subdural abscess, and intracranial abscess. Patients who are suspected of having these conditions require hospital admission for evaluation, which includes neurosurgery consultation, CT of the brain, and lumbar puncture for diagnosis and culture (as long as there is no evidence of significant supratentorial pressure).

Treatment

General - Medical treatment is typically administered in an outpatient setting for both COM/CSOM and cholesteatoma. The goals are to reduce or eliminate infection if possible. Medical treatment consists of keeping water out of the ear, reducing the amount of debris in the ear canal with frequent debridement in the office, and application of topical antibiotic agents *(4)*. Systemic antibiotic treatment is usually less helpful than topical agents since these agents typically provide a much higher concentration of antibiotic at the site of infection. Due to the microbiology of chronic ear disease, which differs significantly from that of acute otitis media, agents that are effective include aminoglycosides and quinolones. Aminoglycoside ear drops such as neomycin/polymyxin B or gentamicin continue to be used, but due to the concern regarding ototoxicity and the advent of the non-ototoxic and effective topical quinolone agents, flouroquinolone ear drops are being used more frequently *(5)*. In the United States, the only FDA-approved topical medication for COM/CSOM is ofloxacin (Floxin Otic™). There is a combination dexamethasone/ciprofloxacin agent (CiproDex™) that is FDA-approved for post-tympanostomy tube otorrhea. There are currently no FDA-approved topical agents for cholesteatoma, so most physicians use one of the available topical agents as an off-label treatment.

Otorrhea can often be eliminated in cases of COM/CSOM and some cases of cholesteatoma. The infection may not cease with medical treatment alone, due to chronically infected squamous debris within the cholesteatoma where the host's immune mechanisms and antibiotics cannot penetrate. There are some cases of COM/CSOM that never clear up solely with medical treatment for reasons that are unknown.

Surgical treatment (COM/CSOM) – The decision to proceed with surgery is based on symptomatology and the child's health status. In many cases, surgical treatment is essentially elective and is performed to improve hearing and decrease or eliminate the recurrent otorrhea and other bothersome symptoms. Because of a concern regarding further ossicular damage and possible complications in cases of very frequent or persistent infection and otorrhea, surgical treatment is strongly recommended in most children. The goal of surgical treatment is to make the ear free of infection, the so-called safe ear.

There are two schools of thought regarding the optimal surgical treatment - tympanoplasty alone or tympanoplasty with mastoidectomy. Some surgeons believe that patients with COM/CSOM have infection most likely due to the presence of the TM perforation, and tympanoplasty, an outpatient procedure that involves repairing the TM perforation, is the best surgical treatment. Other surgeons believe that there is a nidus of chronic infection within the mastoid that should be removed with the mastoidectomy procedure at the same time as the tympanoplasty. There are studies that indicate that either treatment option is successful, but there are only a few studies comparing the relative efficacy of the two procedures *(6,7)*. In cases of damage to the ossicles, an ossicular chain reconstruction (repair of the ossicles using the patient's own bone or prosthetic implant) is usually performed at the same time.

Surgical treatment (cholesteatoma) – Due to the higher risk of destructive processes in the ear and more serious complications, surgical treatment is more frequently recommended than in COM/CSOM. The goal of surgical treatment is to make the ear free of infection and cholesteatoma, the so-called safe ear. The great challenge is not only to remove all the cholesteatoma but to keep it from recurring, since surgery does not necessarily eliminate the risk factors such as eustachian tube dysfunction or other unknown factors that caused the initial cholesteatoma to form in the first place.

The typical surgical procedure includes a tympanoplasty with or without mastoidectomy, depending on the extent of the cholesteatoma. The surgery for cholesteatoma is typically more extensive and complicated than for COM/CSOM. After complete cholesteatoma removal, all areas at risk for forming a recurrent cholesteatoma, such as areas of the TM, are typically strengthened with a stiff material such as cartilage to prevent skin retractions. In some cases, the ear canal may need to be removed in order to eliminate all cholesteatoma, resulting in a mastoid cavity. This surgery is called the canal-wall-down (CWD) or modified radical mastoidectomy. In this procedure, the middle ear space and TM are preserved or reconstructed, allowing for preservation or reconstruction of the hearing mechanism. In rare cases of very severe disease, the radical mastoidectomy is performed, in which case the middle ear is obliterated. A significant advantage of the CWD procedure is that it "exteriorizes" the areas where cholesteatoma form and grow, such as the epitympanum and mastoid. These areas now become accessible during the office examination and any potential cholesteatoma development can be removed by simple mastoid cavity debridement in the office. A disadvantage of the CWD procedure is that these children can be more susceptible to otorrhea, especially with water exposure. In many cases, the ossicular chain is damaged by disease or needs to be disrupted and/or removed in order to eliminate all of the cholesteatoma. The surgical objectives can in some cases be achieved with the canal-wall-up (CWU) approach with opening of the facial recess if the surgical anatomy is favorable. This surgery does not result in an open mastoid cavity, so there is a significant risk of cholesteatoma recurrence. A planned second surgery is often performed to check for residual cholesteatoma and/or to perform the ossicular chain reconstruction after the infectious disease has been well-controlled. A more detailed discussion of the surgical treatment is beyond the scope of this chapter and can be found elsewhere *(8)*.

Outcome

Hearing – The hearing function typically improves as a result of tympanoplasty, as repair of the TM perforation restores most or all of its function. If an ossicular chain reconstruction is performed, the outcomes are, on average, not as good as having the native ossicles, but significant improvement is possible. There are many factors that relate to the overall hearing results, including the severity of disease, functional status of the remaining ossicles, and the development of recurrent disease. The postoperative hearing results appear to have a positive correlation to the preoperative hearing level; that is, the better the hearing level preoperatively, the better the hearing results tend to be after surgery.

Recurrence of TM perforation and otorrhea – The overall success rate of TM perforation closure is very good, with results ranging from 90 to 100% after 1 year *(9–12)*. The success rate tends to decrease over longer periods of observation *(13)*.

Recurrence of AOM – It is important to realize that some children with COM/CSOM are still at risk for developing AOM and COME. Some children with successful closure of the TM may develop AOM or COME, requiring further medical treatment or ventilation tube placement.

Recurrence of cholesteatoma – The long-term control of cholesteatoma continues to be problematic. The recurrence rate of cholesteatoma, including both recidivistic (disease left behind during surgery) and recurrent disease (new formation of cholesteatoma) may be as high as 20–30% over 10 years *(14,15)*. The high recurrence rate likely relates to incomplete understanding of the pathophysiology of the disease etiology and inability to correct surgically any suspected etiologies such as eustachian tube dysfunction. The best surgical efforts to date involve complete removal of the cholesteatoma and reinforcement or exteriorization of areas susceptible to forming another cholesteatoma. It is therefore imperative that patients with cholesteatoma be monitored over many years for recurrent disease with office evaluation and CT scans in selected cases.

Conclusion

Chronic ear disease, which includes COM/CSOM and cholesteatoma, is a condition that is not common in the developed world but can cause significant morbidity, including recurrent or persistent otorrhea, hearing loss, and other more serious sequelae. The diagnosis can be made with a good history, physical examination, and in some cases CT imaging. Medical treatment in the form of ototopical antibiotic agents can typically reduce the level of inflammatory and infectious disease, but surgery in the form of tympanoplasty with or without mastoidectomy is typically needed for definitive treatment. Even after successful treatment, patients require long-term follow-up since there is a significant incidence of disease recurrence.

References

1. Verma AK, Vohra A, Maitra A, et al. Epidemiology of chronic suppurative otitis media and deafness in a rural area and developing an intervention strategy. Indian J Pediatr. 1995;62:725–729.
2. Cohen D, Tamir D. The prevalence of middle ear pathologies in Jerusalem school children. Am J Otol. 1989;10:456–459.
3. Antonelli PJ, Garside JA, Mancuso AA, et al. Computed tomography and the diagnosis of coalescent mastoiditis. Otolaryngol Head Neck Surg. 1999;120:350–354.
4. Hannley MT, Denneny JC 3rd, Holzer SS. Use of ototopical antibiotics in treating 3 common ear diseases. Otolaryngol Head Neck Surg. 2000;122:934–940.
5. Roland PS, Stewart MG, et al. Consensus panel on role of potentially ototoxic antibiotics for topical middle ear use: introduction, methodology, and recommendations. Otolaryngol Head Neck Surg. 2004;130(3 Suppl):S51–S56.
6. Balyan FR, Celikkanat S, Aslan A, et al. Mastoidectomy in noncholesteatomatous chronic suppurative otitis media: is it necessary? Otolaryngol Head Neck Surg. 1997;117: 592–595.
7. Mishiro Y, Sakagami M, Takahashi Y, et al. Tympanoplasty with and without mastoidectomy for non-cholesteatomatous chronic otitis media. Eur Arch Otorhinolaryngol. 2001;258:13–15.
8. Chang CYJ. Cholesteatoma. In Lalwani AK (Ed). Current Diagnosis & Treatment in Otolarynology – Head & Neck Surgery. New York: McGraw-Hill. 2004:707–714.
9. Rizer FM. Overlay versus underlay tympanoplasty. Part II: The study. Laryngoscope 1997;107:26–36.
10. Cueva RA. Areolar temporalis fascia: a reliable graft for tympanoplasty. Am J Otol. 1999; 20:709–711.
11. Chang CY, Gray LC. Pressed scar tissue for tympanic membrane grafting in revision tympanoplasty. Otolaryngol Head Neck Surg. 2005;132:30–36.
12. Vartiainen E, Nuutinen J. Success and pitfalls in myringoplasty: follow-up study of 404 cases. Am J Otol. 1993;14:301–305.
13. Rickers J, Petersen CG, Pedersen CB, Ovesen T. Long-term follow-up evaluation of mastoidectomy in children with non-cholesteatomatous chronic suppurative otitis media. Int J Pediatr Otorhinolaryngol. 2006;70:711–715.
14. Lau T, Tos M. Cholesteatoma in children: recurrence related to observation period. Am J Otolaryngol. 1987;8:364–375.
15. Parisier SC, Hanson MB, Han JC, Cohen AJ, Selkin BA. Pediatric cholesteatoma: an individualized, single-stage approach. Otolaryngol Head Neck Surg. 1996;115:107–114.

Congenital Hearing Loss (Sensorineural and Conductive)

Anthony A. Mikulec

Key Points

- Screening is the cornerstone of effective treatment.
- Genetic testing is proving increasingly useful in the evaluation of congenital sensorineural hearing loss.
- Cochlear implantation of children with bilateral profound sensorineural hearing loss between ages 1 and 2 yields the best long-term results, with the majority of children entering a mainstream grade school.
- Children with atresia can be rehabilitated with bone conducting hearing aids, a bone conducting osseointegrated implant (Baha), or with surgical atresia repair in cases with a favorable temporal bone CT scan.

Keywords: Congenital hearing loss • Sensorineural hearing loss • Cochlear implantation • Aural atresia

Introduction

Congenital hearing loss represents a spectrum of underlying pathologies including environmental and genetic causes. Early identification is needed to maximize rehabilitation and has been facilitated by systematic newborn hearing screening programs. Oral deaf schools, audiologists, and otolaryngologists work together to intensively rehabilitate a hearing-impaired child in the early years of life with the goal of entering the child into the mainstream educational process as soon as possible.

A.A. Mikulec
Otologic and Neurotologic Surgery, Department of Otolaryngology – Head and Neck Surgery, Saint Louis University School of Medicine, St Louis, MO, USA
e-mail: mikuleca@slu.edu

Definitions

Congenital – related to gestation or birth of the child
Sensorineural hearing loss – loss of hearing attributable to the cochlea, cochlear nerve, or brain
Conductive hearing loss – loss of hearing attributed to impaired transmission of sound to the cochlea
Atresia – absence of the external auditory canal, often with associated middle ear abnormalities
Microtia – absence (anotia) or malformation of the outer ear

Prevalence

Congenital sensorineural hearing loss – occurs in 1:500 to 1:2,000 births and 90% of deaf children are born to hearing parents.
Microtia – occurs in 1 to 4:10,000 births and is associated with atresia about 70% of the time. The more severe the microtia, the greater the risk of atresia.
Atresia – occurs in 1 to 4:10,000 births. Atresia without associated microtia is uncommon.
Congenital conductive hearing loss not due to atresia or otitis media and its sequelae is rare.

Diagnosis

Newborn hearing screening is the key to early identification of hearing loss and is now either mandated by law or commonly practiced in most advanced nations. Testing algorithms vary but generally include automated versions of otoacoustic emission testing (OAE),

R.B. Mitchell and K.D. Pereira (eds.), *Pediatric Otolaryngology for the Clinician*,
DOI: 10.1007/978-1-60327-127-1_10, © Humana Press, a part of Springer Science + Business Media, LLC 2009

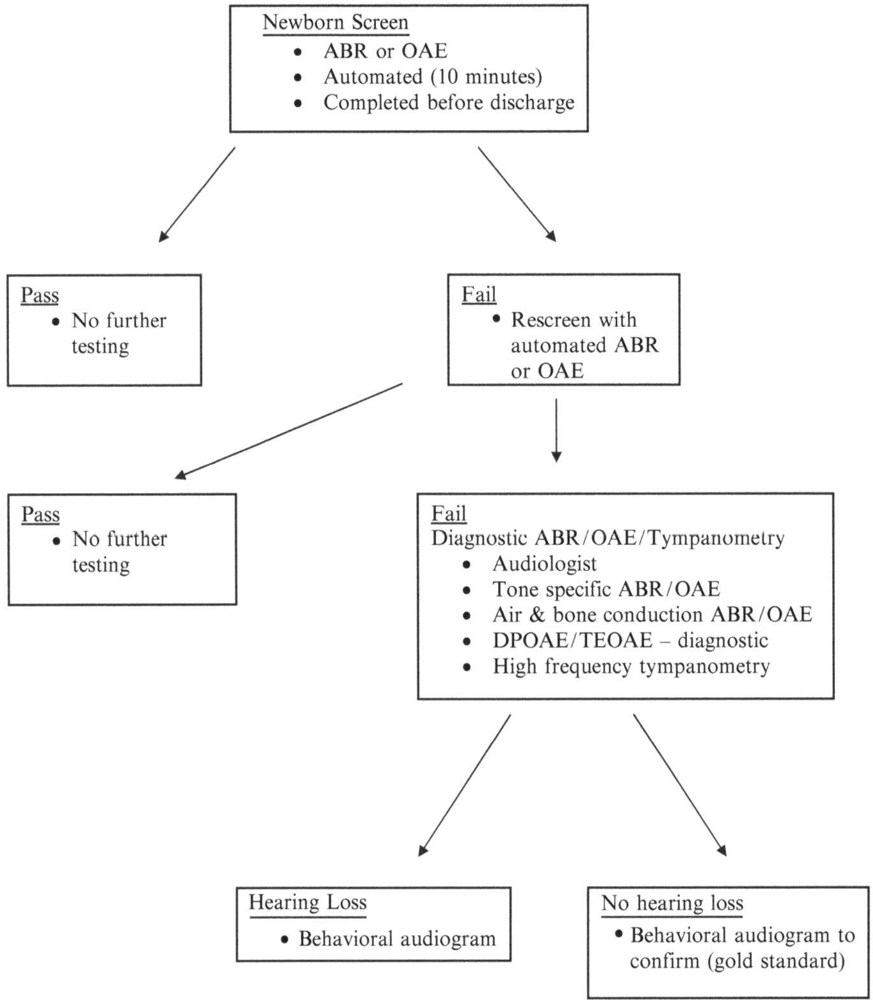

Fig. 1 Sample newborn hearing screening flow diagram. ***ABR*** auditory brainstem response; ***OAE*** otoacoustic emissions; ***DPOAE*** distortion product otoacoustic emissions; ***TEOAE*** transient otoacoustic emissions

automated brainstem response (ABR) testing, or both (Fig. 1). Once a child with hearing loss is identified through screening, a referral is made for further audiometric analysis and otolaryngology evaluation. The most common cause of a failed newborn hearing screening is otitis media with effusion.

Prelingual hearing loss occurs before the onset of speech while postlingual hearing loss occurs after the onset of speech. About 50% of congenital bilateral sensorineural hearing loss is environmental, most commonly due to primary maternal cytomegalovirus (CMV). The other 50% are genetic, of which about 15% are syndromic and 85% are nonsyndromic (Fig. 2). The pneumonic "TORCH" is helpful for remembering environmental causes of congenital hearing loss: toxoplasmosis, rubella, cytomegalovirus, and herpes. Cytomegalovirus is a member of the herpes family of DNA-enveloped viruses and is transmitted across the placenta, in breast milk, and within the birth canal and is present in both semen and cervical secretions. Eighty percent of adults have antibody to CMV. Damage to the fetus requires a previously uninfected mother who sustains primary infection during pregnancy. A common scenario is a mother with one or more previous children who is CMV antibody negative and who becomes infected during a subsequent pregnancy, presumably through the asymptomatic shedding of CMV in saliva and urine of her own children, who have acquired CMV from playmates. Postnatal CMV infection is generally benign, but 20% of infants infected with CMV during gestation will show signs of deafness, microcephaly, and mental retardation.

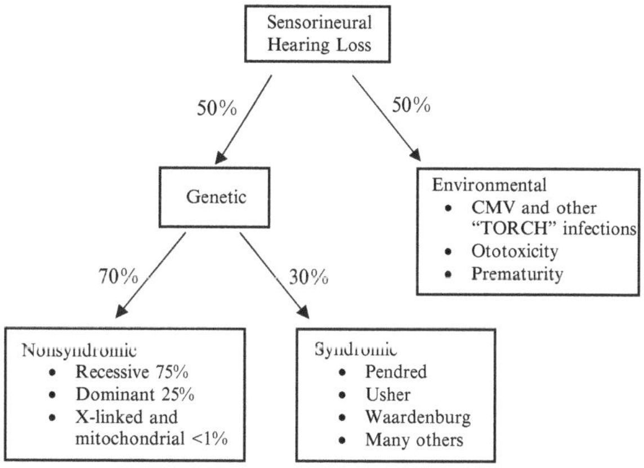

Fig. 2 Causes of congenital sensorineural hearing loss

Sensorineural hearing loss not clearly due to infection or environmental factors is increasingly referred for genetic evaluation, replacing a myriad of diagnostic tests. Over a hundred genes resulting in nonsyndromic hearing impairment have been identified, with DFNA (the acronym DFN comes from DeaFNess) denoting loci for autosomal dominant deafness genes, DFNB for autosomal recessive deafness genes, and DFN for X-linked deafness genes. The GJB2 gene, which codes for the gap junction protein Connexin 26, is the most common abnormality found; identification of a defect in this gene precludes the need for further diagnostics and predicts that progression of hearing loss is unlikely. Genetic screening assists in identification of syndromes that are not clinically apparent and can be useful for family planning if the parents are considering having more children. Computerized tomography or MRI of the temporal bone is obtained to evaluate for inner ear abnormalities such as Mondini dyslapsia (too few cochlear turns), enlarged vestibular aqueduct, or in preparation for cochlear implantation.

Careful clinical evaluation allows identification of associated syndromes, which often have atypical facial features. For example, Usher syndrome is genetically heterogeneous and features four subtypes with varying degrees of the following: sensorineural hearing loss, vestibular dysfunction, and retinitis pigmentosa leading to progressive deafness and blindness. Pendred syndrome constitutes 5–10% of congenital deafness, making it the most common form of syndromic hearing loss. This disorder is autosomal recessive with prelingual hearing loss associated with radiographic abnormalities (enlarged vestibular aqueduct or Mondini dysplasia) and failure of iodine organification which results in goiter at the time of puberty.

Some congenital hearing losses have onset and progression during the first years of life. Such children have postlingual hearing loss and will have passed the newborn hearing screen but the deficit comes to light through later audiometric evaluation, either on parental or physician suspicion of reduced hearing or through a failed school hearing test. These children should be fitted with amplification and proceed to cochlear implantation if needed. Children with Down's syndrome are prone to Eustachian tube dysfunction and recurrent effusions, often necessitating multiple tympanostomy tube placements. Middle ear abnormalities may be present and a progressive mixed hearing loss may develop.

Research has shown a genetic predisposition to hearing loss associated with exposure to noise or ototoxins such as gentamicin and cisplatin. For the purposes of classification, such losses are not generally considered congenital.

Atresia of the outer ear canal results in a 60 dB conductive hearing loss. For children born with atresia, clinical evaluation for associated syndromes, such as Treacher-Collins, is performed and genetic testing considered. Treacher-Collins syndrome is autosomal dominant with manifestations including atresia with resultant conductive hearing loss, microtia, malar hypoplasia, hypoplastic mandible, coloboma, and downturned palpebral fissures. Congenital conductive hearing loss is usually due to atresia or otitis media and its sequelae. Less common causes of congenital conductive hearing loss include congenital stapes fixation and other ossicular malformations. Of note, children with Turner's syndrome may have conductive hearing loss due to ossicular abnormalities which are amenable to surgical repair.

Treatment

Bilateral Sensorineural Hearing Loss

Initial treatment involves amplification; if hearing loss is profound, then proceed to cochlear implantation, either unilateral or bilateral. Even if a child is an implant candidate, amplification should be pursued first as this allows the child to have some neural stimulation allowing for formation of central connections in the brain and habituates the child to reliable device use. The duration of amplification varies among implant surgeons, but a period of 3–6 months is common. In general, the earlier implantation is performed, the better the hearing and speech outcome. A CT scan or MRI is performed prior to implantation to assess for cochlear abnormalities that might necessitate a modified approach or nonstandard implant. Children with enlarged vestibular aqueducts are restricted from contact sports to prevent transmission of concussive forces from the CSF through the patent vestibular aqueduct with resultant step-wise hearing decrement. Bilateral implantation of children has gained increasing favor with the second implant yielding better functional results if it is performed before age 6. Simultaneous bilateral implantation has also been performed and may be an option for some children. Risks of cochlear implantation include facial palsy, device failure, and device extrusion. All children should receive pneumococcal vaccination prior to implantation and the rate of meningitis in implanted children with normal cochlea now approaches that of the unimplanted population. As over 95% of deaf children are born to hearing parents, most of these children are rehabilitated into the mainstream community. Deaf parents of deaf children may desire their child to enter deaf culture with rehabilitation through the use of signing and may eschew cochlear implantation.

Unilateral Sensorineural Hearing Loss

Treatment depends on the degree of hearing loss in the affected ear. For children with mild to severe losses, amplification is used. Children with a profound unilateral loss (dead ear) and a normal contralateral ear might be candidates for a Baha implant (see below) at an age when they can participate in the decision-making process. Both groups are treated with preferential classroom seating with the good ear toward the teacher, with consideration of an FM system (the teacher speaks into a microphone that transmits wirelessly to the child's receiver) and/or a hearing aid.

Bilateral Conductive Hearing Loss Due To Atresia

Options include bone-conducted hearing aids, the Baha implant (an osseointegrated transcutaneous implant utilizing bone conduction), or surgical repair of the atresia. A bone-conducting hearing aid placed on a hard or soft head band is the first intervention in a child with bilateral atresia and is usually fitted within the first year. A single bone-conducting aid can stimulate both cochlea by sound propogation through the skull. Around age 5, atresia repair or Baha implantation can be considered. The Baha implant utilizes growth of bone into a small, specially treated transcutaneous screw placed in the skull to provide reliable long-term bone conduction. Placement of the implant is usually performed in two short outpatient procedures in children, spaced 3–6 months apart, to allow osseointegration of the implant prior to attachment of the sound processor. In adults or older children, the procedure may be performed in one stage. The same osseointegrated implants can also be used to provide a reliable anchor for a prosthetic ear. Candidacy for atresia repair is based on careful review of a temporal bone CT scan for prediction of surgical outcome; a commonly used criteria being the Jahrsdoerfer scale. Surgical atresia repair, which is technically difficult and puts the facial nerve at risk, is generally contemplated if minimal abnormalities are present predicting a high likelihood of significant improvement in conductive hearing loss. Due to its simplicity and safety, Baha implantation is increasingly supplanting surgical atresia repair. If a microtia is associated with the atresia, the microtia is repaired first, generally after age 6, to provide a virgin vascular bed for plastic surgical repair. Fully implantable hearing aids are being used on an investigational basis in children with atresias and may provide an attractive rehabilitative option in the future.

Unilateral Conductive Hearing Loss Due To Atresia

Associated microtia repair can begin around age 6, and is performed before atresia repair. The appropriateness and timing of unilateral atresia repair remains debated; waiting until the child can fully participate in the decision-making process may be worthwhile. In the interim, a traditional hearing aid, unilateral bone-conducted aid, or Baha implant can be considered. The goal of interval amplification is to provide auditory input to the cochlea to allow development of central connections, increasing the probability of effective binaural hearing.

Conductive Hearing Loss Not Due To Atresia or Otitis Media

Options include amplification and consideration of surgical intervention based on CT scan findings. The Baha implant can also be an option. The timing of surgical intervention for children with bilateral otosclerosis or stapes fixation remains controversial; most authors advocate waiting until the child can participate in the decision-making process and fully understand the attendant risk of a profound sensorineural hearing loss. Children with unilateral stapes fixation are offered surgery once they reach adulthood. Children with persistent otitis media are treated with tympanostomy tube placement.

Outcome

Bilateral Sensorineural Hearing Loss

Functional outcomes are dependent on the child's comorbidities and the degree of cochlear anomaly. Children without other significant abnormalities who are implanted in at least one ear before age 2 can usually enter mainstream education before age 7. As cochlear implant technology progresses and the age of implantation decreases, functional results improve. Bilateral implantation, either simultaneous or sequential, provides improvement in discrimination of speech in noise and can aid in sound localization.

Unilateral Sensorineural or Conductive Hearing Loss

Educational and functional outcomes approximate that of the normal population. Patients with unilateral atresia may be offered surgery later in life but can find adjustment to binaural hearing difficulty if the atretic ear has not previously been stimulated with a bone-conducted hearing aid.

Bilateral Conductive Hearing Loss Due To Atresia

Children without significant comorbidities who receive appropriate amplification with a bone-conducting hearing aid or Baha implant should develop normal hearing and speech. In the absence of significant underlying sensorineural hearing loss, the Baha implant can provide normal hearing. The results of atresia repair depend largely on the underlying architecture of the temporal bone. Traditional hearing aids can be utilized when atresia repair does not provide sufficient hearing improvement.

References/Bibliography

1. Castilla EE, Orioloi IM. Prevalence rates of microtia in South America. Int J Epidemiol 1986;12:364–368.
2. Kochar A, Hildebrand MS, Smith RJ. Clinical aspects of hereditary hearing loss. Genet Med 2007;9(7):393–408.
3. Jackler RK. Congenital malformation of the inner ear. In: Cummings CW, et al., eds. Otoalryngology Head and Neck Surgery, Pediatric Volume. St. Louis: Mosby, 1998:418–438.
4. McKinnon BJ, Jahrsdoerfer RA. Congenital auricular atresia: update on options for intervention and timing of repair. Otolaryngol Clin North Am 2002;35:877–890.
5. Stelmachowicz PG, Gorga MP. Audiology: early identification and management of hearing loss. In: Cummings CW, et al., eds. Otolaryngology Head and Neck Surgery, Pediatric Volume. St. Louis: Mosby, 1998:401–417.

Implantable Hearing Devices

Yisgav Shapira and Thomas J. Balkany

Key Points

- Four types of implantable hearing devices exist, each with its specific indication.
- Cochlear implants (CI) are intended for severe to profound sensorineural hearing loss. Patients implanted at a young age may achieve speech and language skills comparable to normal hearing children.
- Bone-anchored hearing aids (BAHA) are intended for conductive hearing loss not amenable to reconstruction or amplification, and for single-sided deafness. Children are usually implanted in two stages.
- Implantable middle ear devices (IMED) are currently not approved for children. They are intended for moderate to moderately severe sensorineural hearing loss.
- Auditory brainstem implants (ABI) are indicated for profoundly deaf patients with an abnormal cochleae or cochlear nerves who are not otherwise candidates for CI. In the USA, only children above 12 years of age with neurofibromatosis type 2 (NF2) are approved for ABI.

Keywords: Cochlear implant • Bone-anchored hearing aid • Implantable middle ear devices • Auditory brainstem implant

Y. Shapira
Department of Otolaryngology, University of Miami Ear Institute, Miami, FL, USA

T.J. Balkany (✉)
Department of Otolaryngology, Miller School of Medicine, University of Miami Ear Institute, Miami, FL, USA
e-mail: TBalkany@med.miami.edu

Introduction

Congenital hearing loss is estimated to occur in 3–5 of every 1,000 births, many of whom can benefit from implantable hearing devices. Cochlear implants (CI) for severe to profound sensorineural hearing loss (SNHL) and bone-anchored hearing aids (BAHA) for certain conductive hearing losses or single-sided deafness are available for children. Implantable middle ear devices and auditory brainstem implants may become available for children in the near future. The indications for each are briefly presented in Table 1.

Cochlear Implants (CI)

The CI replaces the function of the lost hair cells by converting the mechanical energy of sound into electrical energy capable of exciting the cochlear nerve (CN) ***(1,2)***.

CIs have seen tremendous development over the past 25 years. Microspeech processors, minimally traumatic multicontact electrode arrays and improved surgical technique have resulted in improved performance. As a result, children are routinely being implanted under 1 year of age with consistently better results ***(3)***. More than 100,000 people worldwide have received cochlear implants; approximately half were children.

Structure and Principle of the Cochlear Implant

CIs consist of a wearable external speech processor (SP) and a surgically implanted cochlear stimulator (ICS) (Fig. 1). The SP transduces incoming sound into

R.B. Mitchell and K.D. Pereira (eds.), *Pediatric Otolaryngology for the Clinician*,
DOI: 10.1007/978-1-60327-127-1_11, © Humana Press, a part of Springer Science + Business Media, LLC 2009

Table 1 Implantable hearing devices and their indications

Bone-anchored hearing aid (BAHA)	Moderate to severe unilateral or bilateral conductive hearing loss Single-sided deafness
Implantable middle ear devices (IMED)	Bilateral moderate to moderately severe sensorineural hearing loss
Cochlear implants (CI)	Bilateral severe to profound sensorineural hearing loss
Auditory brainstem implant (ABI)	Bilateral profound sensorineural hearing loss with lack of a cochlear nerve Only in neurofibromatosis type 2 in the USA

Table 2 Current selection criteria for pediatric cochlear implantation

1. Age > 12 months (unless ossifying)
2. Severe-to-profound bilateral sensorineural hearing loss
3. Benefit from hearing aids less than that expected from CIs
4. No medical contraindications to undergoing general anesthesia
5. Family support, motivation, and appropriate expectations
6. Rehabilitation support for development of oral language, speech, and hearing

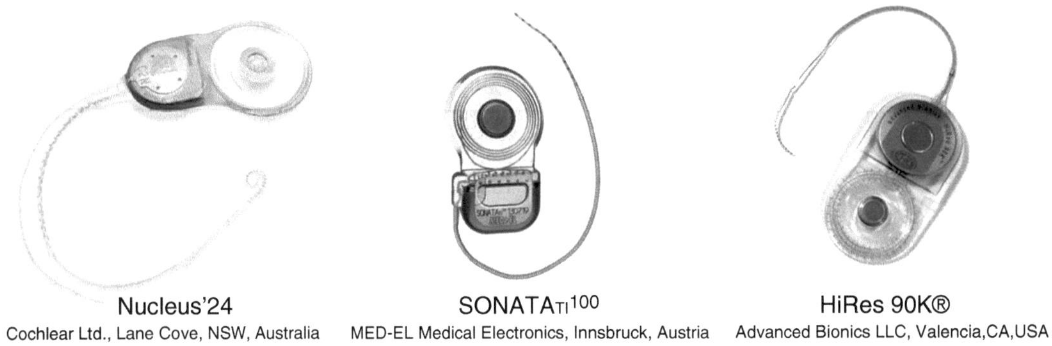

Fig. 1 Cochlear implants

electrical signals and transmits the information to the ICS via the radio-frequency transmitting coil. The ICS further processes the signal and distributes it to the electrode array *(2)*.

The three major devices are depicted in Fig. 1.

Candidacy

Candidacy criteria for cochlear implantation have evolved dramatically as technological advances and newer surgical techniques have resulted in improved outcomes. The Food and Drug Administration (FDA) now approves cochlear implantation in children older than 12 months of age but in many centers children as young as 6 months old are routinely implanted despite lack of FDA approval. Medical and radiological criteria have been expanded to include children with cochlear dysplasia, multiple developmental delays, and certain systemic medical conditions *(4,5)*. Unchanged, however, are requirements for strong family commitment, appropriate expectations, and an oral educational setting. In older children and teenagers, especially those who use sign language, the child's motivation in addition to parental desires should be evaluated *(3)*. Absolute contraindications include agenesis of the inner ear (Michel deformity), absence of the cochlear nerve, and systemic illness precluding anesthesia or surgery. Table 2 summarizes the current criteria for cochlear implantation in children.

Preoperative Evaluation

Audiology

Audiologic evaluation is the primary means of determining candidacy for cochlear implantation. Each ear is evaluated separately in both unaided and aided conditions. This process may prove to be extremely difficult in the young prelingual child, and may require repeated visits to an experienced implant audiologist *(3)*.

Because performance of an infant in a sound booth and on auditory brain responses (ABR) are not a reliable means of determining the need for CI, a hearing aid trial and intensive auditory verbal therapy ("diagnostic therapy") is mandatory unless ossification is noted. An essential element of diagnostic therapy is parental involvement, overseen by the therapist, to ensure continuous, at-home follow-through of therapy procedures. Absence of appropriate progress while participating in such therapy is a strong indication of inadequate auditory input *(3)*. Assessment of parental expectations, support, and compliance with the therapy process are important aspects of the evaluation of the young child.

Imaging

For prelingually deaf children MRI is considered the primary imaging modality, including high resolution T2 axial and coronal views of the internal auditory canal (IAC) with sagital reconstructions (i.e., CISS sequence). The four nerves of the IAC may be visualized and the cochlear nerve followed to the modiolus. MRI is also useful in identifying early cochlear ossification and primary brain abnormalities.

Medical Considerations

Children with CIs do not have a higher prevalence or increased severity of acute otitis media *(3,6,7)*. However, CI candidates with recurrent or chronic otitis media should be treated aggressively prior to implantation. Once the infection is under control, implantation may proceed, even with a ventilating tube in place *(3)*. For meningitis prophylaxis, the Center for Disease Control and Prevention (2002) recommends that CI recipients should receive age-appropriate vaccination against pneumococcal disease. These individuals should receive the 7-valent pneumococcal conjugate (Prevnar®) if under the age of 2, the 23-valent pneumococcal polysaccharide (Pneumovax® and Pnu-Imune®) vaccine if over the age of 5, or both if between the age of 2 and 5 *(8)*.

Ear Selection

Factors used to determine implantation are shown in Table 3. It is preferable to implant a ear which has

Table 3 Considerations for selecting the ear for cochlear implantation

Hearing	Choose better ear: – Anacoustic opposite ear – Disuse > 10 years opposite ear – Neither ear useful Choose worse ear: – Good residual in both ears
Imaging	Absolute contraindications: – Aplasia – Absent auditory nerve Choose better ear: – Ossification – Dysplasia – Facial or vascular anomaly – Pneumatization
Medical	Choose better ear: – Recurrent otitis media – Prior ear surgery
Other	Timing – Most recently deafened – Language – Choose right ear

some residual hearing and which has been used with amplification in the recent past *(3)*. However, ear selection should be individualized and no simple rule to always implant the better or worse hearing ear is valid.

Surgery

Surgical Procedure

CI surgery is performed in the out-patient setting under general anesthesia with continuous facial nerve monitoring. Antibiotics are given intravenously 30 min prior to incision. A 4–5-cm postauricular cut is made to the level of the temporalis/subcutaneous fascia. A pocket is developed postero-superiorly and an anteriorly based pericranial flap elevated. A bony seat and tie-down holes may be created or pericranial sutures may be used to secure the ICS. A complete mastoidectomy and facial recess approach allow access to the cochlear promontory and a cochleostomy is fashioned anterior-inferior to the round window membrane. The ICS is placed into the pocket and the electrode is inserted into the cochleostomy. Device-specific training is necessary for each type of implant. Surgery usually takes 1.5–2 h, and the patient is typically discharged on the day of surgery. Alternative techniques have been described accessing the promontory through a combined mastoid-atticotomy and tympanomeatal approach *(9–11)*.

Complications

Cochlear implantation carries the same risks as any mastoid surgery plus certain additional possible complications. Serious complications are rare and a complete list is shown in Table 4 *(7,10,12)*. The most common indication for revision surgery is device malfunction *(3,13)*.

Habilitation

If cochlear implantation is to be maximally successful, auditory-oral education, with a strong emphasis on oral communication and auditory development throughout childhood, is essential *(2,3)*.

Ethical Considerations

The Deaf community has claimed that deaf children are not disabled, that deaf culture can supply them with all social needs and education, and that implanting deaf children will diminish deaf society *(3)*. However, over 90% of deaf children are born to hearing parents, and for these parents there is often a strong desire for their deaf child to learn to hear and speak. Many in deaf culture oppose the right of these parents to decide whether or not their child should receive a CI. Nonetheless, parents have the responsibility to determine the best interests of their child, and their right to choose has a sound ethical basis. In recent years opposition to CI has declined and many organizations, such as the National Association of the Deaf and Gallaudet University, are moderating their opposition to the implantation of children.

Table 4 Possible complications in cochlear implant surgery

Infection	Wound infection
	Flap necrosis
	Purulent labyrinthitis
	Meningitis
Bleeding	Surgical field
	Epidural
Inner ear injury	Loss of residual hearing
	Dizziness/vertigo
	Perilymphatic fistula
Device related	Device malfunction
	Malpositioning
	Electrode extrusion
	Device migration
Nerve injury	Facial palsy/paresis
	Chorda tympani nerve injury
Other	Cerebrospinal fluid (CSF) leak
	Tympanic membrane perforation
	Cholesteatoma

Outcomes

With the advancement of CI technology there has been a progressive improvement in performance achieved by cochlear implant recipients. For prelingually deaf children, cochlear implantation by the age of 12 months is associated with the best results *(14–17)*.

Recent studies have shown that implanted children acquire language at a rate equal to that of normal hearing children (12-month growth in 12 months) in contrast to nonimplanted deaf children who acquire linguistic skills at half that rate at best. Although language and speech production skills improve in all implanted children, those children who are trained to use aural/oral communication perform at a higher level and achieve results faster than those children who use total communication *(2,3)*. Prelingually deaf children implanted at a young age achieve a 74% reading ability compared to age-matched hearing children, which represents a significant improvement compared to nonimplanted deaf children *(17)*.

Bone-Anchored Hearing Aid (BAHA)

The BAHA system (Cochlear Ltd., Lane Cove, NSW, Australia) combines a sound processor with a small titanium fixture implanted behind the ear that allows sound conduction through the bone rather than via the middle ear. The middle ear and external ear are bypassed, and both cochleae are stimulated *(2,18–20)*. Development of this device followed advances in titanium osteointegration technology *(20,21)*. The BAHA has now been in use for 30 years, and more than 25,000 patients have been implanted. BAHA is FDA-approved for children

5 years and older. However, in many centers in the USA and elsewhere, children as young as 13 months have been successfully implanted with the device *(18)*.

Structure and Principle of BAHA

The system is composed of a titanium fixture surgically implanted into the skull, a transcutaneous abutment, and an external sound processor (Fig. 2). The sound processor is coupled to the abutment via a plastic snap. Sound is picked up by the microphone and transformed by the processor into vibration which is transferred through the skull to both cochleae. Both ear-level and body-worn processors are available.

Candidacy

Candidacy criteria and considerations are detailed in. For conductive hearing loss, the size of the air-bone gap is of no significance.

Surgery

A postauricular skin flap is elevated and subcutaneous tissue is removed to the level of pericranium. A small area of pericranium is removed and a pilot bone hole is drilled 3–4-mm deep. The titanium, self-tapping screw with percutaneous attachment is then inserted and the flap returned, sutured in position, and covered with a light pressure dressing. The external processor is first used within 6–12 weeks for healthy adults. A two-step procedure, keeping the skin flap intact over the screw for 3 months or more may be necessary in young children or in cases suspected of poor healing *(22)*.

Complications

Major complications with BAHA surgery are rare. However, skin complications such as partial necrosis, inflammation, or infection around the implant may occur in over 10% of recipients in spite of proper

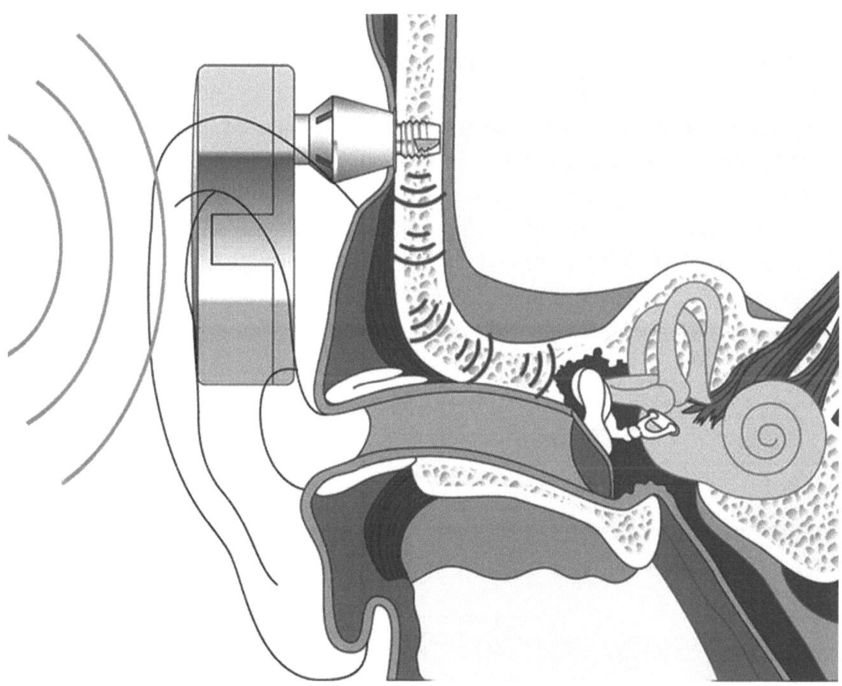

Fig. 2 Bone-anchored hearing aid

surgical technique. In most cases, conservative local care, with or without systemic medication, resolves the problem. In unusual cases, the implant does not integrate, or osteomyelitis occurs requiring the implant to be removed to allow healing *(1)*.

Follow-up

Routine weekly visits should be performed until proper healing of the implant site is observed. Patients and/or care-takers should be instructed on the importance of daily routine cleaning of the implant site. Certain sports which may involve direct head contact should be avoided. Swimming is allowed without the sound processor attached.

The titanium screw is MRI-compatible but the sound processor must be removed when performing an MRI.

Outcomes

For pure conductive hearing loss, the BAHA achieves closure of the air-bone gap to within 10 dB in 80% of patients *(18,22–24)*. Speech reception thresholds improve to an average of 30 dB. However, patient satisfaction is decreased in cases of mixed loss, especially when the sensorineural component is greater than 20 dB.

For single-sided deafness, results are available for adults only *(25,26)*. Quality-of-life questionnaires in several studies have shown a very high overall patient satisfaction compared to nonaided patients or to the contralateral routing of signal (CROS) hearing aids *(26,27)*.

Implantable Middle Ear Devices

Implantable middle ear devices (IMED) directly vibrate the ossicular chain, thereby reducing the occlusion effect and feedback problems. They are intended for patients who suffer from moderate to severe sensorineural hearing loss with normal middle ear function. Early manufacturer-supported studies suggest that amplification is not greater than conventional hearing aids but that compliance may be improved *(1,28–30)*.

The Vibrant Soundbridge (MED-EL Corporation, Innsbruck, Austria) is approved by the FDA for use in adults. The Esteem (Envoy Medical Corporation, Saint Paul, MN) and the Carina (Otologics, LLC, Boulder, CO) devices have approval in Europe and are under FDA investigational trials. The first is an electromagnetic, partially implantable device and the latter two are fully implantable piezoelectric devices *(28,29,31)* (Fig. 3). It is likely that these devices will be used in children after more data are available from trials involving adults.

Auditory Brainstem Implant (ABI)

Auditory brainstem implants (ABIs) electrically stimulate the cochlear nucleus and are used in profoundly deaf patients who would be CI candidates, but have lost the auditory nerve during removal of bilateral acoustic neuromas. The externally worn speech processor and the implanted receiver/stimulator are identical to those of the CI. However, the electrode array is implanted on the surface of the cochlear nucleus in the brainstem through the lateral recess of the fourth ventricle, thus bypassing the inner ear and auditory nerve

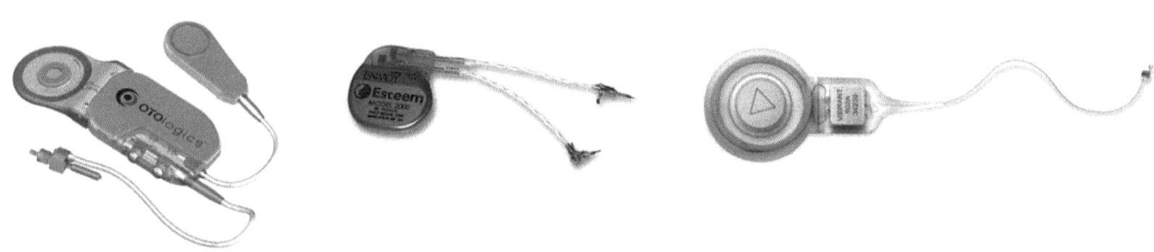

Fig. 3 Implantable middle ear devices

(32). Candidates are NF2 patients 12 years and older, but in other countries, patients as young as 14 months have been implanted for a variety of reasons *(33)*. The risks of surgery involving the brainstem are substantial and NF2 patients typically do not achieve open-set speech perception *(32,33)*.

References

1. Weber PC. Medical and surgical considerations for implantable hearing prosthetic devices. Am J Audiol. 2002; 11(2): 134–138.
2. Eshraghi AA, Waltzman SB, Feghali JG, Van De Water TR, Cohen NL. Hearing aids, bone-anchored hearing aids and cochlear implants. In: Van De Water TR, Staecker H, eds. Otolaryngology: Basic Science and Clinical Review. New York: Thieme Medical Publishers, 2006: 385–394.
3. Balkany TJ, Hodges AV, Eshraghi AA, Butts S, Bricker K, Lingvai J, Polak M, King J. Cochlear implants in children--a review. Acta Otolaryngol. 2002; 122(4): 356–362.
4. Luntz M, Balkany TJ, Hodges AV. Cochlear implants in children with congenital inner ear malformations. Arch Otolaryngol Head Neck Surg. 1997; 123: 974–977.
5. Luntz M, Balkany TJ, Hodges AV. Surgical technique for implantation of malformed inner ear. Am J Otol. 1997; 18: 66–67.
6. Migirov L, Yakirevitch A, Kronenberg J. Surgical and medical complications following cochlear implantation: comparison of two surgical approaches. ORL J Otorhinolaryngol Relat Spec. 2006; 68(4): 213–219.
7. Postelmans JT, Cleffken B, Stokroos RJ. Post-operative complications of cochlear implantation in adults and children: five years' experience in Maastricht. J Laryngol Otol. 2007; 121(4): 318–323.
8. Dodson KM, Maiberger PG, Sismanis A. Intracranial complications of cochlear implantation. Otol Neurotol. 2007; 28(4): 459–462.
9. Kronenberg J, Baumgartner W, Migirov L, Dagan T, Hildesheimer M. The suprameatal approach: an alternative surgical approach to cochlear implantation. Otol Neurotol. 2004; 25(1): 41–44.
10. Migirov L, Taitelbaum-Swead R, Hildesheimer M, Kronenberg J. Revision surgeries in cochlear implant patients: a review of 45 cases. Eur Arch Otorhinolaryngol. 2007; 264(1): 3–7.
11. Muller J. Technical devices for hearing-impaired individuals: cochlear implants and brain stem implants: developments of the last decade. In: GMS Curr Top Otorhinolaryngol Head Neck Surg 2005; 4: Doc04. Accessed August 14, 2007, at: http://www.egms.de/en/journals/cto/2005–4/cto000010.shtml.
12. Stratigouleas ED, Perry BP, King SM, Syms CA. Complication rate of minimally invasive cochlear implantation. Otolaryngol Head Neck Surg. 2006; 135(3): 383–386.
13. Kempf HG, Johann K, Lenarz T. Complications in pediatric cochlear implant surgery. Eur Arch Otorhinolaryngol. 1999; 256(3): 128–132.
14. Uziel AS, Sillon M, Vieu A, Artieres F, Piron JP, Daures JP, Mondain M. Ten-year follow-up of a consecutive series of children with multichannel cochlear implants. Otol Neurotol. 2007; 28(5): 615–628.
15. Staller S, Parkinson A, Arcaroli J, Arndt P. Pediatric outcomes with the nucleus 24 contour: North American clinical trial. Ann Otol Rhinol Laryngol Suppl. 2002; 189: 56–61.
16. Osberger MJ, Zimmerman-Phillips S, Koch DB. Cochlear implant candidacy and performance trends in children. Ann Otol Rhinol Laryngol Suppl. 2002; 189: 62–65.
17. Rubinstein JT. Paediatric cochlear implantation: prosthetic hearing and language development. Lancet. 2002; 360(9331): 483–485.
18. Davids T, Gordon KA, Clutton D, Papsin BC. Bone-anchored hearing aids in infants and children younger than 5 years. Arch Otolaryngol Head Neck Surg. 2007; 133(1): 51–55.
19. Lloyd S, Almeyda J, Sirimanna KS, Albert DM, Bailey CM. Updated surgical experience with bone-anchored hearing aids in children. J Laryngol Otol. 2007; 9: 1–6.
20. Snik AF, Mylanus EA, Cremers CW. The bone-anchored hearing aid: a solution for previously unresolved otologic problems. Otolaryngol Clin North Am. 2001; 34(2): 365–372.
21. Spitzer JB, Ghossaini SN, Wazen JJ. Evolving applications in the use of bone-anchored hearing aids. Am J Audiol. 2002; 11(2): 96–103.
22. Priwin C, Jönsson R, Hultcrantz M, Granström G. BAHA in children and adolescents with unilateral or bilateral conductive hearing loss: a study of outcome. Int J Pediatr Otorhinolaryngol. 2007; 71(1): 135–145.
23. Seemann R, Liu R, Di Toppa J. Results of pediatric bone-anchored hearing aid implantation. J Otolaryngol. 2004; 33(2): 71–74.
24. Tjellstrom A, Hakansson B, Granstrom G. Bone-anchored hearing aids: current status in adults and children. Otolaryngol Clin North Am. 2001; 34(2): 337–364.
25. Lin LM, Bowditch S, Anderson MJ, May B, Cox KM, Niparko JK. Amplification in the rehabilitation of unilateral deafness: speech in noise and directional hearing effects with bone-anchored hearing and contralateral routing of signal amplification. Otol Neurotol. 2006; 27(2): 172–182.
26. Niparko JK, Cox KM, Lustig LR. Comparison of the bone anchored hearing aid implantable hearing device with contralateral routing of offside signal amplification in the rehabilitation of unilateral deafness. Otol Neurotol. 2003; 24(1): 73–78.
27. Johnson CE, Danhauer JL, Reith AC, Latiolais LN. A systematic review of the nonacoustic benefits of bone-anchored hearing Aids. Ear Hear. 2006; 27(6): 703–713.
28. Backous, DD, Duke, W. Implantable middle ear hearing devices: current state of technology and market challenges. Curr Opin Otolaryngol Head Neck Surg. 2006; 14(5): 314–318.
29. Leuwer R, Müller J. Restoration of hearing by hearing aids. In: GMS Curr Top Otorhinolaryngol Head Neck Surg 2005; 4: Doc03. Accessed August 14, 2007, at: http://www.egms.de/en/journals/cto/2005-4/cto000009.shtml.

30. Shohet JA. Implantable Hearing Devices. In: emedicine. Accessed August 8, 2007, at: http://www.emedicine.com/ent/topic479.htm.
31. Jenkins H, Pergola N, Kasic J. Intraoperative ossicular loading with the Otologics fully implantable hearing device. Acta Oto-Laryngologica. 2007; 127: 360–364.
32. Rauschecker JP, Shannon RV. Sending sound to the brain. Science. 2002; 295(5557): 1025–1029.
33. Colletti V. Auditory outcomes in tumor vs. nontumor patients fitted with auditory brainstem implants. In: Møller AR, ed. Cochlear and Brainstem Implants. Adv Otorhinolaryngol. Basel, Karger, 2006, vol 64, pp 167–185.

Rhinology

Pediatric Facial Fractures

T.J. O-Lee and Peter J. Koltai

Key Points

- Falls, motor vehicle accidents, and sports-related activities are the leading causes of facial trauma in children.
- Children below 6 years of age suffer more orbital roof and skull fractures than facial fractures due to proportionally larger cranial volume.
- Nasal and dentoalveolar fractures are the most common facial fractures in children. Nasal septal hematoma need to be detected early and drained promptly to avoid complications.
- Mandible fractures are the most common facial fractures treated in the hospital setting. Intermaxillary fixation is limited to 2–3 weeks and is followed by 6–8 weeks of using guiding elastic bands.
- It is often necessary to overcorrect nasoethmoid fracture-induced telecanthus to obtain long-term satisfactory results.
- Rib or calvarial bone grafts are preferred over alloplastic materials in the reconstruction of pediatric bony defects.

Keywords: Pediatric • Facial fracture • Mandible • Nasal fracture • Intermaxillary fixation • Facial growth • Orbital fracture

T.J. O-Lee and P.J. Koltai (✉)
Department of Otolaryngology, Head and Neck Surgery, Division of Pediatric Otolaryngology, Head and Neck Surgery, Stanford University School of Medicine, Stanford, CA, USA

Introduction

Trauma is the leading cause of death in children in the United States. Each year approximately 15,000 children die and about 100,000 become permanently disabled due to trauma-related injuries. Medical care for these injuries is valued at over $15 billion annually ***(1)***. Despite these staggering numbers, pediatric facial trauma is relatively rare. Pediatric maxillofacial injuries account for approximately 5% of all fractures, with reported incidence ranging between 1.5 and 15% ***(2–6)***. Children under 5 years have a significantly lower risk of facial fractures ranging from 1 to 1.5% ***(7)***. With increasing age, the incidence of facial fracture also increases, ultimately reaching the pattern and frequency of adult trauma victims around late adolescence ***(7)***.

Great advances have been made in the management of pediatric facial fractures during recent decades. The specific techniques used for reconstruction in children must accommodate their developing anatomy, rapid healing, immature psychology, and potential for deformity as a consequence of altered facial growth ***(7)***. The prevalence of CT scans makes accurate diagnosis of facial fractures possible in most instances ***(8,9)***. Rigid internal fixation has been successfully adapted to pediatric cases from our knowledge of managing facial fractures in adults, though with careful modification. Open reduction and rigid internal fixation are indicated for severely displaced fractures. Primary bone grafting is preferred over secondary reconstruction. Alloplastic materials should be avoided when possible ***(10)***.

Associated injuries are a common feature of childhood maxillofacial trauma. Neurologic and orthopedic injuries were seen in 30% of children with facial fractures, which reinforce the importance of a complete

R.B. Mitchell and K.D. Pereira (eds.), *Pediatric Otolaryngology for the Clinician*,
DOI: 10.1007/978-1-60327-127-1_12, © Humana Press, a part of Springer Science + Business Media, LLC 2009

initial assessment of a child with facial trauma and highlights the dilemma with regard to the timing of the reconstruction because of the rapid healing of bony injuries in children *(7)*.

Etiology

To understand the cause of pediatric facial fractures, two separate issues need to be addressed: (1) the traumatic event that results in injury to a child's face and (2) the unique anatomic features of the pediatric facial skeleton that predispose it to a pattern of observed injuries *(7)*.

Falls, motor vehicle accidents (MVA), and sports-related injuries are the most common causes of facial fractures in children *(11)*. Falls are low-velocity injuries that commonly affect young children below the age of 6 *(11)*. While prevalent, falls rarely produce serious injuries. On the other extreme, MVAs produce high-velocity forces that often cause devastating injuries. MVAs are the leading cause of death in children after the perinatal period and the incidence of MVA-related maxillofacial injuries increases with age *(12)*. Improved vehicle safety features (padded dash boards, collapsible steering columns, air-bags, child safety seats) and enforcement of safety belt laws have led to a significant decrease in the incidence and severity of MVA-related facial fractures *(13–15)*. Most sports-related facial fractures occur in children 10–14 years of age. As motor skills improve from childhood to adolescence, an increase in activity level and outdoor exposure makes older children more susceptible to sports-related traumatic injuries *(16)*.

A young child's face has characteristics that make fractures less likely to happen. Facial soft tissue of children is relatively thicker, which protects the underlying bony framework. The bony structures are soft and elastic with relative thickness and strength not weakened by the paranasal sinuses. In addition, immature bone has greater elasticity caused by thin cortical plates and a greater proportion of cancellous bone. This elasticity is also the reason that greenstick fractures occur more frequently in children. The presence of unerupted teeth in the maxilla and mandible are the final features that make pediatric faces more resistant to fracture *(17)*.

Facial Growth

At birth, the ratio between cranial volume and facial volume is 8:1, where as in adults, this ratio is 2.5:1. Eighty percent of cranial growth occurs during the first years of life. Only after the first 2 years of life will the rate of facial growth begin to exceed that of skull growth. The orbit and the brain are near growth completion by age 7; however, lower facial growth continues into the early 20s. The consequence of the retruded position of the face relative to the skull is an important reason for the lower incidence of midface and mandibular fractures and higher incidence of orbital roof and cranial injuries in young children. Fractures below the orbits generally occur after the age of 7 and are not associated with cranial injuries, whereas orbital roof and cranial injuries are most commonly seen in children less than 5 years old *(18)*.

The possibilities of growth disturbances after facial fractures need to be considered when planning treatment. Injuries to certain vulnerable sites, such as the nasal septum, head of the condyle, and the multiple suture sites of the midface, may adversely affect future facial growth *(7)*. Growth potential may serve to improve long-term results with compensatory condylar growth after condylar fractures. Children with deciduous and mixed dentition also demonstrate some capacity for spontaneous occlusal readjustment as deciduous teeth are shed and permanent dentition erupts *(11)*.

Sites of Injury

Nasal fractures are by far the most common facial bone injuries in children followed by dentoalveolar injuries. Theses fractures are usually treated in an out-patient setting without surgical intervention. Exact statistics regarding incidence and treatment are difficult to obtain since records are typically not as well kept as for hospitalized patients *(17)*.

Fractures of the mandible are the most common facial fractures requiring hospitalization. They account for 30–50% of all pediatric facial fractures when nasal fractures are excluded *(17,19,20)*. Because pediatric condyles are highly vascularized and the thin necks are poorly resistant to impact forces, the most vulnerable part of the pediatric mandible is the condyle. More than 50% of pediatric mandibular fractures involve one of the condyles whereas only 30% of adult cases show condylar involvement ***(21)***. As the patient matures, the frequency of symphyseal, body, and ramus fractures increases.

Midfacial fractures are rare in children. They usually result from high-impact, high-velocity forces such as MVAs. Orbital fractures are the most common accounting for 20–25% of pediatric fractures. Zygomaticomalar complex (ZMC) fractures are seen in 10–15%, and LeFort maxillary fractures are seen in 5–10%. Orbital roof fractures occur in very young children whose frontal sinuses are still underdeveloped. These are often associated with skull injuries ***(2–4,18)***.

Management

Nasal Fractures

The initial examination of a child with a nasal fracture may be very limited by midfacial swelling. Several days are required for the swelling to subside before the true extent of the deformity can be appreciated. Conversely, immediate intranasal examination is important to detect the presence of a septal hematoma. Unilateral nasal obstruction is the hallmark of septal hematoma and can be observed on anterior rhinoscopy as an obvious purple bulge on one side of the nose. The bulge is compressible with a cotton tip applicator and does not shrink with topical vasoconstriction. A septal hematoma requires immediate evacuation upon detection. An untreated hematoma can become a thick, scarred, and obstructive septum. And if the hematoma becomes infected, the resulting loss of cartilage can cause a saddle nose deformity ***(10)***.

In cases of nasal fracture without septal hematoma, the patient is asked to return 3–4 days after injury, when a more accurate examination is possible. If a cosmetic deformity or a fixed nasal obstruction is detected, then definitive surgical management is undertaken. Closed reduction of the bony fracture can be performed with intranasal instrumentation and bimanual external manipulation. If significant dislocations are present or if the injury is more than 2 weeks old, then open reduction may be necessary.

Mandible Fractures

Clinical signs of mandibular fractures may include displacement of the fragments, mobility, swelling, mucosal tears, limited mouth opening, malocclusion, and pain. Clinical suspicion of a fracture is confirmed by either a panorex X-ray, a complete mandible series, or by CT scans. CTs are especially helpful in condylar fractures to help determine three-dimensional displacement of the condyles.

Immobilization is difficult before 2 years of age because of incomplete eruption of the deciduous teeth; however, later growth and remodeling frequently compensate for less-than-ideal postinjury alignment. The primary teeth, which have firm roots between 2 and 5 years of age, can be used for splints and arch bars. Deciduous roots are resorbed between 6 and 12 years of age; hence arch bars may need extra support from circum-mandibular wiring and piriform aperture suspension. Permanent teeth are safe anchors for fixation after 13 years of age ***(10)***.

The central question in the management of pediatric condylar fracture is whether the patient needs immobilization. Although minimally invasive endoscopic open reduction with internal fixation (ORIF) is gaining popularity in the management of adult condylar fractures, most authors still advocate conservative management when it comes to pediatric cases ***(11,22)***. If the patient has normal occlusion and normal mandibular movement, a soft diet and movement exercises are sufficient. However, if open-bite deformities with retrusion of the mandible and movement limitation are present, then a brief period of immobilization, lasting 2–3 weeks, followed by the use of guiding elastics is more likely to yield normal function ***(10)***.

Displaced symphysis fractures can be treated by ORIF through an intraoral incision after the permanent incisors have erupted at age 6 or older ***(11)***. ORIF in parasymphyseal fractures is possible once the buds of the canines have moved up from the mandibular border after age 9. In body fractures, the inferior mandibular border can be plated when the buds of the permanent premolar and molar have migrated superiorly toward the alveolus.

Frequent postoperative follow-up is necessary to detect and treat early complications such as infection, malocclusion, malunion, or nonunion. Late complications such as damage to permanent teeth, temporomandibular joint (TMJ) dysfunction, or midface deformity with facial asymmetry also need attention and possible treatments.

Nasoethmoid Complex Fractures

In nasoethmoid fractures, the integrity of the medial canthal ligament must be assessed. This is done by inserting a hemostat into the nose toward the medial orbital rim under general anesthesia. Mobility of the underlying fragments suggests that the bone with the medial canthal ligament has been displaced. Reconstruction of the nasal maxillary buttress and possibly transnasal wiring may then be necessary *(10)*. Measurement of soft-tissue intercanthal distance is difficult since ethnic, racial, and gender variations can significantly impact its values. Nevertheless, the average intercanthal distance at 4 years of age is approximately 25 mm, by age 12 it is 28 mm, and by adulthood approximately 30 mm. Near-adult intercanthal distance is achieved at a very early age and an easy mistake is to set the intercanthal distance too wide. Intercanthal distances 5 mm more than the average values tend to be indicative of displaced fractures of the nasoethmoidal complex with a measurement of 10 mm confirming this diagnosis. Attempts should not be made to narrow the distance between the eyes or project the nose of a child excessively.

Zygomaticomalar Complex Fractures

Zygomaticomalar (ZMC) fractures are uncommon before the age of 5 years and parallel the pneumatization of the maxillary sinus. Surgical correction of ZMC fractures is indicated when bony displacement is present. Adequate exposure is essential as correction is achieved by a process called triangulation *(7)*. Three key sites need to be directly visualized: (1) the frontozygomatic suture, (2) infraorbital rim, and (3) anterior zygomaticomaxillary buttress. Access can be achieved via the lateral upper eyelid incision, the lower eyelid infraciliary or transconjuctival incision, and the transoral buccal sulcus incision *(7)*. Contrary to adults, one-point fixation at the frontozygomatic suture may suffice in children because of shorter lever arm forces from the frontozygomatic suture to the infraorbital rim.

Orbital Floor Fractures

The treatment of isolated blowout fractures is symptom dependent. If persistent enophthalmos, extraocular muscle restriction, or pain on movement of the eye is present, then surgical exploration is indicated. Large fractures are also routinely explored as well as fractures with obvious muscle entrapment as evident on CT. Absorbable gelatin film is usually sufficient for reconstructing small defects of the floor; however, large disruptions are best repaired with calvarial bone grafts.

Orbital Roof Fractures

Pediatric orbital roof fractures are different than those of adults. They occur more frequently due to the lack of frontal sinus penumatization. Children have a craniofacial ratio of 8:1 at birth, compared to 2.5:1 in adults, and thus expose more of their cranium and skull base to potential injuries. Most orbital roof fractures, particularly those that are nondisplaced or with fragments displaced superiorly (blowout fractures) can be safely observed in the acute setting. Treatments should be directed by the presence of symptoms, such as extraocular muscle entrapment, enophthalmos, exophthalmos, diplopia, vision changes, or dystopia. Large blowin fractures have a higher chance for late onset complications; therefore surgical thresholds should be lower. Depending on the extent and location of the orbital roof fracture, various approaches are available to access the area of interest. Cooperation between neurosurgery, ophthalmology, and head and neck surgery are essential to optimize the care for these children.

Conclusion

Children of all ages can be afflicted by facial trauma, often resulting in functional and cosmetic deficits. The factor that differentiates the treatment of pediatric facial fractures from those of adults is facial growth. A thorough understanding of pediatric skull and facial growth enables us to focus our search for subtle fractures in the most age-appropriate locations. Anticipation of mandibular growth facilitates repair because most injuries can be treated with intermaxillary fixation. Unerupted dentition requires careful selection of fixation methods and cautious screw placement if rigid fixation is ultimately required. The modern rigid plating systems have greatly enhanced the surgeons' ability to reconstruct facial fractures in a three-dimensional fashion. Depending on the site of injury, a multidisciplinary team approach can ensure that injuries to organ systems around the face are cared for in an optimal manner.

References

1. Rowe IM, Fonkalsrud EW, O'Neil JA, et al.: The injured child. *In* Essentials of Pediatric Surgery. St. Louis, Mosby, 1995
2. Gussack GS, Lutterman A, Rodgers K, et al.: Pediatric maxillofacial trauma: unique features in diagnosis and treatment. Laryngoscope 97:925–930, 1987
3. Kaban LB: Diagnosis and treatment of fractures of the facial bones in children 1943–1993. J Oral Maxillofac Surg 51:722–729, 1993
4. Koltai PJ, Rabkin D, Hoehn J: Rigid fixation of facial fractures in children. J Craniomaxillofac Trauma 1:32–42, 1995
5. McGraw BL, Cole RR: Pediatric maxillofacial trauma. Arch Otolaryngol Head Neck Surg 116:41–45, 1990
6. Rowe NL: Fractures of the facial skeleton in children. J Oral Surg 26:505–515, 1967
7. Koltai PJ, Rabkin D: Management of facial trauma in children. Pediatr Clin North Am 43:1253–1275, 1996
8. Holland AJ, Broome C, Steinberg A, Cass DT: Facial fractures in children. Pediatr Emerg Care 17:157–160, 2001
9. Posnick JC, Wells M, Pron GE: Pediatric facial fractures: evolving patterns of treatment. J Oral Maxillofac Surg 51:836–844, 1993
10. Koltai PJ: Pediatric facial fractures. *In* Bailey Head and Neck Surgery-Otolaryngology. Philadelphia, Lippincott, 2001
11. Zimmermann CE, Troulis MJ, Kaban LB: Pediatric facial fractures: recent advances in prevention, diagnosis and management. Int J Oral Maxillofac Surg 35:2–13, 2006
12. Statistics NCfH. Natl Vital Stat Rep 49:16–29, 2001
13. Adam CD, Januszkiewcz JS, Judson J: Changing patterns of severe craniomaxillofacial trauma in Auckland over eight years. Aust N Z J Surg 70:401–404, 2000
14. Reath DB, Kirby J, Lynch M, Maull KI: Injury and cost comparison of restrained and unrestrained motor vehicle crash victims. J Trauma 29:1173–1176, 1989
15. Tyroch AH, Kaups KL, Sue LP, ODonnell-Nicol S: Pediatric restraint use in motor vehicle collisions: reduction of deaths without contribution to injury. Arch Surg 135:1173–1176, 2000
16. Iizuka T, Thoren H, Annino DJ, et al.: Midfacial fractures in pediatric patients. Frequency, characteristics and causes. Arch Otolaryngol Head Neck Surg 121:1355–1371, 1995
17. Koltai PJ: Maxillofacial injuries in children. In Smith JD, Bumstead R (eds): Pediatric Facial Plastic and Reconstructive surgery. New York, Raven Press, 1993
18. McGraw BL, Cole RR: Pediatric maxillofacial trauma. Age-related variations in injury. Arch Otolaryngol Head Neck Surg 116:41–45, 1990
19. Hardt N, Gottsauner A: The treatment of mandibular fractures in children. J Craniomaxillofac Surg 21:214–219, 1993
20. Thoren H, Iizuka T, Hallikainen D, et al.: Different patterns of mandibular fractures in children: An analysis of 220 fractures in 157 patients. J Craniomaxillofac Surg 20:292–296, 1992
21. Kaban LB, Mulliken JB, Murray JE. Facial fractures in children: an analysis of 122 fractures in 109 patients. Plast Reconstr Surg 59:15–20, 1977
22. Troulis MJ, Kaban LB. Endoscopic approach to the ramus/condyle unit: clinical applications. J Oral Maxillofac Surg 59:503–509, 2001

Pediatric Epistaxis

Cherie L. Booth and K. Christopher McMains

Key Points

- The most common cause of epistaxis in the pediatric population is digital trauma.
- Behavioral, environmental, congenital, hereditary, systemic, and neoplastic conditions may contribute to epistaxis in this population.
- History and physical examination is the mainstay of diagnosis.
- Taking care to allay patient anxiety can improve yield of the physical examination.

Keywords: Epistaxis • Pediatric • Nasal • Vascular • Surgical • Genetic • Bleeding

Introduction

Epistaxis in children is a very common condition but is rare before 2 years of age *(1)*. It is usually a minor problem secondary to mucosal irritation and excoriation in the anterior septal or Little's area (Kiesselbach's plexus) *(2)*. Thirty percent of all children aged 0–5 years, 56% of those aged 6–10 years, and 64% of those aged 11–15 years, have had at least one episode of epistaxis in their lifetime *(3)*. However, the warning signs of a serious underlying disease must be recognized to ensure appropriate management and treatment. This chapter will review the relevant anatomy, differential diagnosis, work-up, and treatment of important causes of epistaxis in the pediatric population.

C.L. Booth and K.C. McMains (✉)
Department of Otolaryngology/Head and Neck Surgery, University of Texas Health Science Center at San Antonio, San Antonio, TX, USA
e-mail: mcmains@uthscsa.edu

Anatomy

It is important to understand the anatomy and blood supply in the nasal cavity to properly evaluate and manage a child with epistaxis. From a clinical perspective, epistaxis is usually classified as either anterior or posterior, with significant differences in the clinical presentation and prognosis of each, reflecting the anatomy of the blood supply of the nose *(4)*. Anterior bleeds most commonly arise from Little's area on the anterior region of the nasal septum at Kiesselbach's plexus. Posterior bleeding usually originates from the sphenopalatine artery distribution, which supplies the majority of the lateral wall and the posterior septum *(5)*.

The nasal cavity has an abundant blood supply from terminal branches of both the internal and external carotid arteries. In the majority of children, spontaneous hemorrhage is almost always venous and originates from the anterior region of the nasal septum, where a number of arteries anastomose with each other forming a plexus of vessels (Kiesselbach's plexus) under thin mucosa (Fig. 1) *(1)*. Recently, a detailed study of the vasculature of Little's area involving microdissections of the nasal septum in 24 cadaveric specimens found that the arteries of the anterior septum form a consistent arterial anastomotic triangle, consisting of large, thin-walled vessels supplied by the terminal branches of the sphenopalatine (external carotid distribution) and anterior ethmoidal (internal carotid distribution) and the superior labial arteries (external carotid distribution) *(6)*.

The blood supply to the lateral nasal wall below the middle turbinate is from the sphenopalatine artery, a distal branch of the external carotid artery (Fig. 2).

R.B. Mitchell and K.D. Pereira (eds.), *Pediatric Otolaryngology for the Clinician*,
DOI: 10.1007/978-1-60327-127-1_13,

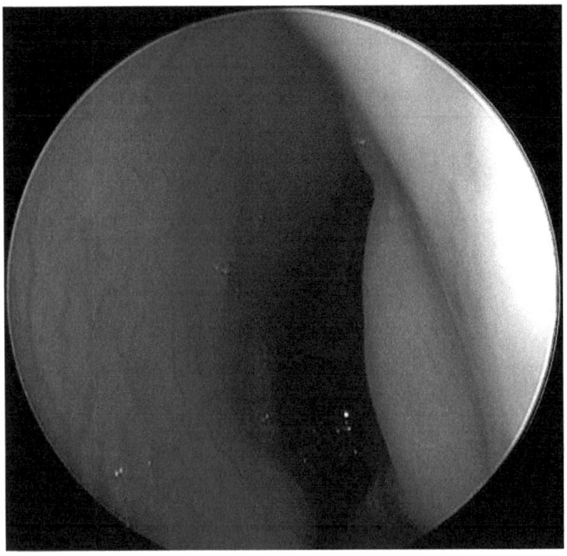

Fig. 1 Endoscopic view of the left anterior nasal septum. Note the prominent vessels interdigitating in Little's area to form Kiesselbach's plexus. (*Picture courtesy of Dr. William D. Clark, MD*)

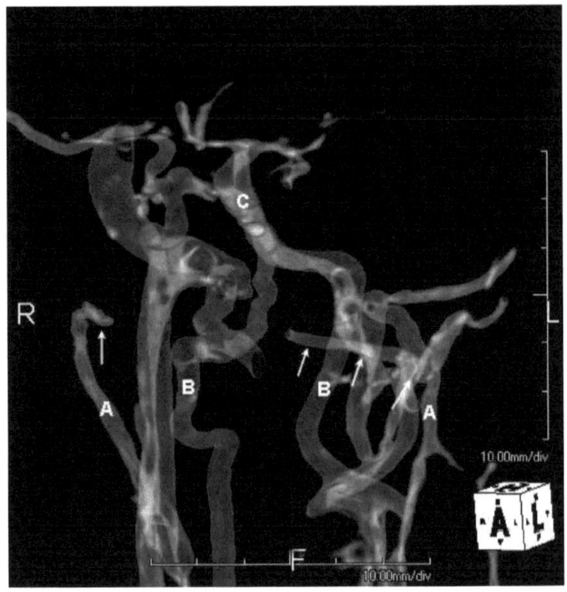

Fig. 2 Digitally subtracted CT angiogram demonstrating the vessels supplying the sino-nasal region: (**a**) external carotid artery (ECA), (**b**) internal carotid artery and (**c**) basilar artery. (*Arrows* demonstrate the Internal maxillary arteries). (*Image courtesy of Christian Stallworth, MD*)

Disruption of this artery is responsible for most cases of posterior epistaxis *(7)*. The sphenopalatine artery enters the nasal cavity through the sphenopalatine foramen. It then divides into the nasopalatine artery and the posterior superior branch of the sphenopalatine artery *(8)*. The nasopalatine courses postero-medially over the face of the sphenoid to supply the nasal septum. The posterior superior branch of the sphenopalatine supplies the middle and inferior turbinates *(8)*. The mucosa of the lateral nasal wall above the middle turbinate is supplied by the anterior and posterior ethmoidal arteries (Fig. 3) *(7)*.

Pathophysiology

Risk factors and causes of epistaxis can be divided into local and systemic etiologies *(8)*.

In only a small number of cases can epistaxis in children be attributed to a well-defined primary cause. In the majority of cases, bleeding arises from a normal vessel. The terms "spontaneous" or "idiopathic" epistaxis have therefore been used to describe this most common category of epistaxis *(1)*.

Childhood recurrent idiopathic epistaxis is usually attributed to crusting, nasal vestibulitis, and/or digital trauma, although in many cases no direct cause can be established *(3,9)*. The incidence of idiopathic epistaxis in all ages is highest during the winter months in northern climates, when upper respiratory tract infections are more frequent and when indoor humidity decreases to low levels at both home and in the work place due to central and radiant heater use *(10)*. Changes from a cold outside environment to a warm dry one may cause variation of the normal nasal cycle, sinonasal congestion, engorgement of the nasal mucosa, and epistaxis. Epistaxis is also common in hot dry climates with low humidity *(1)*. Allergic rhinitis can predispose patients to epistaxis because the nasal mucosa becomes inflamed and friable *(11)*.

By far, the most common cause of anterior epistaxis in the pediatric population is digital trauma. Irritation of the nasal mucosa leading to nose picking may result from low relative humidity, especially during the winter months. Lack of moisture causes drying, crusting, and bleeding *(5)*. Bleeding often results from Little's area being exposed to dry air or minor trauma. The subsequent crusts and scabs can then cause itching, which in turn leads children to traumatize the area again by picking and rubbing *(1)*.

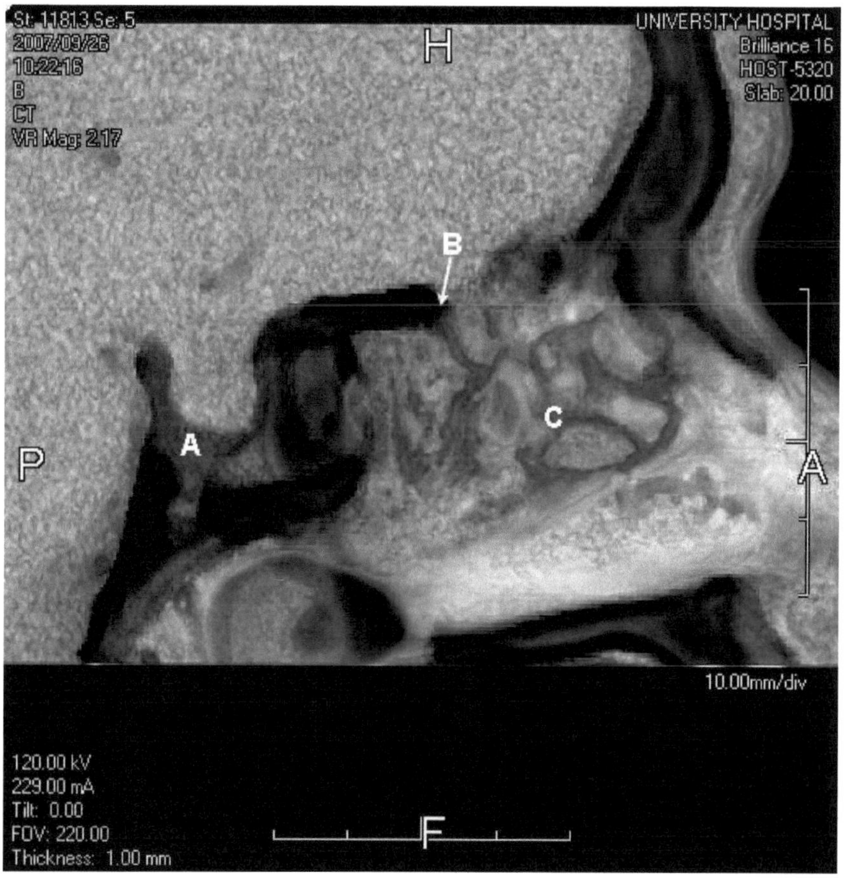

Fig. 3 Modified sagittal CT image demonstrating (**a**) internal carotid artery (ICA), (**b**) anterior ethmoid artery (a distal branch of the ICA) and (**c**) Keisselbach's Plexus. (*Modification courtesy of Christian Stallworth, MD*)

Systemic etiologies of epistaxis include coagulation disorders, vascular diseases, congenital disorders, systemic infections, and neoplasms. Coagulation deficits or disorders include von Willebrand disease, idiopathic thrombocytopenic purpura (ITP), thrombocytopenia, hemophilia, factor deficiencies, vitamin deficiencies (A, D, C, E, or K), leukemia, and other acquired and congenital coagulopathies. Vascular diseases in children include hereditary hemorrhagic telangiectasia (HHT), collagen abnormalities, and other types of vasculitis *(5,8)*. Systemic infections include typhoid fever, unilateral nasal diphtheria, congenital syphilis, pertussis, malaria, rheumatic fever, influenza, dengue fever, measles, and varicella *(5)*. Majority of these infections are very rare if not nonexistent in the western world.

For recurrent epistaxis that is not amenable to conservative treatment and is associated with nasal obstruction or significant lymphadenopathy, neoplasms must be ruled out. Neoplasms that can cause epistaxis include rhabdomyosarcoma, lymphoma, juvenile nasopharyngeal angiofibroma, epidermoid carcinomas, nasal papilloma, adenocarcinoma, esthesioneuroblastoma, and hemangioma. Vascular malformations such as aneurysms should also be excluded *(8)*.

Diagnosis

Initial evaluation of a child with epistaxis involves a "primary survey" with special attention to hemodynamic stability and potential airway compromise. Vital signs and laboratory studies should be reviewed *(8)*. Persistent tachycardia must be recognized as an early indicator of significant blood loss requiring intravenous fluid and, potentially, transfusion. Altered vital signs can be a very late and ominous sign in children.

Once stability is assured, a complete history can be obtained. Important questions include the frequency of epistaxis, anterior/posterior predominance, duration, amount, the proportion of the child's life that has included nosebleeds, and whether one side predominates *(12)*.

A thorough medical and family history is required to determine if there is a related medical condition or potential familial bleeding disorder. A thorough medication history should be obtained to identify all medicines with effects on vessels or coagulation.

A thorough head and neck examination should follow. Ideally, this would include anterior rhinoscopy and fiberoptic examination. The child's anxiety and poor cooperation may limit the examination. Some children may not even tolerate an anterior rhinoscopy with a nasal speculum and may only allow a nasal exam with an otoscopic speculum. To maximize the information gathered through physical examination, any large clots should be removed carefully by suction.

It is important to examine the remainder of the head and neck as well as the other areas of the body. Significant findings include a hemotympanum, active bleeding in the posterior pharynx, and petechiae. Constant dripping of blood in the posterior pharynx may signify a posterior rather than an anterior bleed. The oral cavity and the palate should also be examined to determine if petechiae or ecchymosis is present, suggesting an underlying coagulation disorder. The skin should also be examined for evidence of bruises or petechiae that may indicate an underlying hematologic abnormality or nonaccidental injury *(13)*.

Differential Diagnosis

As previously stated, the majority of childhood epistaxis is usually a combination of digital trauma and decreased humidity usually during the winter months. However, there are several systemic disorders seen in patients with recurrent epistaxis. This section reviews the most common systemic diseases resulting in pediatric epistaxis. Many other coagulation or hematologic diseases may contribute but are beyond the scope of this chapter.

Von Willebrand Disease

As many as 5–10% of children with recurrent nosebleeds may have mild, previously undiagnosed von Willebrand's disease (vWd) ***(14,15)***. First described in 1926, vWD has an estimated frequency of 1% and is believed to be one of the most common inherited disorders of bleeding in humans ***(16,17)***. vWD tends to present in infancy and childhood. It primarily involves the mucous membranes, with epistaxis being the most common symptom ***(18)***. Clinically, it is characterized by spontaneous bleeding from mucous membranes, excessive bleeding from wounds, and menorrhagia. The disease is usually autosomal dominant but several autosomal recessive variants have been identified ***(19)***. Overall, more than 20 variants of vWD have been described.

vWD is characterized by a triad of laboratory abnormalities: a prolonged bleeding time, a deficiency of factor VIII (von Willebrand factor slows breakdown of factor VIII), and an impaired platelet adhesiveness with a normal platelet count ***(16,17)***. Laboratory abnormalities tend to fluctuate throughout the course of the disease, at times falling within the normal range. Therefore, sequential testing is often required in order to establish the diagnosis.

Hemophilia

Hemophilia A is considered the most common hereditary bleeding disorder. It is caused by a reduction in the amount or activity of factor VIII. This protein serves as a cofactor for the activation of factor X in the coagulation cascade *(17)*. Hemophilia A is inherited as an X-linked recessive trait, and thus it occurs in males and in homozygous females *(17)*. Approximately 30% of patients diagnosed with hemophilia A have no family history and are presumed to represent new mutations. Hemophilia A can exhibit a wide range of clinical severity. In all symptomatic cases, there is a tendency toward easy bruising and massive hemorrhage after trauma or operative procedures. On physical examination, petechiae are not often seen *(17)*.

Laboratory values usually demonstrate a normal bleeding time and platelet count, with a prolonged PTT and a normal PT. These tests point to an abnormality of the intrinsic coagulation pathway. To accurately diagnose the disease, factor VIII assays are required. Treatment includes symptomatic treatment of bleeding and the infusion of factor VIII, currently derived from human plasma, introducing the risk of bloodborne pathogen infection.

Hemophilia B is also known as Christmas disease and is a severe factor IX deficiency. Clinically, it is indistinguishable from hemophilia A. The laboratory values are identical to hemophilia A except that a factor IX assay is required. In about 14% of patients with hemophilia B, factor IX is present but is nonfunctional. Treatment is similar to hemophilia A, but with factor IX replacement.

Hereditary Hemorrhagic Telangiectasia (HHT)

Hereditary hemorrhagic telangiectasia is also known as Osler-Weber-Rendu syndrome. It is an autosomal dominant disease with incomplete penetrance characterized by dermal, mucosal, and visceral telangiectasia as well as pulmonary, hepatic, GI, and cerebral arteriovenous malformations *(20)*. The incidence is 2–4 per 100,000 *(8)*. Due to lack of smooth muscle and elastic tissue in the vascular endothelium, dilated capillaries and veins, present from birth, are distributed widely over the skin and mucous membranes. The most common manifestation of HHT is recurrent epistaxis, occurring in up to 90% of children *(21)*. Although widely variable, the average onset of epistaxis is about 12 years old and patients average about 18 episodes of epistaxis per month *(18)*. Because these patients have recurrent, severe episodes of epistaxis, they can undergo dozens of blood transfusions over their lifetime. Severe gastrointestinal, hepatic, pulmonary, or cerebral arteriovenous malformations can be present and must be investigated at the time of diagnosis and periodically throughout their lifetime *(8)*.

Juvenile Nasopharyngeal Angiofibroma (JNA)

Juvenile nasopharyngeal angiofibromas (JNAs) account for less than 0.5% of all head and neck tumors. JNAs are extremely vascular, benign neoplasms seen almost exclusively in the nasopharynx of adolescent males. Controversy exists as to the exact cause and site of origin of JNAs. They are slow-growing lesions that initially expand intranasally and to the pterygomaxillary space, and may eventually invade the infratemporal fossa, orbit, and middle cranial fossa *(22)*. JNAs commonly present with a triad of unilateral nasal obstruction, epistaxis, and nasopharyngeal mass. Facial swelling, proptosis, cranial neuropathy, massive hemorrhage, and headaches can also be seen at presentation *(22)*.

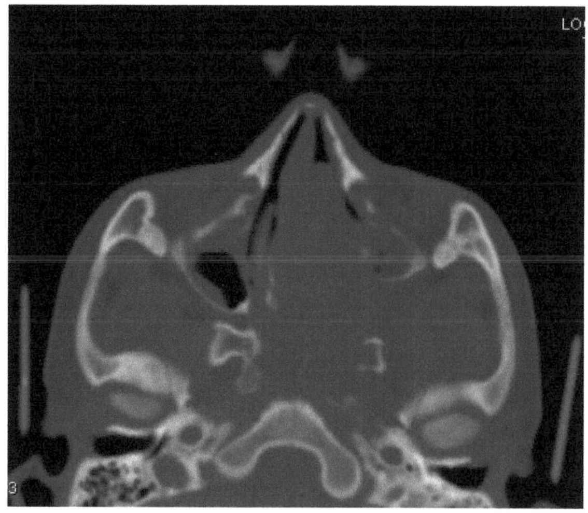

Fig. 4 Axial CT scan of a patient with a juvenile nasopharyngeal angiofibroma (JNA). Note expansion of the pterygopalatine fossa on the *left*

Appropriate imaging studies should be performed for evaluation. These may include CT (Fig. 4), MRI (Fig. 5), and/or angiography. The treatment of choice is surgical excision. Both open and endoscopic techniques have been described. The surgical approach should be based on several considerations, including size and extent of the lesion and the surgeon's experience. Due to the vascularity of the tumor and the potential for extensive blood loss during surgical excision, preoperative angiography with embolization of the external carotid system should be considered.

Glanzmann's Thrombasthenia

Glanzmann's thrombasthenia (GT) is a rare, autosomal recessive hemorrhagic disorder. It is characterized by chronic nonthrombocytopenic purpura, a prolonged

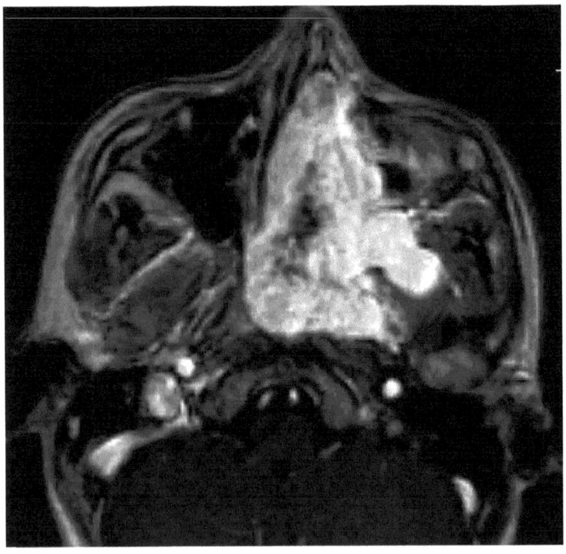

Fig. 5 T-1 weighted, contrast-enhanced MRI scan of a patient with a JNA. Note the lateral extension into the infratemporal fossa

bleeding time, and deficient platelet aggregation *(23)*. GT is caused by deficiencies in two platelet membrane glycoproteins, Iib and IIIa, that are involved in platelet aggregation and clot retraction *(24)*. Clinically, purpura usually begins in infancy and bleeding in early childhood. GT follows a characteristic pattern of recurrent, spontaneous mucosal and cutaneous hemorrhage *(25)*. The natural disease progression results in a decrease in bleeding episodes as one approaches adulthood. Laboratory studies demonstrate a normal platelet count, prothrombin time, and partial thromboplastin time. An increased bleeding time of more than 10 min and markedly reduced clot retraction is seen. Platelet aggregation studies in response to collagen, epinephrine, thrombin, 5-hydroxytryptamine, and ADP are abnormal, while normal aggregation in response to ristocetin is seen.

Work-Up

Epistaxis is the most common bleeding symptom and may signal the presence of a coagulopathy *(26)*. A full hematologic evaluation is indicated with severe, recurrent epistaxis, family history of bleeding, and/or abnormal screening laboratory evaluations *(12)*. Laboratory studies are not needed for a single episode of epistaxis or for infrequent recurrences especially with a history of nose picking or trauma to the nose. Initial screening includes a hemoglobin and hematocrit, platelet count, bleeding time, prothrombin time, partial thromboplastin time, and ristocetin cofactor activity. If these studies are abnormal, consultation with a pediatric hematologist should be considered for further treatment and/or management.

If the patient has nasal airway obstruction, significant lymphadenopathy or other physical exam findings suggestive of a neoplasm, imaging should be performed. Plain radiographs of the sinuses lack sufficient diagnostic detail. CT of the sinuses with contrast is indicated for initial evaluation but additional imaging including MRI and angiography may be necessary to guide management decisions.

Treatment

Treatment of epistaxis largely depends on the cause, severity, and location of the epistaxis. This can range from conservative medical management to aggressive surgical treatment. Contributing systemic disorders should be aggressively managed while procedural intervention is considered.

Medical management of recurrent, self-limiting epistaxis usually includes keeping the nasal cavity moist either with an emollient or an antibiotic ointment. Other conservative measures can include increasing the humidity of the ambient air with the use of a bedside humidifier and avoiding digital trauma to the nasal cavity and aggressive treatment of allergic diseases.

If conservative measures and treatment of systemic disease do not control epistaxis, intervention is indicated. The surgical procedures are based on the source of epistaxis. It is important to determine whether the patient is suffering from anterior or posterior epistaxis as this will guide you as to which vessels may be involved and the appropriate surgical approach if needed. Nasal cauterization with silver nitrate is often sufficient for anterior epistaxis if tolerated by the patient. If chemical cautery fails, or is poorly tolerated, evaluation under anesthesia (EUA) of the nasal cavity is recommended. This can involve electrocautery and/or packing with bioresorbable materials. If a posterior source of bleeding is suspected, EUA is indicated to identify the specific location of the bleeding with posterior packing. Surgical approaches include a septoplasty, internal maxillary and ethmoid artery ligations, transantral internal maxillary artery ligation, and transnasal endoscopic sphenopalatine artery ligation (TESPAL). The description of the surgical procedures is beyond the scope of this text. It should be noted that the transantral internal maxillary artery ligation is contraindicated in the pediatric population because of the risk of injury to the unerupted teeth ***(8)***. Arterial embolization of vessels in the external carotid distribution can be utilized if appropriate facilities and skilled staff are available. Posterior packing requires admission and observation in a monitored setting due to the risk of airway compromise.

Management of HHT requires unique approaches not normally required for other causes of epistaxis. Commonly used therapeutic approaches for controlling epistaxis in HHT include cauterization, septal dermoplasty, hormonal therapy with estrogen or progesterone, and laser ablation ***(18)***. Septal dermoplasty was originally described by Saunders in 1960. In the performance of septal dermoplasty, the fragile mucosa of the anterior nasal chamber is removed and replaced with a split thickness skin graft. This graft represents a more resistant lining, and better protection against trauma and subsequent epistaxis ***(16)***. This procedure has traditionally been performed through a lateral rhinotomy but recently has been described through endoscopic techniques. Laser coagulation of telangiectasias requires laser energy delivered in a wavelength absorbed by the heme molecule, such as the pulse dye or KTP laser.

Conclusion

Careful history and physical examination is the mainstay of diagnosing the causes of epistaxis in children. The physician must closely attend to behavioral, environmental, congenital, hereditary, systemic, and neoplastic conditions that may contribute to epistaxis. Additionally, a child's anxiety may limit the evaluation in the office, leading to increased reliance on imaging. Vital signs in children remain well compensated until late in the progression of fluid abnormalities and may mask pending hematologic decompensation. Laboratory studies may be helpful in diagnosing contributing conditions in patients with severe or recurrent disease. Successful treatment relies on accurate identification of the location and cofactors exacerbating epistaxis.

References

1. The Cochrane Database of Systemic Reviews: Interventions for Recurrent Idiopathic Epistaxis in Children.
2. Boat JF, Doeshuk CF, Stern RC, et al. Diseases of the respiratory system. In: WD Nelson (ed.) Textbook of Pediatrics. WB Saunders Co., Philadelphia, p. 1012, 1983.
3. Petruson B. Epistaxis. Acta Otolaryngol Suppl 1974; 317: 1–73.
4. Pope LE, Hobbs CG. Epistaxis: an update on current management. Postgrad Med J 2005; 81: 309–314.
5. Wolff, Ruth RN. Pediatric epistaxis. Nurse Pract 1982; 7(10): 12–17.
6. Chiu T, Dunn JS. An anatomical study of the arteries of the anterior nasal septum. Otolaryngol Head Neck Surg 2006; 14: 33–36.
7. Douglas R, Wormald PJ. Update on epistaxis. Curr Opin Otolaryngol-Head Neck Surg 2007; 15: 180–183.
8. Massick D, Tobin EJ. Epistaxis. In: CW Cummings (Ed.). Cummings Otolaryngology Head and Neck Surgery. Cummings Textbook (4th edition). Elsevier Mosby Inc., Philadelphia, pp. 942–961, 2005.
9. Guarisco JL, Graham 3rd HD. Epistaxis in children: causes, diagnosis and treatment. Ear Nose Throat J 1989; 68: 522–538.
10. Nunez DA, McClymont LG, Evans RA. Epistaxis: a study of the relationship with weather. Clin Otolaryngol 1990; 15: 49–51.
11. Watkinson JC, Epistaxis. In: Kerr AG, Mackay IS, TR Bull (Eds.). Scott-Brown's Otolaryngology (6th edition), Volume 4: Rhinology. Butterworth-Heinemann, Oxford, pp. 4/18/1–19, 1997.
12. Sandoval C, Dong S, et al. Clinical and laboratory features of 178 children with recurrent epistaxis. J Pediatr Hematol/Oncol 2002; 24(1): 47–49.
13. Gluckman W, et al. Epistaxis eMedicine. (http://emedicine.medscape.com/article/994459-overview).
14. Katsanis E, Koon-Hung L, Hsu E, Li M, Lillcrap D. Prevalence and significance of mild bleeding disorders in children with recurrent epistaxis. J Pediatr 1988; 113: 73–76.
15. Kiley V, Stuart JJ, Johnson CA. Coagulation studies in children with isolated recurrent epistaxis. J Pediatr 1982; 100: 579–581.
16. Leston Jr. JA, Birck HG. Septal dermoplasty for von Willdebrand's disease in children. Laryngoscope 1973; 83(7): 1078–1083.
17. Cotran RS, Kumar V, Collins T. Red cells and bleeding disorders. In: Robbins Pathologic Basis of Disease (6th edition). WB Saunders Company, Philadelphia, pp. 638–640, 1999.
18. Abildgaard CF, et al. Von Willebrand's disease: a comparative study of diagnostic tests. J Pediatr 1968; 73: 355.

19. Ewenstein BM. Von Willebrand disease. Annu Rev Med 1997; 4: 525.
20. Aassar OS, Friedman CM, White RI. The natural history of epistaxis in hereditary hemorrhagic telangiectasia. Laryngoscope 1991; 101: 977–980.
21. Bird RM, Hammarsten JF, Marshall RA, et al. A family reunion: a study of hereditary hemorrhagic telangiectasia. N Engl J Med 1957; 257: 105–109.
22. Enepekides DJ. Recent advances in the treatment of juvenile angiofibroma. Curr Opin Otolaryngol Head Neck Surg 2004; 12: 495–499.
23. McMillan CW. Platelet and vascular disorders. In: DR Miller (Ed.). Blood Diseases of Infancy and Childhood. CV Mosby Co., St Louis, pp. 829–830, 1984.
24. Phillips DR, Agin PP. Platelet membrane defects in Glanzmann's thrombasthenia. Evidence for decreased amounts of two major glycoproteins. J Clin Invest 1977; 60: 535–545.
25. Guarisco JL, et al. Limited septoplasty as treatment for recurrent epistaxis in a child with Glanzmann's thrombasthenia. Laryngoscope 1987; 97: 336–338.
26. Werner EJ. Von Willebrand disease in children and adolescents. Pediatr Clin North Am 1996; 43: 683–707.

Nasal Obstruction in the Neonate

Stacey Leigh Smith and Kevin D. Pereira

Key Points

- Neonates are obligatory nasal breathers.
- Severe nasal obstruction presents with *cyclical* cyanosis relieved by crying.
- Rhinitis is the main cause of neonatal nasal obstruction.
- Choanal atresia, pyriform aperture stenosis, and congenital nasal masses must be ruled out when evaluating neonatal nasal airway obstruction.
- Birth trauma can result in septal deformities or septal hematoma.
- Iatrogenic nasal scarring can be avoided by careful instrumentation.
- Conservative treatment such as nasal humidification, topical decongestants, and intraoral devices are used for mild cases of obstruction.
- Surgical intervention is necessary for severe or bilateral obstruction.

Keywords: Neonate • Nasal • Obstruction • Airway • Congenital • Pyriform • Choanae

S.L. Smith
Department of Otolaryngology-Head and Neck Surgery, University of Texas, Health Science Center at San Antonio, San Antonio, TX, USA

K.D. Pereira (✉)
Department of Otorhinolaryngology – Head and Neck Surgery, University of Maryland School of Medicine, Baltimore, MD, USA
e-mail: kevindpereira@gmail.com

Neonatal Nasal Development and Physiology

Nasal airway obstruction is a potentially life-threatening condition in the newborn. Due to the high position of the larynx, a relatively large tongue, and the immaturity of the central nervous system, neonates are obligatory nasal breathers. Mouth breathing is not learned until at least 6–8 weeks after birth, although some neonates require up to 6 months. Because of this, nasal obstruction in neonates can produce severe respiratory distress and cyanosis immediately after birth. However, when the infant cries, the respiratory distress is relieved due to air passage through the mouth *(1)*. Nasal resistance is very high in neonates when compared with the remainder of the airway. Due to this resistance and the relatively smaller size of the nasal cavity and choanae, even a small decrease in the dimensions of the nasal cavity can cause significant symptoms of airway obstruction.

Normal nasal dimensions in the newborn (Table 1) have been studied using computerized tomographic (CT) images. Solvis et al. *(2)* reported the normal diameter of the nasal air space of a full-term newborn to be in the range of 3–10 mm. At roughly 40 mm in depth, the neonatal nasal airway has a volume of approximately 1.0 cm^3 and its narrowest portion is about 8 mm into the nostril. The minimal cross-sectional area at this location is approximately 0.1 cm^2, while the mean posterior cross-sectional area is 0.3 cm^2*(3–5)*. Using intraoperative measurement of posterior nasal choanae in children, Sweeney et al. *(6)* determined that a linear relationship exists between age and average choanal size, with choanae enlarging at a rate of 0.208 mm per year. A study using CT scan measurements indicated that the mean choanal width was approximately 4.85 mm + (0.04 × age in weeks) *(7)*.

R.B. Mitchell and K.D. Pereira (eds.), *Pediatric Otolaryngology for the Clinician*,
DOI: 10.1007/978-1-60327-127-1_14,

Table 1 Normal nasal dimensions in newborn

Dimension	Mm
Length	30
Anterior bony width	13
Anterior mucosal width	9
Middle mucosal width	8
Posterior bony width	14.5
Each choana	5.7

Signs and Symptoms of Nasal Airway Obstruction

Neonates with nasal airway obstruction present with clinical findings that depend on the extent and location of the obstruction. Mild respiratory distress as evidenced by noisy breathing and circumoral cyanosis while feeding may represent less severe obstruction or nasal congestion. Complete nasal obstruction results in a critical respiratory response manifested by episodic apnea, cyclical respiratory distress, and cyanosis relieved by crying. These events can be life threatening.

Effects of Nasal Airway Obstruction

Feeding in the neonate depends on a patent airway of adequate dimensions. If the nasal cavity is obstructed, a neonate will often aspirate during feeding. This can lead to both failure to thrive and, rarely, sudden death.

Nasal airway obstruction can also affect craniofacial development. Using plain radiographs with Caldwell projections, Koga et al. *(8)* compared the nasal and facial width and interorbital distance of patients with congenital bony nasal stenosis versus normal infants. They determined that the nasal width and facial width of patients with nasal stenosis was significantly narrower than those of normal infants, but the intraorbital distance was not. They also found that nasal width is equal to or smaller than intraorbital distance in nasal stenosis patients, but nasal width is larger than intraorbital distance in normal infants.

Diagnostic Workup

Nasal obstruction should be included in the differential diagnosis of a child with cyclical cyanosis once cardiopulmonary causes have been ruled out. Anterior rhinoscopic examination should be part of the routine newborn examination. Historical methods of evaluation for nasal obstruction include observing a cotton wisp placed below the nostril, listening for nasal breath sounds using a stethoscope, or looking for misting on a mirror *(9)*. Traditionally, failure to pass a nasogastric tube 3–4-mm thick or a 6 French red rubber catheter through the nose and into the nasopharynx (at least 32 mm) raises the suspicion of nasal obstruction and possible choanal atresia.

The nasal passages can be divided into three anatomic regions: pyriform aperture, middle nasal cavity, and posterior choanae. Nasal masses are best studied using both CT and MRI. CT better delineates the bony anatomy of the nose and skull base, whereas MRI more accurately differentiates soft tissue and can demonstrate intracranial extension. CT scanning can confirm the diagnosis of nasal obstruction and can assist with surgical planning. A HRCT scan with thin axial cuts through the nasal cavity can demonstrate the level and side of nasal airway obstruction as well as the nature of the obstruction (bony or membranous). Measurements should be performed at the level of the maximum transverse diameter of the pyriform aperture and the posterior choanae.

Acoustic rhinometry can produce a graphic presentation of the nasal airway geometry, describing both the size and location of the obstruction. Acoustic rhinometric measurements were shown to be a comparable tool to CT scan measurements in the diagnosis of congenital choanal malformations *(10)*. Nasal endoscopy can also assist with establishing the diagnosis. However, it is not a reliable measure of the degree and location of the obstruction and can lead to mucosal damage.

Differential Diagnosis

The differential diagnosis of nasal obstruction in the neonate is limited. The most common cause of nasal dyspnea in the neonate is rhinitis (Table 2).

Congenital

Choanal atresia is an uncommon but well-recognized cause of respiratory distress in the neonate, with an incidence of 1 in 7,000–8,000 births. It is twice as common in females as in males. It results from a unilateral or bilateral atretic plate at the posterior aperture of the nose. Patients with unilateral atresia may not present until later in life; those with bilateral atresia present as newborns with cyclic cyanosis relieved by crying. Classic theories of the cause of choanal atresia include persistence of the oro-nasal (nasobuccal) membrane, failure of the oro-pharyngeal (buccopharyngeal) membrane to recanalize or persistence of epithelial plugs. The atretic plate is bounded superiorly by the sphenoid, laterally by the pterygoids, medially by the thickened vomer, and inferiorly by the horizontal portion of the palatine bones (Fig. 1a,b). About 70% of choanal malformations can be classified as a mixture of bony and membranous obstruction, whereas 30% are from purely bony obstruction. Approximately 30–40% of cases are bilateral ***(11)***. Choanal atresia can be diagnosed if the posterior choanal orifice measures <0.34 cm unilaterally. In roughly 50% of cases, choanal atresia is associated with other congenital anomalies, which require full investigation and genetic counseling. Specifically, choanal atresia is a manifestation of CHARGE syndrome (coloboma, congenital heart defects, choanal atresia, retarded physical and neuromotor development, genital hypoplasia, and ear anomalies).

Table 2 Differential diagnosis

Congenital	Acquired
Choanal atresia	Septal deformations
Nasal pyriform aperture stenosis	Septal hematoma
Craniofacial anomalies	Iatrogenic nasal synechiae
Anterior skull base defects	
Developmental nasal anomalies	
Nasal lacrimal duct obstruction	

Congenital nasal pyriform aperture stenosis (CNPAS) is a rare form of nasal obstruction. The pyriform aperture is the narrowest, most anterior bony portion of the nasal airway and is bounded superiorly by the nasal bones, laterally by the nasal process of the maxilla, and inferiorly by the premaxilla and the anterior nasal spine (Fig. 2). A decrease in its cross-sectional area will significantly increase nasal airway resistance ***(12)***. It is caused by excessive growth of the medial nasal process of the maxilla that leads to the narrowing of the bony part of the nasal cavity ***(13)***. Association with single central maxillary incisor (megaincisor) is high. It is thought that CNPAS may be a microform of holoprosencephaly. Diagnosis can be made by physical exam, but is confirmed when CT scan reveals overgrowth and medial displacement of the nasal process of the maxilla while the posterior nasal choanae are normal caliber ***(13)***. In a term infant, the pyriform aperture is considered to be stenotic when either the maximum transverse diameter is less than or equal to 3 mm or when the pyriform aperture width is less than 8 mm ***(12)***.

Nasal stenosis is often associated with *congenital anomalies* or syndromes such as mandibulofacial dysostosis, craniosynostosis, holoprosencephaly, Crouzon's syndrome, and Apert syndrome. It is thought that nasal stenosis might be more prominent in patients with congenital anomalies than in isolated cases ***(8)***.

Congenital anterior skull base defects causing nasal obstruction are rare clinical entities, occurring in only 1 in 30,000 live births. The development of these masses occur during the early stages of gestation if dural projections fail to involute and begin to herniate

a **b**

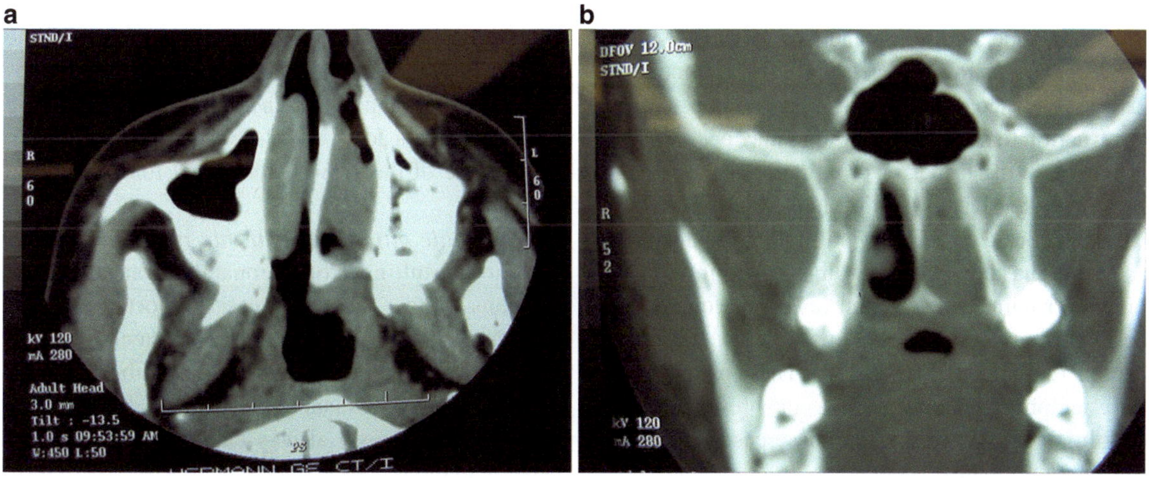

Fig. 1 Choanal atresia

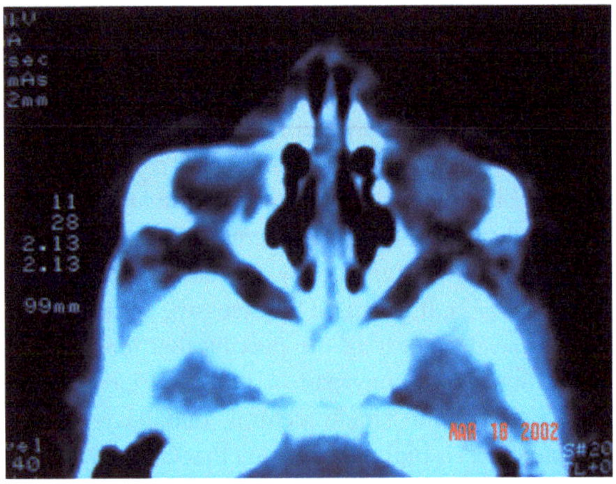

Fig. 2 Congenital pyriform aperture stenosis

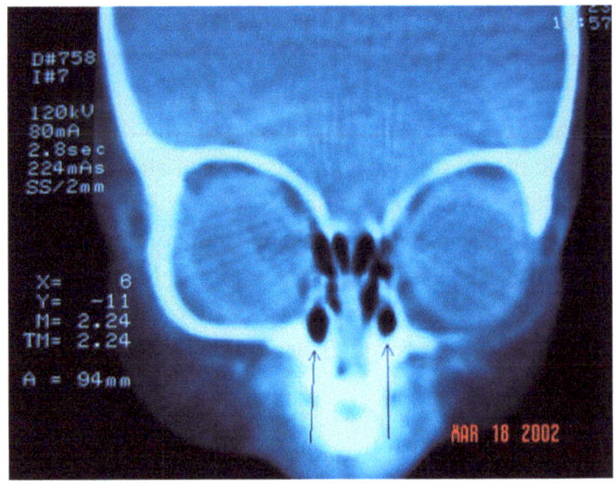

Fig. 3 Congenital nasolacrimal duct cysts

through the foramen cecum anteriorly. These midline defects can be divided into three major groups based on their tissue of origin (neurogenic, ectoderm, and endoderm). They are also classified as occipital, frontonasal, or basal depending on their location *(14)*. Dermoids, encephaloceles, and gliomas are the most common midline nasal masses in the neonatal population *(15)*.

Developmental nasal anomalies occur once in every 20,000–40,000 births and may be derived from ectodermal, mesodermal, or neurodermal tissue. In a review article of a 10-year experience managing developmental nasal anomalies, Morgan et al. *(16)* describe treating nasopharyngeal cysts, hairy polyps, meningoencephalocoeles, gliomatas, dermoids, capillary hemangiomatas, fibromas, fibromyxomas, mucoceles, granulomas, lipomas, nasal aplasias, nasal clefts, and nasal webs. Other rare neonatal nasal masses include chordomas and hamartomas *(17,18)*.

Nasal lacrimal duct obstruction is an uncommon cause of neonatal nasal airway obstruction. Obstruction to the lacrimal system may occur distally at the valve of Hasner or proximally at the valve of Rosenmueller. Distal dilation may result in an intranasal mucocele of the lacrimal duct, which presents as an intranasal cystic mass close to the inferior turbinate. Proximal dilation can result in a dacrocystocele, presenting as a cystic mass below the medial canthal region of the eye (Fig. 3). These patients often have epiphora, dacryocystitis, or preseptal/orbital cellulitis *(19)*. Up to 85% of these cases resolve by the age of 9 months.

Acquired

Nasal septal deformations have been found in up to 18% of newborns. Children born by spontaneous vaginal delivery have a higher likelihood of septal deviations than those delivered by Caesarean section. Anterior dislocation of the septum off the maxillary crest has been associated with trauma in the birth canal, while combined anterior and posterior septal deformities usually occur due to transmitted intrauterine forces during fetal skull molding. When accompanied by mucosal edema, a septal deviation can lead to total nasal obstruction in a neonate. In order to prevent nasal obstruction and future systemic complications, neonates found to have septal deformity should undergo surgical repositioning, although deviations of the cartilaginous septum often undergo spontaneous straightening during the first days of life *(20)*. Nasal septal abscess can result from an infected hematoma of the septum. In a short term, it can cause sagging and widening of the nasal pyramid and impair breathing. If not treated, it can lead to septal destruction, resulting in disturbance of the growth, form, and function of the nose *(21)*.

Iatrogenic intranasal synechia is a serious complication resulting from neonatal intranasal interventions (Fig. 4). One case report describes complete nasal obstruction due to synechia caused by intranasal catheters used for continuous positive airway pressure. Nasal dilators used for patients with narrowed nasal airway can also contribute to synechiae *(22)*.

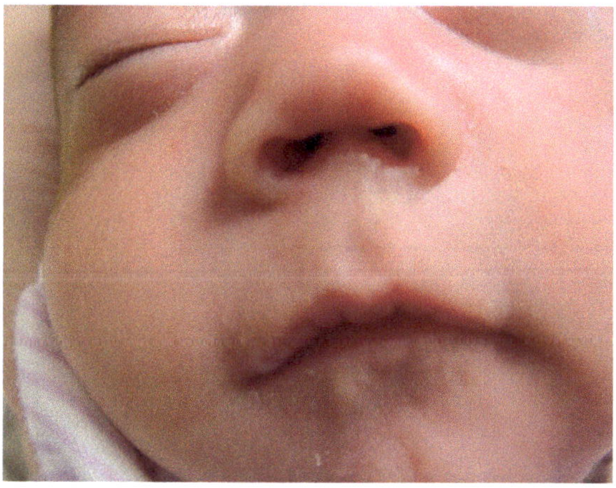

Fig. 4 Iatrogenic nasal obstruction – a complication of CPAP prongs causing pressure necrosis of the columella

Management

Management of neonatal nasal airway obstruction should be based on the severity of symptoms (Fig. 5). Topical treatment and nasal stenting should be performed in patients with mild symptoms. Saline nasal drops or sprays along with gentle bulb suction can wash out crusts and mucus and facilitate mucociliary clearance. Topical steroid drops may be used for more severe symptoms of rhinitis. In general, ophthalmic preparations of topical steroids in low strength used for 5–7 days provide significant relief of nasal obstruction. Antibiotic therapy covering streptococcus and staphylococcus should be instituted if purulent secretions are seen. Patients with more severe symptoms may require immediate intubation and ventilation. For patients with sleep apnea, repeated intubations, failure of extubation, feeding difficulties with cyanosis, and unresponsiveness to continuous positive airway pressure, surgery should be considered. Surgical management should also be considered when relief of nasal obstruction could not be reached with medical treatment within 10–15 days. The objectives of surgical correction include securing a patent nasal airway, reducing the risk of stenosis, and preventing the need for revision.

Historically, many approaches have been used to repair choanal atresia including transnasal, transantral, transpalatal, and transseptal. Unilateral atresia repair is generally delayed to allow development, reducing the risk of postoperative stenosis. Bilateral atresia requires urgent correction, but these patients can be temporized by training the infant to mouth-breathe through an oral appliance. Until recently, the transpalatal technique was the method preferred by most surgeons, as it provides good visualization and has high success rates. This approach is associated with increased morbidity, palatal fistulas, and risks of cross-bite. Purely transnasal techniques often require prolonged stenting and have higher rates of restenosis. However, with the rigid endoscopes and powered instrumentation, a transnasal endoscopic approach is now considered the surgical technique of choice to treat choanal atresia ***(10,23)***. The key points to any surgical approach include removing and shortening the posterior bony septum and removing both the lateral pterygoid plate and the superior-lateral nasal wall. During surgery, care must be taken to avoid damage to the periosteum, nasal mucosa, tooth buds, nasolacrimal duct, and normal bony structure. Many surgeons still use postoperative stents; however, these can create local infections, pain, formation of granulation tissue, nasal synechiae, and alar retraction.

Treatment of pyriform aperture stenosis is based on severity. Mild cases can often be managed conservatively with lavage, home apnea monitoring, and indwelling oral appliances such as a McGovern nipple. Surgical treatment of severe cases is done transnasally or through a sublabial approach. Redundant bone and soft tissue of the nasal process of the maxilla are removed with a curette or burr. Nasal stents are used postoperatively to keep the aperture patent and are typically removed 7 days after the procedure.

Definitive management of congenital midline nasal masses is surgical. If intracranial extension exists, neurosurgeons must be involved. These masses which originate from anterior skull base defects have traditionally been repaired with bifrontal craniotomy approaches, but can be successfully repaired with transnasal endoscopic techniques. Nasal obstruction, cosmetic deformity, craniofacial development, risk of meningitis, and intracranial complications are important considerations in the management of these lesions ***(15,18)***.

Treatment modalities of nasal lacrimal obstruction and mucocele include applying a warm cloth over the nasal vestibule, instillation of topical vasoconstrictor nose drops, removal of the cyst with a microdebrider, and endoscopic marsupilization of the larger intranasal mucoceles.

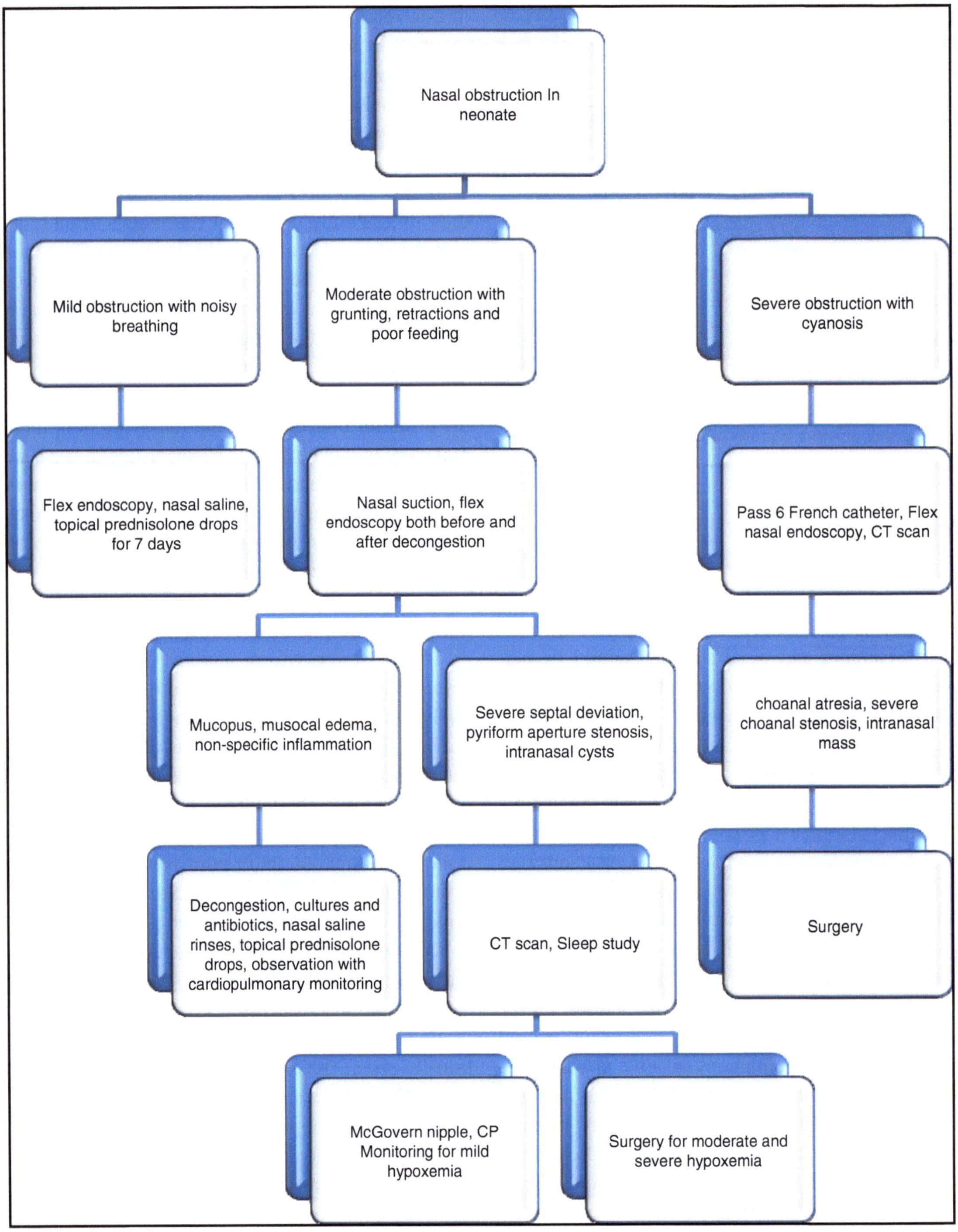

Fig. 5 Diagnostic workup and treatment

Conclusions

Because of obligatory nasal breathing, any type of nasal obstruction can be life threatening in neonates. A succinct differential diagnosis should be kept in mind when evaluating neonates with nasal obstruction. A variety of medical and surgical treatments allow for management of this problem.

References

1. Richardson MA, Osguthorpe JD. Surgical management of choanal atresia. *Laryngoscope*. 1988;98:915–918.
2. Solvis TL, Renfro B, Watts FB. Choanal atresia: precise CT evaluation. *Radiology*. 1985;155:345–348.
3. Buenting JE, Dalston RM, Drake AF. Nasal cavity area in term infants determined by acoustic rhinometry. *Laryngoscope*. 1994;104:1439–1445.
4. Djupesland PG, Lyholm B. Nasal airway dimensions in term neonates measured by continuous wide-band noise acoustic rhinometry. *Acta Otolaryngol*. 1997;117:424–432.
5. Pederson OF, Berkowitz R, Yamagiwa M, et al. Nasal cavity dimensions in the newborn measured by acoustic reflections. *Laryngoscope*. 1994;104:1023–1028.
6. Sweeney KD, Deskin RW, Hokanson JA, Thompson CP, Yoo JK. Establishment of normal values of nasal choanal size in children: comparison of nasal choanal size in children with and without symptoms of nasal obstruction. *Int J Pediatr Otorhinolaryngol*. 1997;29:51–57.
7. Corsten MJ, Bernard PA, Udjus K, et al. Nasal fossa dimensions in normal and nasally obstructed neonates and infants: preliminary study. *Int J Pediatr Otorhinolaryngol*. 1996;36:23–30.
8. Koga K, Kawashiro N, Araki A, et al. Radiographic diagnosis of congenital bony nasal stenosis. *Int J Pediatr Otorhinolaryngol*. 2001;59:29–39.
9. Benjamin B. Evaluation of choanal atresia. *Ann Otol Rhinol Laryngol*. 1985;94:429–432.
10. Djupesland P, Kaastad E, Franzen G. Acoustic rhinometry in the evaluation of congenital choanal malformations. *Int J Pediatr Otorhinolaryngol*. 1997;41:319–337.
11. Brown OE, Pownell P, Manning SC. Choanal atresia: a new anatomic classification and clinical management applications. *Laryngoscope*. 1996;106:97–101.
12. Osovsky M, Aizer-Danon A, Horev G. Congenital pyriform aperture stenosis. *Pediatr Radiol*. 2007;37:97–99.
13. Brown OE, Myer CM III, Manning SC. Congenital nasal pyriform aperture stenosis. *Laryngoscope*. 1989;99:86–91.
14. Hughes GB, Sharpino G, Hunt W, et al. Management of the congenital midline nasal masses: a review. *Head Neck Surg*. 1980;2:222–233.
15. Kanowitz SJ, Bernstein JM. Pediatric meningoencephaloceles and nasal obstruction: a case for endoscopic repair. *Int J Pediatr Otorhinolaryngol*. 2006;70:2087–2092.
16. Morgan DW, Evans JNG. Developmental nasal anomalies. *J Laryngol Otol*. 1990;104:394–403.
17. Tao ZZ, Chen SM, Liu JF, Huang XL, Zhou L. Paranasal sinuses chordoma in pediatric patient: a case report and literature review. *Int J Pediatr Otorhinolaryngol*. 2005;69:1415–1418.
18. Terris MH, Billman GF, Pransky SM. Nasal hamartoma: case report and review of the literature. *Int J Pediatr Otorhinolaryngol*. 1993;28(1):83–88.
19. Brachlow A, Schwartz RH, Bahadori RS. Intranasal mucocele of the nasolacrimal duct: an important cause of neonatal nasal obstruction. *Clin Pediatr.* 2004;43:479–481.
20. Kawalski H, Spiewak P. How septum deformations in the newborns occur. *Int J Pediatr Otorhinolaryngol*. 1998;44:23–30.
21. Dispenza C, Saraniti C, Dispenza F, et al. Management of nasal septal abscess in childhood: our experience. *Int J Pediatr Otorhinolaryngol*. 2004;68:1417–1421.
22. DeRowe A, Landsberg R, Fishman G, et al. Neonatal iatrogenic nasal obstruction. *Int J Pediatr Otorhinolaryngol*. 2004;68:613–617.
23. Van Den Abbeele T, Francois M, Narcy P. Transnasal endoscopic treatment of choanal atresia without prolonged stenting. *Arch Otolaryngol Head Neck Surg*. 2002;128:936–940.

The Pediatric Allergic Nose

Thomas Sanford

Key Points

- Allergic rhinitis (AR) is one of the most common ailments that can involve the pediatric upper airway with a prevalence of 20–40%.
- AR is closely related to asthma and atopic dermatitis.
- Along with the airway symptoms, AR also has an effect on the cognitive performance of a child.
- Diagnosis of AR is made by a combination of history and physical examination in combination with allergy testing. Allergy testing is done in vivo (skin testing) or in vitro (Rast testing).
- Treatment of AR can include allergen avoidance, pharmacotherapy, and immunotherapy. All three of these therapies are effective and safe.

Keywords: Allergy • Rhinitis • Child

Introduction

Nasal symptoms are one of the most common complaints in the pediatric population. It is estimated that about 50% of rhinitis is atopic in nature. AR is the most common atopic disease and one of the most frequent chronic conditions of children *(1)*. It is interesting that these figures apply primarily to industrialized nations and are less prevalent in underdeveloped countries. The factors that cause these differences are not clear, but likely involve genetic and environmental mechanisms. One possible explanation for the differences in these respective populations is the "Hygiene" hypothesis. The "Hygiene" hypothesis stems from the observation that AR and other atopic diseases are less common in children from large families, where they are more likely to be exposed to a greater number of infectious agents from their siblings, as compared to children from small families. Whether exposure to antigenic and infectious agents early in life is protective against AR remains controversial. Recent studies have reported that other immunologic diseases such as inflammatory bowel disease, multiple sclerosis, and type 1diabetes are not less common in children from large families or children with early antigen exposure *(2)*. As our understanding of the immunological processes of AR and the physiology of the nose and upper airway increase so will our treatment paradigms.

Pathophysiology

AR in children is inherited through multiple genes from both parents. The genotype of the AR child leads to inflammation of the upper airway. The principal cause of inflammation is the result of IgE-mediated pathways. However, it is also likely that non-IgE pathways may play a role *(3)*. Patients with AR are found to have an increase in TH2 lymphocytes, cells that support and enhance the production of IgE through release of cytokines (IL-4, IL-5, IL-13) and other mediators. Increased levels of specific IgE are then produced by repeated exposure to antigens (dust, pollen, mold, danders, and others). This process is termed sensitization. After a child is sensitized, exposure to an antigen will cause mast cell release of multiple mediators resulting in inflammation. The allergic response is divided into two principal time points termed early and late phases. The early phase is triggered by binding of antigen to

T. Sanford
Department of Otolaryngology – Head and Neck Surgery, Saint Louis University School of Medicine, St Louis, MO, USA
e-mail: tsanfor2@slu.edu

R.B. Mitchell and K.D. Pereira (eds.), *Pediatric Otolaryngology for the Clinician*,
DOI: 10.1007/978-1-60327-127-1_15, © Humana Press, a part of Springer Science + Business Media, LLC 2009

IgE-coated mast cells causing degranulation of the mast cells. Degranulation releases preformed compounds (histamine, tryptase, chymase, heprin, and others). Prostaglandins and leukotrienes are also released during the early-phase reaction. These early-phase compounds can cause vessel swelling and leakage, and irritation of sensory nerves resulting in symptoms of AR. The late-phase reaction occurs more than 4 h after antigen binding. The late phase is composed of cellular migration into region of inflammation. Eosinophils, neutrophils, basophils, macrophages, and T cells migrate to the area and can cause regional changes. They also produce compounds that result in systemic symptoms such as fatigue and inability to concentrate.

Diagnosis

Clinical Course of Atopy and Rhinitis

One of the common reasons for a child to visit the physician is chronic nasal airway symptoms. The challenge for the physician is to find the underlying cause and therapy for the child. Infectious causes are the most common reason for acute rhinitis in children. Between the ages of 2 and 6, the average child has six infections per year with each lasting 7–10 days, unless a secondary infection occurs, extending the duration to 2–3 weeks *(4)*. Recurrent infections can mimic the chronic process of AR. Immunologic deficiencies can increase the frequency and length of rhinologic infections. Structural causes for rhinitis should be evaluated which include foreign bodies, choanal atresia, nasal polyps, nasal tumors, and septal deviation. Physiologic causes for rhinitis in children include ciliary dyskinesia, reflux, and cystic fibrosis. Drugs can lead to rhinitis in children, the most common being topical decongestants. If the above causes of rhinitis are ruled out, then the physician can consider atopy and AR as the cause of the child's chronic nasal symptoms.

It is useful to keep in mind the age-related manifestations of AR and atopy in children. This is often referred to as the "Allergic March." It is rare for a child younger than 2 years to demonstrate AR. Eczema is usually the first manifestation of atopy beginning at age 1, peaking by age 5, and then declining during school age. Asthma also begins early with a peak of incidence at age 8 years and declining during early adolescence. AR is less common in early childhood but increases and peaks by the teenage years *(4)*.

History

A complete history is integral to the diagnosis of allergic rhinitis. To diagnose AR, the physician should evaluate the symptoms and comorbidities of the child. Table 1 is a list of the frequent signs, symptoms, and comorbidities of children with AR. A set of questions directed at these areas should be used as a screening device to raise suspicion for a diagnosis of AR.

Children with AR frequently have school absences and experience disruption of sleep with associated fatigue and impaired concentration. Their ability to perform well in school and extracurricular activities is also affected. These challenges can cause emotional problems, isolation, and poor self-esteem.

Family history can also support the diagnosis of AR. If both parents are affected by atopic disease, there is a 50% chance that the child will have AR. The percentage risk increases to 70% if the parent's symptoms are of the same type with greater severity.

Physical Exam

The physical examination can vary but the following symptoms are often identified. Children with AR often

Table 1 Allergic rhinitis: signs, symptoms, and comorbidities

Nasal:	Itching
	Congestion
	Rhinorhea
	Epistaxis
	Micronosmia
Eye:	Itching
	Conjunctival edema
	Hyperemia
Ear:	Chronic effusion
	Chronic otitis
Airway:	Cough
	Throat clearing
	Asthma
Skin:	Atopic dermatitis
Behavior:	Sleep disorders
	Chronic fatigue
	Problems at school

clear their throats and develop a habit of rubbing their nose and eyes. Their voice is often hyponasal and mildly hoarse. The "allergic salute" is a common finding and is the result of rubbing the nose with the palm of the hand causing a horizontal crease on the distal one third of the nasal dorsum (Fig. 1a). AR can often cause venous congestion of the midface resulting in periorbital findings: swelling of the lower eyelid will cause creases in the lid termed "Dennies lines" (Fig. 1b). The lower eyelid can also become swollen and darkened giving the appearance of lower lid injury termed "allergic shiners," as demonstrated in Fig. 1c. Children with AR are often mouth breathers and this can lead to facial deformities with a high arched palate and malocclusion. The nasal examination will reveal large turbinates blocking the nasal airway trapping nasal secretions. Ear examination may show evidence of negative pressure and chronic middle ear effusion. The skin should be evaluated for atopic dermatitis especially in the malar regions of the face and the flexor regions of the arms and legs.

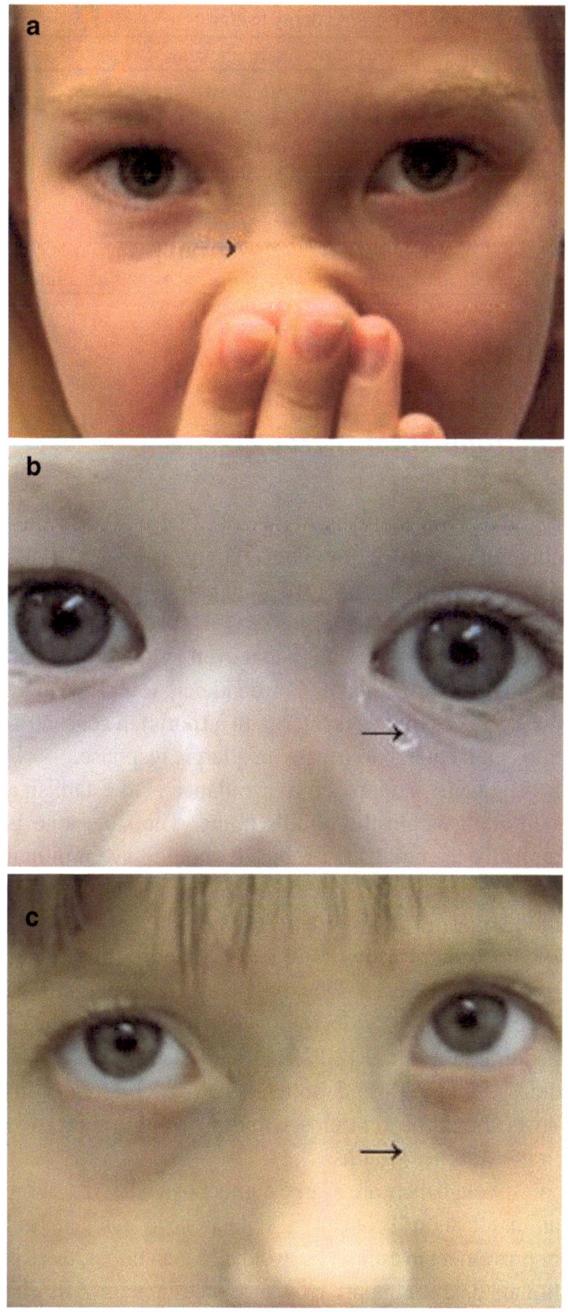

Fig. 1 (**a**) Ten-year-old demonstrating allergic salute, *arrow* on dorsal crease. (**b**) Three-year-old with Dennies lines, *arrow* on lines. (**c**) Six-year-old with allergic shiners, *arrow* on shiner

Diagnostic Tests

Total serum IgE and eosinophil count are not specific-enough tests to be used as part of the routine work-up. If a child with nasal symptoms has a history and physical examination consistent with an allergic cause, the physician has two options. Either treat the process empirically or evaluate the child by testing with in-vitro or in-vivo methods. Allergy testing can identify antigens the child is sensitive to and help in formulating a treatment plan for the child. Table 2 lists and compares the two major testing techniques for atopy. Each technique has its own advantages and the respective applications will vary depending on the needs of the child. For example, a child at risk of anaphylaxis due to a strong history of allergy would be most safely tested by serum techniques. However, skin testing is considered the gold standard. Skin testing is done using prick or intradermal methods. Intradermal testing is frequently applied with multiple concentrations of antigens and can be useful when planning desensitization therapy. Skin and serum testing is usually done as a screen with one or two representative antigens from the common groups of antigens. A larger number of antigens can be tested if there are clinical indications or injection therapy is being planned. It is useful to remember that positive reactions to antigens, either strong or weak, with either skin or serum testing do not predict how a child will respond to therapy.

Table 2 Comparisons of allergy testing

Skin testing	Serum testing
Prick/Intradermal	IgE (Rast)
Multiple needle sticks	Single needle stick
Results immediate	Delay
Anaphylaxis possible	No anaphylaxis
Works on complex antigens	Less sensitive to complex antigens
Affected by skin conditions	Not affected by skin conditions
Affected by antihistamines	Not affected by antihistamines

AR Therapy

Environmental Therapy

Avoidance of allergens is the first line of therapy for children with AR. The common allergens (pollen, mold, danders, and dust mites) are often ubiquitous and therefore hard to avoid. During peak seasons, pollen and mold counts can be so high that even indoor counts can be clinically significant. Cat dander is found in many public places (movie theaters and airports) in concentrations high enough to trigger an allergic response.

The general approach to avoidance is to establish a safe zone within the child's home. The safe zone is typically the child's bedroom. It should have minimal cloth and carpeting to decrease antigens and minimize the habitat for dust mites. The humidity of the room should be kept below 50% and bed and pillow coverings should be used. Dust mite antigen concentrations have been shown to decrease with frequent washing of bedding in water at 130°F and with the use of arachnicides. For mold- and pollen-sensitive children, windows should be kept closed and air-conditioning used in the summer months.

Although there are a large number of studies that show an association between a reduction in antigen and improvement in asthma by avoidance techniques, there is limited data to support avoidance measures for AR. The physician should keep this in mind when recommending life style changes for children with AR. The modest gains of lifestyle change such as limiting outdoor activities may have greater negative psychosocial effects.

Pharmacotherapy

The pharmacology therapy of AR can be quite effective. There are five major categories and multiple forms of medication, including many over-the-counter medications available. The five categories of medications are antihistamines, intranasal steroids, leukotriene inhibitors, decongestants, and mast cell stabilizers. These medications can be given simultaneously and are often found in paired mixtures. A child with refractory symptoms can often benefit from application of multiple classes of therapy. It is useful to carefully review with the parents what medicines have been tried and if they were effective, as this can guide the physician during treatment modification.

Histamine is the central mediator for the inflammatory pathways of AR. There are many histamine receptors distributed throughout the body including the respiratory tract, the gastrointestinal tract, and brain. The binding of histamine to its receptor will cause vascular and nerve ending changes in the lining of the nose leading to the symptoms of AR. Antihistamines bind to the histamine receptors and block many of the physiological responses to histamine. Table 3 lists the commonly used antihistamines, the FDA-approved age limits, and doses. Antihistamines can be delivered orally or topically.

The antihistamines can be categorized into two forms designated as 1st and 2nd generation drugs. The major feature distinguishing the two groups is the lipophilic nature of the compounds. The 1st generation drugs are more lipophilic rendering them more likely to cross the blood–brain barrier and result in CNS symptoms like sedation. They have a shorter half-life of 6–12 h and are usually used twice per day. The selectivity of 1st generation drugs is less stringent leading to more side effects. For these reasons, 1st generation drugs are usually used as acute short-term therapy such as over-the-counter medications.

The 2nd generation antihistamines are considered first-line therapy for children with AR. Their advantage comes from a longer half-life and decreased side effects. Because the 2nd generation drugs are more selective, they are less likely to bind to antiserotinergic, anticholinergic, and alpha-adrenergic receptors. Five 2nd generation medications are currently available in the USA. All five medications have been shown to be effective in children as long-term therapy. Desloratadine, Loratadine, and Fexofenadine are nonsedating at the recommended doses. Desloratadine and Loratadine can be sedating at higher than recommended doses. Azelastine and Cetirizine have mild risk of sedation at their recommended doses. Azelastine is available in an intranasal and intraocular form.

Table 3 Antihistamines

Name/generation	Age: Dose	Route	Sedation
Chlorpheniemine/1st	2–6 years: 1 mg q 6 h 6–12 years: 2 mg q 6 h >12 years: adult dose	Oral	Yes
Diphenhydramine/1st	3–12 years: 5 mg/kg/day divided tid /qid >12 years: adult dose	Oral	Yes
Hydroxyzine/1st	<6 years: 25 mg divided tid/qid 6–12 years: 50 mg divided tid/qid >12 years: adult dose	Oral	Yes
Fexofenadine/2nd	6–12 years: 30 mg bid >12 years: adult dose	Oral	No
Loradtadine/2nd	2–5 years: 5 mg q daily >5 years: adult dose	Oral	No
Desloratadine/2nd	>12 years: adult dose	Oral	No
Cetirizine/2nd	6–12 months: 2.5 mg q daily 12–24 months: 2.5 mg q bid 2–5 years: 2.5–5 mg q bid >6 years: 5–10 mg q daily	Oral	Some
Azelastine/2nd	>3 years: 1 drop each eye bid >12 years: adult dose	Opthalmic	Some
Azelastine/2nd	5–11 years: 1 puff each nostril daily >12 years: adult dose	Nasal	Some

The 2nd generation antihistamines work well for most of the symptoms of AR except for nasal congestion. Most of the 2nd generation antihistamines are available in combination with the decongestant pseudoephederine to improve control of nasal congestion. All antihistamines will work best if taken before antigen exposure; however, they have also been shown to work in an acute setting *(5)*.

Intranasal corticosteroids are also considered a first-line therapy for children with AR. Intranasal steroids improve symptoms of AR including sneezing, rhinorrhea, itching, and congestion. Table 4 lists the common intranasal steroids currently available in the USA for AR treatment. Multiple studies have compared the different nasal steroids and have found them very similar in efficacy for AR symptoms. The onset of action for intranasal steroids is longer than that for antihistamines since the primary molecular pathway for their action is through intranuclear control of gene expression. The onset of action is 8–12 h depending on the compound and symptom measured. The optimal response to intranasal steroid is at 4–7 days. Topical steroids have been shown to be equal or superior to antihistamines with or without decongestants for the treatment of AR in multiple studies and for long-term use *(4, 5)*. The most common side effects are nasal burning, sneezing, smell and taste disturbance, and epistaxsis. These are usually mild and resolve when treatment is stopped. Nasal perforation and increase in intraocular pressure are rare.

One concern with pediatric use of intranasal steroid is the possibility of growth delay. Controlled clinical studies have shown that use of intranasal steroids (beclomethsone) can affect growth velocity *(6)*. Other studies with newer intranasal agents have not demonstrated an effect on growth. Currently, the FDA has labeled intranasal steroids with a warning that they may cause growth suppression. It is recommended that if long-term intranasal steroid is to be used one should consider use of a steroid with lower bioavailability, and the child's growth should be monitored at regular intervals.

Leukotrienes are potent inflammatory agents that when blocked decrease the symptoms of AR. Leukotrienes are released by inflammatory cells during allergic reactions. Increased levels of leukotrienes have been isolated from nasal secretions in patients with AR. Antileukotriene agents block enzymatic synthesis or their receptors thereby inhibiting the inflammatory response. The leukotriene receptor antagonist Montelukast has been shown to be effective and safe for the treatment of AR in children. Like the antihistamines, the leukotrienes improve many symptoms including ocular symptoms and have an additional positive effect on nasal congestion. The leukotriene agents have similar effectiveness to antihistamines but are less effective than intranasal steroids *(7)*.

Table 4 Intranasal steroids

Steroid name	Age: Dose	Dose per spray	Onset	Bioavailability
Beclomethasone/Becanase	>6 years: 168–336 μg/day bid	42 μg	3 days	17%
Budesonide/Rhinocort	6–11 years: 64–128 μg/day >12 years: 64–256 μg/day	32 μg	24 h	11%
Mometasone/Nasonex	3–11 years: 100 μg/day >12 years: 200 μg/day	50 μg	12–24 h	<0.1%
Triamcinolone acetonide/Nasocort	6–11 years: 220 μg/day >12 years: 220–440/day	55 μg	24 h	22%
Flunisolide/Nasarel	6–14 years: 25–200 μg/day bid >14 years: 200–400 μg/day bid	25 μg	4–7 days	20–50%
Fluticasone propionate/Flonase	>4–11 years: 100–200 μg/day bid >12 years: 200–300 μg/day bid	50 μg	12–24 h	<2%
Fluticasone furoate/Veramyst	2–11 years: 55 μg/day 12 years: 110 μg/day	27.5 μg	24 h	<0.5%

Decongestants come in oral and topical forms. They primarily act on the α-adrenergic receptors in the nasal mucosa and vasculature. Because the decongestants are not anti-inflammatory, they work best in combination with other medicines such as antihistamines. The topical form has a rapid onset of action and can be helpful in the treatment of acute congestion. However, prolonged use can lead to rebound nasal congestion. Oral agents can cause CNS stimulation with resulting insomnia and hyperactivity in as many as one third of children *(8)*.

Mast cell stabilizers are another drug class that can be effective in the treatment of AR. These drugs cause a stabilization of the mast cell membrane thereby blocking the degranulation of the cells and the release of inflammatory mediators. Because these drugs do not have other anti-inflammatory properties, to be most effective, they are best given as prophylactics 1–2 weeks prior to antigen exposure. The topical agent cromolyn sodium is available in an over-the-counter form and has a very safe profile for children. Cromolyn sodium preforms at a lower level when compared to antihistamine or intranasal steroids and has a short duration of action requiring a dosage of 4–6 times per day *(6)*.

Omalizumab is a recombinant monoclonal anti-IgE antibody that can be effective for both asthma and AR. Its mechanism of action is blocking IgE interaction with mast cells and basophils, as well as lowering of serum IgE levels. Initial studies have shown an improvement in nasal symptoms and decrease in antihistamine use with Omalizumab *(9)*. The FDA currently limits the labeling of this medication for use in children with moderate to severe asthma. Future studies are needed to evaluate the safety and cost effectiveness of this drug.

Immunotherapy

If the child with AR does not respond or tolerate environmental and pharmacological therapies, then immunotherapy should be considered. Research in animals and humans has begun to uncover the mechanisms by which immunotherapy (injection therapy) works. Regular exposure to antigens by injections causes an antigen-specific selection of T-lymphocytes which down regulate production of IgE-producing B-cells. Multiple studies have demonstrated the improvement of symptoms and quality of life as well as a decrease in medication reliance in AR patients treated with immunotherapy *(10)*. In addition, it has been shown that specific immunotherapy can support long-term prevention of asthma in children with AR *(11)*. The potential benefits of immunotherapy have to be weighed against the risk of anaphylaxis and the pain and inconvenience of weekly shots. Immunotherapy, if successful, is usually given for 3–5 years.

There has been a growing interest in sublingual delivery of antigen as a method for the treatment of AR. Sublingual therapy has the benefits of being less invasive with decreased risk of anaphylaxis, therefore allowing for self administration. The practice of sublingual therapy in the USA has been limited. However, a recent European meta-analysis of 577 patients concluded that sublingual therapy can be effective in children with AR *(12)*. Further studies will be required to confirm the role of sublingual therapy as well as the dosing concentrations and schedules for treatment of AR.

References

1. Bousquet J, et al. Allergic rhinitis and its impact on asthma (ARIA). In Collaboration with the World Health Organization. Allergy 2006; 61: 814–855.
2. Beiger RS. Allergic and nonallergic rhinitis: classification and pathogenesis Part. II. Non-allergic rhinitis. Am J Rhinology 1989; 3: 113–139.
3. Guarner F, et al. Mechanisms of disease: the hygiene hypothesis revisited. Nat Clin Pract Gastroenterol Hepatol 2006; 3: 275–284.
4. Meltzer EO. Allergic rhinitis: managing the pediatric spectrum. Allergy Asthma Proc 2006; 27: 2–8.
5. Dykewicz MS, et al. Diagnosis and management of rhinitis: complete guidelines of the Joint Task Force of Practice Parameters in Allergy, Asthma, and Immunology. Ann Allergy Asthma Immmunol 1998; 81: 478–518.
6. Skoner DP, et al. Detection of growth suppression in children during treatment with intranasal beclomethasone diproionate. Pediatrics 2000; 105(2): E23.
7. Nathan RA. Pharmacotherapy to allergic rhinitis: a critical review of luekotriene receptor antagonists compared with other treatments. Ann Allergy Asthma Immunol 2003; 90: 182–190.
8. Lai L, et al. Pediatric allergic rhinits. Immunol Allergy Clin North Am 2005; 25: 283–299.
9. Casale TB, et al. Omalizumab Seasonal Allergic Rhinitis Trial Group. Effect of omalizumab on symptoms of seasonal allergic rhinitis: a randomized controlled trial. JAMA 2001; 286: 2956–2967.
10. Marple BF, et al. Keys to successful management of patients with allergic rhinitis: focus on patient confidence, compliance, and satisfaction. Otolarygol Head Neck Surg 2007; 136: s107–s124.
11. Niggemann B, et al. Five-year follow-up on the PAT study: specific immunotherapy and long-term prevention of asthma in chidren. Allergy 2006; 61: 855–859.
12. Penagos M, et al. Clinical efficacy of sublingual immunotherapy in the treatment of allergic rhinitis in pediatric patients 3 to 18 years of age: a meta-analysis of randomized, placebo controlled, double-blind trials. Ann Allergy Asthma Immunol 2006; 97: 141–148.

Acute and Chronic Rhinosinusitis

Zoukaa Sargi and Ramzi Younis

Key Points

- Rhinosinusitis is a commonly encountered condition in children. Children average six to eight upper respiratory infections per year, of which 5–10% are complicated by acute rhinosinusitis.
- *Acute rhinosinusitis* (ARS) is a bacterial infection of the sinonasal mucosa lasting up to 4 weeks (28 days). *Chronic rhinosinusitis* (CRS) is a larger spectrum of pathologies, affecting the paranasal sinuses for more than 12 weeks.
- The most common organisms in rhinosinusitis are *Streptococcus pneumoniae, Haemophilus influenzae*, and *Moraxella catarrhalis.*
- Rhinosinusitis is a condition that is managed in most cases by medical treatment. Surgical therapy is required for orbital or intracranial complications of ARS or for children with CRS who remain symptomatic despite maximal medical treatment and optimal control of associated comorbidities.

Keywords: Pediatric sinusitis • Acute rhinosinusitis, Chronic rhinosinusitis • Nasal allergy • Functional endoscopic sinus surgery • Antibiotics • Nasal steroids • Adenoidectomy

Z. Sargi and R. Younis (✉)
Department of Otolaryngology, University of Miami Miller School of Medicine/Sylvester Comprehensive Cancer Center, Miami, FL, USA
e-mail: ryounis@med.miami.edu

Acute and Chronic Rhinosinusitis

Rhinosinusitis is a commonly encountered condition in children. Its true incidence is difficult to measure since upper respiratory infections (URIs) are very common in children and are frequently misdiagnosed as rhinosinusitis. Children average six to eight URIs per year, of which 5–10% are complicated by acute rhinosinusitis *(1)*.

Additionally, respiratory allergy is very prevalent in the pediatric population and plays an important role in the development of rhinosinusitis. The symptoms of respiratory allergy and rhinosinusitis are similar and at times difficult to distinguish from each other.

The ability to diagnose rhinosinusitis and identify and treat associated comorbidities is of great importance for the clinician. In doing so, unnecessary antibiotics are avoided, and rhinosinusitis is treated early enough to prevent potentially life-threatening complications.

Definition and Classification

The most comprehensive review of the definition of rhinosinusitis was reported by a consensus conference convened by five national societies *(2)*. The committee decided to accept the term "rhinosinusitis" because "sinusitis" is almost always accompanied by concurrent nasal airway inflammation, and in many cases, sinusitis is preceded by rhinitis. The adopted definition had been previously developed by the Sinus and Allergy Health Partnership Taskforce and defines rhinosinusitis as a group of disorders characterized by inflammation of the mucosa of the nose and the paranasal sinuses *(3)*.

R.B. Mitchell and K.D. Pereira (eds.), *Pediatric Otolaryngology for the Clinician,*
DOI: 10.1007/978-1-60327-127-1_16, © Humana Press, a part of Springer Science + Business Media, LLC 2009

Rhinosinusitis is typically divided into three types: acute, subacute, and chronic, based on the duration of the symptoms. Two other conditions, recurrent acute rhinosinusitis and acute exacerbations of chronic rhinosinusitis, are important to consider, since their presence could mean a slightly different treatment.

Acute rhinosinusitis (ARS) is a presumed bacterial infection of the sinonasal mucosa lasting up to 4 weeks (28 days). It is typically believed to be induced by viruses and does not require antibiotics during the first 10–14 days. When infection persists after 14 days, bacteria are suspected and antibiotics are then administered *(2)*.

In early childhood, the only significantly pneumatized sinuses are the maxillary and ethmoid sinuses. Pneumatization of the sphenoid and frontal sinuses occurs around years 6–7, and is completed in early adulthood. One form of ARS, *acute ethmoiditis*, is much more common in the pediatric population and has serious potential orbital and intracranial complications if not recognized at an early stage *(4)*.

Subacute rhinosinusitis is rarely encountered, and lasts for 4–12 weeks. It is commonly the result of a long-lasting ARS in a child with untreated respiratory allergies or a previously undiagnosed chronic rhinosinusitis.

Chronic rhinosinusitis (CRS) is a larger spectrum of pathologies, affecting the paranasal sinuses for more than 12 weeks. It is further divided into CRS without polyps and CRS with polyps, depending on the preoperative fiberoptic exam or on the intraoperative findings. In these cases, many underlying factors can contribute to the sinus disease. Identifying and treating these factors is thus a very important element in the management of CRS.

Pathophysiology

The most significant factor in the pathophysiology of rhinosinusitis is *impaired drainage* of the sinuses through the ostia. A sinus ostium is a small opening that allows the sinus cavity to communicate directly or indirectly with the nasal airway. It allows for a natural drainage pathway for the secreted mucous provided the ciliary function of the epithelium and the characteristics of the secretions are within normal limits. Mucosal swelling blocks the ostium, causing pooling of secretions in the sinus cavity and creates an optimal environment for bacterial growth. Subsequently, inflammatory mediators as well as anaerobic changes within the sinus can perpetuate the mucosal disease, leading to chronic conditions.

URIs are the most common predisposing factor for ARS in children. Viral-induced inflammation and edema lead to obstruction of the ostia and stasis of secretions. Additionally, viral infection can also impair the ciliary function. Since symptoms of cold overlap those of rhinosinusitis, the duration of symptoms plays a very important role in the diagnosis of ARS. It is agreed that if cold symptoms (secondary to a viral infection) are not improving by 7–10 days, a sinus bacterial infection (ARS) should seriously be considered *(5)*. The *bacteriology* of ARS is very similar to that of otitis media, with the most common organisms being *Streptococcus pneumoniae, Haemophilus influenzae*, and *Moraxella catarrhalis*.

Rhinosinusitis, like acute otitis media, is more frequently encountered in children who attend *day care* when compared to children in home care *(6)*. This difference seems to be related to the higher number of URIs per year, and is more significant for children younger than 3 years of age *(7)*.

The pathophysiology of CRS is more complex and involves several predisposing factors. One of the most important factors in the development of CRS is *allergic rhinitis* (seasonal or perennial). More than 80% of children with rhinosinusitis have a positive family history of allergy *(8)*. On the other hand, the association of asthma and CRS is well documented, and acute exacerbations of CRS have been linked to asthma exacerbations. Furthermore, treatment of rhinosinusitis significantly improves symptoms and decreases the need for treatment of asthma attacks *(9)*.

Adenoid hypertrophy can cause nasal obstruction and can represent a bacterial reservoir for infections of the sinuses and middle ear. Both factors contribute to the development of rhinosinusitis, and adenoidectomy has been shown to have a beneficial impact in the treatment of CRS in the pediatric population.

Gastroesophageal reflux (Gastronasal reflux) has been shown to play a causative role in rhinosinusitis. Studies suggest that treatment of reflux improves symptoms of CRS and reduces the need for surgery in children *(10)*.

Environmental factors, particularly *passive cigarette smoke exposure,* may cause local irritation and inflammation, affecting the ciliary function and mucociliary clearance. These become even more important when other predisposing conditions such as allergic rhinitis are present *(11)*.

Other less common conditions can also interfere with the normal physiology of the sinuses. *Mechanical obstruction* can be encountered with anatomic abnormalities or variants (septal deviation, choanal atresia, paradoxical middle turbinate) and with nasal foreign bodies. *Impaired mucous clearance* is responsible for CRS in diseases like cystic fibrosis and ciliary dyskinesias. *Immune deficiencies* such as IgA deficiency or IgG subclass deficiency can predispose children to more acute exacerbations of CRS and must be considered when infections recur soon after interruption of adequate antibiotic treatments *(11)*.

Clinical Presentation and Diagnosis

As previously mentioned, acute and chronic rhinosinusitis may mimic other conditions and can easily be misdiagnosed in the pediatric population. *ARS* presents as a URI lasting for more than 10 days or as worsening symptoms after initial improvement. The most common symptoms are rhinorrhea and daytime cough. Occasionally, high-grade fever, purulent nasal discharge, facial pain, or periorbital edema can be encountered. When compared to adults with ARS, children are generally less able to communicate the presence and severity of symptoms. Also, headache is not a common complaint of ARS in children *(12)*.

CRS presents with symptoms that last more than 12 weeks and include a nasal discharge and cough in younger children and nasal congestion and headache in older children *(13)*. These symptoms are very similar to and overlap with those of adenoid hypertrophy. Thus, it is often impossible, based solely on clinical symptoms, to distinguish between these two related conditions.

The *physical examination* is very important and adds significant information to the history. Rhinoscopy is the most helpful part, whether performed with an otoscope or a flexible fiberoptic telescope. It can visualize purulent secretions emanating from the middle meatus, which is highly suggestive of an ARS when symptoms are acute. When a CRS is suspected, the nasal cavity exam is mandatory to rule out or confirm the presence of polyps in the middle meatus. Adenotonsillar hypertrophy should be noted on nasopharyngeal and oropharyngeal exams. Inner canthal areas must be inspected in an effort to rule out an early periorbital cellulitis that may complicate ARS. Otoscopy should always be performed since middle ear disease is frequently encountered in children with acute or chronic rhinosinusitis.

Microbiological and radiological exams are rarely needed for the diagnosis of ARS, whereas computed tomography (CT) scan is essential for the diagnosis of CRS. *Sinus aspiration* for culture is not performed routinely but is reserved for immunocompromised children with severe presentation, complications, or after failure of appropriate medical treatment. *Plain radiographs* of the sinuses (Waters' view) may be adequate for confirming the diagnosis of ARS *(14)*. An air fluid level within the sinus cavity or a unilateral complete opacification in a child with acute symptoms and signs is highly suggestive of ARS. Lateral neck films can be useful in assessing adenoid hypertrophy causing nasal obstruction. A *CT scan* should be performed in ARS when orbital or intracranial complications are suspected. Additionally, a CT scan is essential for the diagnosis of CRS, showing opacification or mucosal thickening in the sinuses and/or middle meatus. In the absence of any sinus mucosal disease on CT scan, CRS is very unlikely and other etiologies must be considered. A CT scan (coronal and axial images in bone and soft tissue windows) is mandatory before sinus surgery, to assess the extent of disease and to show the anatomical landmarks *(12)*. *Magnetic resonance imaging* (MRI) is the best indicator when a neoplasm is suspected, as it helps distinguish between tumor and secretion retention within the sinus cavity. It is also valuable for the diagnosis of intracranial complications. In CRS, however, it can over estimate minimal mucosal disease and thus give false positive results. Other tests are helpful to look for contributing factors and include allergy testing, double-probe pH monitoring to look for gastronasal reflux, and immunoglobulin titers when immune deficiencies are considered.

Management

Rhinosinusitis is a condition that is managed in most cases by medical treatment. Surgical therapy is required for orbital or intracranial complications of ARS or for children with CRS who remain symptomatic despite maximal medical treatment and optimal control of associated comorbidities.

Antimicrobials are the cornerstone of therapy for ARS. Many cases of acute bacterial rhinosinusitis can, however, spontaneously resolve. Nonetheless, the evidence supports the use of antibiotics to increase rates of clinical cure in ARS in children ***(15)***. Conversely, the use of antibiotics in viral infections results in an increase of resistant strains among causative germs.

Numerous *antibiotics* are available for the treatment of ARS ***(16)***. The appropriate choice is dictated by the microbiology as well as the local resistance pattern of the bacteria to different antibiotics ***(17)***. High-dose amoxicillin (45–80 mg/kg/day) with or without clavulanate and second-generation cephalosporins are usually a good empirical treatment for ARS. Macrolides and clindamycin are available alternatives for children allergic to beta-lactams. In the case of a moderate to severe ARS, or when a *Streptococcus Pneumoniae* with reduced susceptibility to penicillin is considered, high-dose amoxicillin (80–90 mg/kg/day) should be used.

Other adjunctive therapies, which lack significant evidence in the treatment of ARS, may be administered in association with antibiotics. These include nasal irrigation, decongestants, antihistamines, and mucolytics. In recurrent ARS, it is also very important to look for underlying causes and manage them effectively (daycare, reflux, allergy, secondhand smoking).

Although an infectious etiology may not always be the causative factor in CRS, the initial treatment of CRS must also include an antibiotic regimen. The same pathogens encountered in ARS (*Streptococcus pneumoniae, Haemophilus influenzae*, and *Moraxella catarrhalis*) are also the most frequent species isolated in CRS. However, with CRS, there is a higher prevalence of anaerobes and *Staphylococcus aureus*. High-dose amoxicillin–clavulanate (80–90 mg/kg/day) and second-generation cephalosporins are good regimens to start with. In the adult population, respiratory fluoroquinolones are also considered as first-choice antibiotics for the treatment of CRS; however, these molecules are generally not approved for use in children.

Another important part in the management of CRS is the long-term treatment of allergy. For this, *nasal steroids* have been shown to improve symptoms and aid in the regression of radiographic abnormalities when given in association with antibiotics ***(18)***. A trial of topical nasal steroids is usually recommended prior to surgical intervention. Concerns related to potential growth suppression in children have been dismissed with the newer generation steroid sprays ***(19)***.

In addition to antibiotics and nasal steroids, *management of risk factors* is very important in CRS since this condition is often multifactorial.

Surgical therapy is reserved for cases where maximal medical treatment has failed. It is aimed to help restore the drainage of the sinuses. *Functional endoscopic sinus surgery* is the gold standard surgery for CRS. However, in children, other factors must be considered. Of these, the role of the adenoids in the pathophysiology of CRS, as mentioned earlier, makes an *adenoidectomy* an important first step in the surgical management of CRS. For children younger than 6 years with mild CT scan changes and without asthma, adenoidectomy is considered the first-line surgical therapy ***(12)***.

Indications for pediatric endoscopic sinus surgery have been defined by an international consensus meeting ***(20)***. The committee decided that only CRS with frequent exacerbations that are nonresponsive to optimal medical treatment should be considered for surgery. This should be done after the exclusion of a noninfectious condition or systemic disease.

Conclusion

Pediatric rhinosinusitis, whether acute or chronic, is a challenging disease, in its diagnosis as well as in its management. It is closely related to two other common problems in children: upper respiratory tract infections and respiratory allergies. Combining information from the clinical history, nasal endoscopy, and CT scans will help define and classify the disease. Bacterial pathogens encountered are comparable to otitis media, the most common organisms being *Streptococcus pneumoniae, Haemophilus influenzae*, and *Moraxella catarrhalis*. Microbiology and radiology investigations are rarely needed to diagnose ARS, but are helpful when complications are suspected. A CT scan is very important for the diagnosis of CRS. Multiple risk factors need to be considered and managed in a child with recurrent ARS or CRS. The treatment remains medical in most cases, with antibiotics and nasal steroids being the preferred method of choice. Controlling the known risk factors is another very important therapeutic goal. Surgery is reserved for carefully selected cases of recurrent ARS or CRS resistant to optimal medical treatment.

References

1. Lieser JD, Derkay CS. Pediatric sinusitis: when do we operate. Curr Opin Otolaryngol Head Neck Surg. 2005; 13(1):60–6.
2. Meltzer EO, Hamilos DL, Hadley JA, et al. Rhinosinusitis: establishing definitions for clinical research and patient care. J Allergy Clin Immunol. 2004;114(6 Suppl):155–212.
3. Benninger MS, Ferguson BJ, Hadley JA, et al. Adult chronic rhinosinusitis: definitions, diagnosis, epidemiology, and pathophysiology. Otolaryngol Head Neck Surg. 2003;129(3 Suppl):S1–32.
4. Francois M, Mariani-Kurkdjian P, Dupont E, et al. Acute ethmoiditis in children, a series of 125 cases. Arch Pediatr. 2006;13(1):6–10.
5. Ramadan HH. Pediatric sinusitis: update. J Otolaryngol. 2005;34(1 Suppl):S14–17.
6. Goldsmith AJ, Rosenfeld RM. Treatment of pediatric sinusitis. Pediatr Clin North Am. 2003;50(2):413–26.
7. Wald ER, Guerra N, Byers C. Frequency and severity of infections in day care: three-year follow-up. J Pediatr. 1991;118(4):509–14.
8. Shapiro GG, Rachelefsky GS. Introduction and definition of sinusitis. J Allergy Clin Immunol. 1992;90(3 Pt 2):417–18.
9. Smart BA, Slavin RG. Rhinosinusitis and pediatric asthma. Immunol Allergy Clin North Am. 2005;25(1):67–82.
10. Bothwell MR, Parsons DS, Talbot A, Barbero GJ, Wilder B. Outcome of reflux therapy on pediatric chronic sinusitis. Otolaryngol Head Neck Surg. 1999;121(3):255–62.
11. Hertler MA, Mitchell RB, Lazar RH. Pathophysiology and etiology of pediatric rhinosinusitis. In: Pediatric Sinusitis and Sinus Surgery. Taylor & Francis, New York 2006.
12. Younis RT. Pediatric endoscopic sinus surgery. In: Pediatric Sinusitis and Sinus Surgery. Taylor & Francis, New York 2006.
13. Lund VJ, Neijens HJ, Clement PA, Lusk R, Stammberger H. The treatment of chronic sinusitis: a controversial issue. Int J Pediatr Otorhinolaryngol. 1995; 32 Suppl:S21–35.
14. Ros SP, Herman BE, Azar-Kia B. Acute sinusitis in children: is the Water's view sufficient. Pediatr Radiol. 1995;25(4):306–7.
15. Morris P, Leach A. Antibiotics for persistent nasal discharge (rhinosinusitis) in children. Cochrane Lib 2003;1:1–26.
16. Benninger MS, Sedory Holzer SE, Lau J. Diagnosis and treatment of uncomplicated acute bacterial rhinosinusitis: summary of the Agency for Health Care Policy and Research evidence-based report. Otolaryngol Head Neck Surg. 2000;122(1):1–7.
17. Felmingham D, White AR, Jacobs MR, Appelbaum PC, Poupard J, Miller LA, Gruneberg RN. The Alexander project: the benefits from a decade of surveillance. J Antimicrob Chemother. 2005;56(2 Suppl):ii3-ii21.
18. Benninger MS, Anon J, Mabry RL. The medical management of rhinosinusitis. Otolaryngol Head Neck Surg. 1997;117(3 Pt 2):S41–9.
19. Benninger MS, Ahmad N, Marple BF. The safety of intranasal steroids. Otolaryngol Head Neck Surg. 2003;129(6): 739–50.
20. Clement PA. Pediatric endoscopic sinus surgery—does it have a future. Int J Pediatr Otorhinolaryngol. 2003;67 (1 Suppl):S209–11.

The Head and Neck

Congenital Head and Neck Masses

John P. Maddolozzo, Sandra Koterski, James W. Schroeder, Jr., and Hau Sin Wong

Key Points

- A thyroglossal duct cyst is the most common congenital neck mass. Its evaluation and diagnosis can be performed with ultrasonongraphy that is noninvasive and cost-effective. A Sistrunk procedure is the recommended surgical resection.
- Branchial cleft anomalies result from abnormal development of the branchial apparatus, forming sinuses, fistulas, or cysts. Second branchial anomalies are the most common, occurring along a tract that extends deep to the second arch structures. The treatment for all branchial anomalies is surgical excision.
- Dermoids and teratomas are composed of one to three germ layer components. Surgical excision is the treatment of choice but needs to be tempered by the relation of the tumor to critical structures.
- Lymphatic malformations have varying histologic and anatomic features that assist in predicting the likely response of these neck masses to various treatment modalities. Single cysts and macrocystic lymphangiomas are most amenable to sclerotherapy, but are also easily treated with surgical resection. Microcystic and cavernous lymphangiomas are less successfully treated with sclerotherapy and/or surgical resection and may need multiple resections.
- Thymic anomalies result from thymic rest cells that are deposited in the neck during development. Thymic cysts are the most common thymic anomalies and often mimic second branchial cleft cysts. Surgical excision is the preferred treatment.
- Fibromatosis coli, which presents in the first few weeks of life, results from edema and fibrosis of the sternocleidomastoid muscle. Spontaneous resolution within the first year of life is the rule, but physical therapy should be initiated if neck rotation is limited.

Keywords: Thyroglossal duct cyst • Branchial anomalies • Lymphatic malformation • Teratoma • Dermoid • Thymic cyst • Fibromatosis coli

Introduction

Head and neck masses are commonly seen in children and require a thorough evaluation *(1, 2)*. The most common cause of head and neck masses in children is lymphadenopathy secondary to infections of the ear, nose, and throat. The second most common head and neck masses in children are congenital lesions *(3, 4)*. Congenital neck masses are more prevalent in children than malignant lesions, although concern about the latter may be the main reason for consultation. Congenital neck masses occur in the following order of frequency: thyroglossal duct cysts, branchial anomalies, teratomas, vascular malformations, and lymphatic malformations. Each of these congenital anomalies has varying histories and presentations. The evaluation and management of these congenital masses will be discussed in further detail in this chapter. Vascular malformations will be discussed in a separate chapter.

J.P. Maddolozzo (✉), S. Koterski, and J.W. Schroeder, Jr.
Division of Pediatric Otolaryngology, Department of Otolaryngology – Head and Neck Surgery, Children's Memorial Hospital of Chicago, Northwestern University Feinberg School of Medicine, Chicago, IL, USA
e-mail: jpmaddolozzo@childrensmemorial.org

H.S. Wong
Children's Hospital of Orange County, University of California – Irvine Medical Center, Orange, CA, USA

R.B. Mitchell and K.D. Pereira (eds.), *Pediatric Otolaryngology for the Clinician*,
DOI: 10.1007/978-1-60327-127-1_17, © Humana Press, a part of Springer Science + Business Media, LLC 2009

Thyroglossal Duct Cyst

Thyroglossal duct cysts (TDCs) are the most common congenital lesions in the neck and are second to cervical adenopathy in the prevalence of pediatric neck masses *(3)*. A TDC results from an aberrant embryology of the thyroid gland. The thyroid gland begins as an anlage of tissue located at the foramen cecum near the base of the tongue. At 3 weeks of gestation, the thyroid anlage descends antero-inferiorly, or through the hyoid bone, to eventually lie just at or below the cricoid cartilage. By weeks 5–8 of gestation, the thyroglossal duct obliterates, leaving the foramen cecum at the base of tongue proximally and the pyramidal lobe of the thyroid gland distally. If the duct fails to obliterate, a cysts persists and is at risk of becoming infected.

The majority of TDCs are detected in the first two decades of life, but they can present at any age. TDCs appear as a midline cervical mass that either lies directly above the hyoid bone or just below it. Their location, however, may vary; approximately one third may present as submental or low cervical masses. Less than 1% of TDCs do not present in the midline of the neck. On physical examination, TDCs appear as smooth, round, firm masses that are approximately 2 cm in diameter (Fig. 1). They may move upward during swallowing or tongue protrusion as a result of their intimate relationship with the hyoid. There is no sex predilection.

The diagnosis is made following a detailed history and physical examination complimented by radiologic studies. Ultrasonography can identify the cyst and confirm the presence of normal thyroid tissue *(5, 6)*. In rare instances, a TDC can represent the patient's only thyroid tissue and thus removal would require the child to be on a lifetime of hormonal supplements. Additional evaluation with thyroid function tests and a radionucleotide thyroid scan can assist in determining the activity of ectopic thyroid tissue.

Knowledge of the thyroid gland's embryology is critical to the treatment of a TDC. Due to its intimate relationship with the hyoid and base of tongue, surgical resection requires complete excision of the cyst with a central portion of the hyoid bone and a cuff of glossal tissue (Fig. 2). This technique was described by Sistrunk *(7)* and has resulted in lower recurrence rates as compared to a simple excision of the cyst alone.

Timely surgical excision is the mainstay of treatment for TDCs as they are prone to infection and ulceration. Once infected, a large incision and drainage is not recommended due to the increased risk of recurrence following a later complete excision of the cyst. Instead, antibiotic therapy with the needle aspiration to

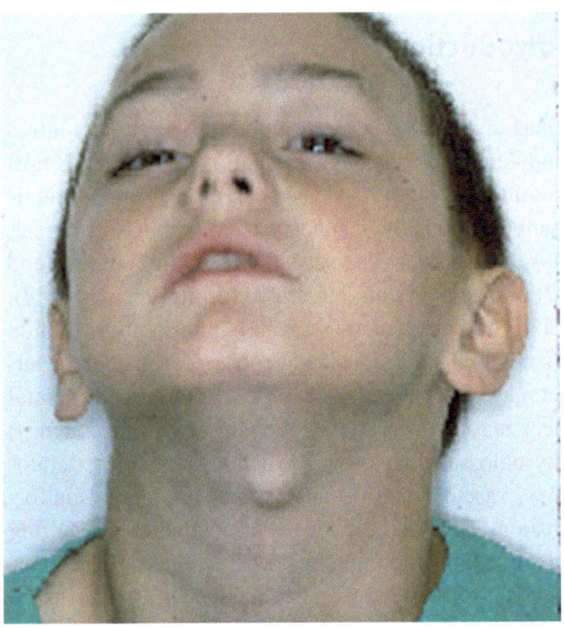

Fig. 1 Typical clinical appearance of a thyroglossal duct cyst

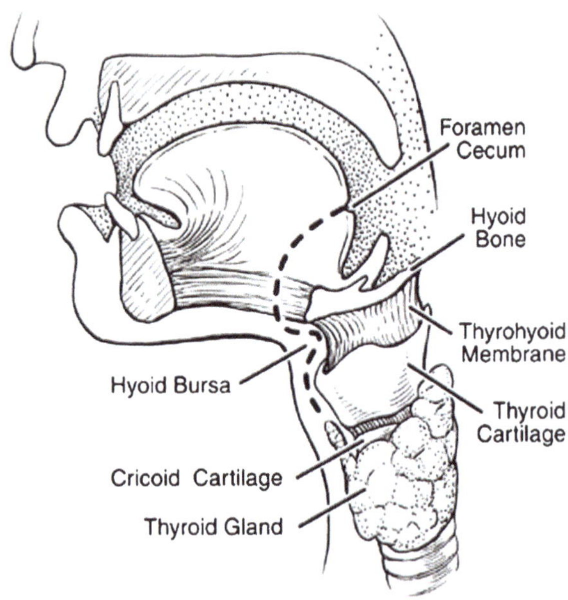

Fig. 2 Course of the thyroglossal duct. Thyroglossalduct cysts can occur anywhere along this pathway

decompress the cyst is advised. In addition, there exists a potential for a TDC to undergo malignant degeneration to form a papillary carcinoma.

Branchial Cleft Anomalies

The branchial apparatus consists of four paired arches, each composed of ectoderm, mesoderm, and endoderm, which develop during weeks 3–7 of fetal life *(8, 9)*. Proper development generates important structures of the head and neck, further described in Table 1. Abnormal development of the branchial apparatus results in branchial cysts, sinuses, and fistulas.

During normal development, ectoderm-lined clefts separate the arches externally. The mesoderm of each arch contains its own unique artery, vein, and skeletal structures. Internally, the arch contains a pouch composed of endoderm. Branchial apparatus abnormalities are thought to arise from the vestiges of branchial clefts, pouches, or both. Logically then a cleft sinus would communicate with the skin, while a pouch sinus would communicate through pharyngeal mucosa. Fistulas, which connect gut to skin, are thought to result from remnants of both clefts and pouches with no interposed mesoderm plate. Cysts are considered to be entrapped remnants of clefts or pouches and usually present as soft, fluctuant neck masses. On examination, sinuses and fistulae are usually evident with associated mucoid secretions. Frequently these abnormalities present with a complicating infection and sometimes with associated abscess formation. It is important to evaluate for possible communication with the aerodigestive tract in such cases. Branchial abnormalities usually present in childhood, but may be seen at any age. No gender predilection has been noted.

Branchial abnormalities are classified by their arch of origin in the branchial apparatus.

First branchial anomalies are duplications of the external auditory canal *(9, 10)*. Work further classified these abnormalities into Type I and Type II. Type I deformities are strictly ectodermal in origin and are usually postauricular. Type II lesions, which are more common, contain ectoderm and mesoderm. They may be located anywhere above the hyoid bone and often have an intimate association with the facial nerve, which makes surgical removal challenging *(11)*.

Second branchial anomalies are the most common and frequently present as a complete fistula. The tract appears anterior to the sternocleidomastoid, passes deep to the second arch structures including the external carotid artery and posterior belly of the digastric. It then passes superficial to third arch structures, including the internal carotid artery and glossopharyngeal nerve, before ending in the tonsillar fossa. Second branchial sinuses follow the same course, but usually end blindly, while cysts are isolated entities that can be found anywhere along the anatomic path described.

Third branchial abnormalities are rare. The tract also starts anterior to the sternocleidomastoid, but then passes posteriorly to the common carotid artery and its bifurcation, as well as the glossopharyngeal nerve. However, the tract remains superficial to the hypoglossal nerve and then enters the digestive tract at the level of the pyriform sinus.

The existence of fourth branchial anomalies has never been conclusively proven. Only 60 cases of fourth branchial abnormalities have been reported, with the first description by Sanborn in 1972 *(12)*.

The treatment for all brachial anomalies is elective surgical excision. Abscess formation should first be treated with incision and drainage followed by a complete course of antibiotics before planning for removal. Excision of the entire tract of the anomaly, using the anatomy described earlier, is necessary for successful excision to prevent recurrence.

Table 1 Designates the branchial arch and its corresponding derivative

Arch	Nerve	Muscle	Skeletal structure	Artery
1	Trigeminal (V)	Muscles of mastication, mylohyoid, anterior digastric, tensor tympani, tensor veli palatini	Malleus, incus, portion of mandible	Maxillary
2	Facial (VII)	Muscles of facial expression, stapedius, stylohyoid, posterior digastric	Stapes, styloid, lesser cornu and upper body of hyoid	Stapedial
3	Glossopharyngeal (IX)	Stylopharyngeus	Greater cornu and lower body of hyoid	Common/internal carotid
4	Superior laryngeal	Pharyngeal constrictors, cricothyroid	Laryngeal cartilages	Right subclavian left aortic arch

Teratoma and Dermoid

Teratomas are a group of tumors that contain all three germ layers. They occur in 1:4000 births, with 1–3.5% affecting the head and neck. The nasopharynx is the most common site of presentation followed by the lateral neck. Three theories have been proposed for the origin of teratomas. The congenital inclusion theory proposes that incomplete closure of embryogenic fusion lines results in the capture of germ layers into ectopic areas. Acquired implantation suggests that skin or mucous membrane with its associated mesodermal components is traumatically implanted into deeper tissues. The third theory proposes that totipotential rest cells from two or three germ layers become isolated and begin independent growth in a disorganized manner.

Teratomas have been classified into four groups: (1) true teratomas, (2) teratoid tumors, (3) epignathi, and (4) dermoid cysts. True teratomas are composed of all three germ layers with differentiation to structures such as teeth and hair within them. Teratoid tumors also are composed of all three germ layers but are poorly differentiated. Epignathi are similar to true teratomas but display reduplicated fetal parts such as limbs. Finally, dermoid cysts, the most common teratomas of the head and neck, are comprised of only one to two germ cell layers.

Teratomas develop in the midline or lateral neck during the second trimester and can rapidly expand. If significant growth occurs before birth, it can cause esophageal and/or airway obstruction. Commonly, mothers present with polyhydramnios and further evaluation is performed with prenatal ultrasonography, CT, or MRI. If airway obstruction is suspected, a coordinated multispeciality approach for the delivery of the infant is necessary. An EXIT (ex utero intrapartum treatment) procedure is arranged to allow for the maintenance of uteroplacental circulation while establishing a safe airway (Fig. 3). A timely surgical excision is then the mainstay of treatment.

A dermoid cyst is the most common teratoma in the head and neck. Although pathologically related to teratomas, dermoid cysts do not contain all three germ cell layers. These cysts occur as a result of entrapment of epithelial components along embryonic fusion lines. Because nasal and orbital dermoids may have intracranial extensions, they should routinely be evaluated with a CT and/or MRI scan prior to excision. Cervical dermoids, conversely, present as painless superficial masses that move with the skin. They will gradually enlarge but rarely will become infected. Ultrasonography or CT assists in additional diagnostic evaluation. A complete surgical excision is necessary because incomplete resection or intraoperative rupture is associated with an increased rate of recurrence.

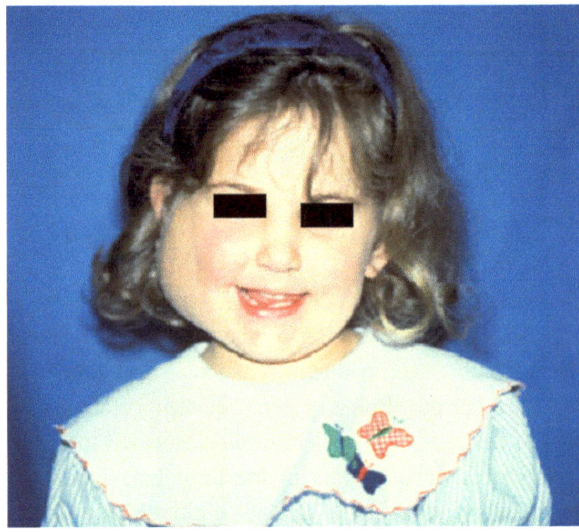

Fig. 3 A newborn with a massive teratoma in the cervicofacial region

Lymphatic Malformation

Lymphatic malformations are either congenital malformations of lymphatic tissues that fail to connect to the normal lymphatic system or growth of primordial lymph channels. They commonly present in the head and neck region, but can also occur throughout the body. Lymphatic malformations have classically been categorized based on the following histologic appearance: capillary lymphangiomas, cavernous lymphangiomas, and cystic hygromas. These histologic categories, however, do not correlate with clinical behavior or therapeutic response. In an attempt to obtain this correlation, Smith et al. *(13)* categorized lymphangiomas based on their response to sclerotherapy by dividing them into macrocystic, microcystic, and mixed. Macrocystic lymphangiomas respond well while microcystic lymphangiomas respond poorly to sclerotherapy. de Serres et al. *(14)* categorized lymphangiomas based on anatomic location into suprahyoid and infrahyoid lesions. This assists the clinician in predicting the prognosis and surgical outcome. Suprahyoid lesions have a poorer prognosis and require multiple surgical resections while infrahyoid lesions tend to be more responsive to single therapy. Most clinicians currently classify lymphangiomas based on the size of cysts and location of the lesion.

Lymphatic malformations can present at birth with the majority appearing by age 2. There is no sex, race, or ethnic predilection. Lymphatic malformations commonly present as painless, soft tissue masses that are slow growing. On physical examination they are fluctuant and can be transilluminated. They may rapidly enlarge with upper respiratory infections and regress with the resolution of the infection. Rarely do they spontaneously involute, but rather usually recur and enlarge. Due to the large size and/or infiltrative nature of lymphangiomas, they can cause an anatomic dysfunction with associated dsyphagia or respiratory compromise as well as a cosmetic problem. Lymphangiomas are best evaluated with either a computerized tomography (CT) or magnetic resonance imaging (MRI) scans that generally reveal a characteristic multiloculated cyst.

Surgical excision is the mainstay of therapy, but it needs to be appropriately timed in young children *(15, 16)*. Aspiration of the malformation can serve as a temporizing measure while waiting for definitive treatment. Preservation of normal structures is encouraged during the resection and multiple-staged procedures may be necessary to remove infiltrative masses while preserving vital structures (Fig. 4). More expeditious resection may be necessary when there is recurrent infection, obstruction of the aerodigestive tract, or significant cosmetic deformity.

Although surgical excision is the main treatment option, additional medical therapy is becoming available. The use of sclerotherapy to create an inflammatory response within the lymphangiomatic cyst and cause and involution of the cyst is currently being investigated *(17–19)*. The following agents are being researched: bleomycin, ethanol *(17)*, tetracycline, and OK-432 *(18)*. OK-432 is a biological preparation containing Streptococcus pyogenes Su strain cells. It is available in the United States in a research capacity. OK-432 is chosen over the other sclerosing agents because it has the advantage of not causing perilesional fibrosis and thus making postsclerosing surgical excision more manageable. Okazaki et al. *(19)* compared the success rate and complications between other sclerosing agents and OK-432. Sclerotherapy was not as effective as previous reports suggested and also not as effective as surgical excision. However, they were optimistic about the role of sclerotherapy and OK-432 in treating large single

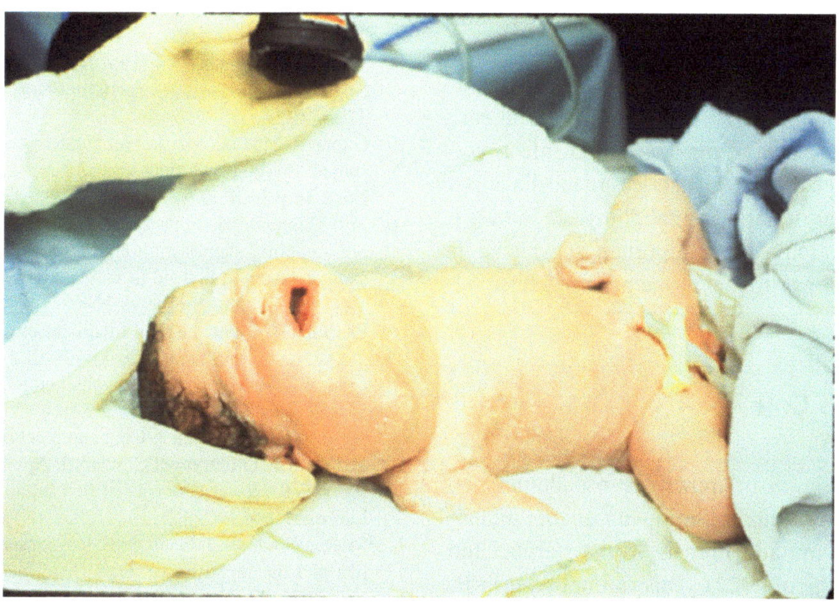

Fig. 4 A child with lymphangioma of the parotid gland (pre-op view)

cysts and macrocystic lymphagiomas *(19)*. Thus, for single and macrocystic lymphangiomas, surgical excision or sclerotherapy are options, while microcystic and cavernous lymphangiomas may be better treated with surgical excision.

Thymic Anomalies

Thymic tissue is an uncommon source of pediatric neck masses, but it should be considered in the differential diagnosis. Thymic cysts, ectopic cervical thymus, and cervical thymoma have all been described in the neck, with thymic cysts being most common *(20, 21)*. During embryological development, the thymus traverses the neck between weeks 6 and 8 prior to entering the mediastinum. Thymic rests may be deposited along the path from the angle of mandible to the midline of the neck descending between the common carotid artery and the vagus nerve.

Thymic cysts often mimic second branchial cleft cysts or lymphatic malformations. They present as a painless neck swelling and a male predominance has been reported. These cysts are found more frequently in the lower neck and within the carotid sheath. A preoperative CT or ultrasound examination may reveal the cystic nature of the lesion and may alert the surgeon to the possibility of a thymic anomaly, but the definitive diagnostic test is histopathological examination. Excision is the preferred treatment.

Fewer than 100 cases of ectopic cervical thymus have been reported *(8, 20)*. They usually present early in life with hyperplasia of the tissue after infection or vaccination. Often these neck masses are misdiagnosed as lymphatic malformations, rhabdomyosarcomas, or low-flow hemangiomas. It is important to evaluate the child for mediastinal thymic tissue prior to excision.

Fibromatosis Coli

Fibromatosis coli, also known as pseudotumor of infancy or sternocleidomastoid tumor of infancy, results from edema and fibrosis of the sternocleidomastoid with torticolis *(22)*. This is important in the consideration of congenital neck masses because infants present most commonly between birth and 3 weeks of age with a hard, mobile mass within the sternocleidomastoid. The mass is usually nontender and ultrasound imaging is diagnostic. Treatment is conservative with 50–70% resolving spontaneously within the first year of life. If neck rotation is limited, early physical therapy should be initiated to prevent plagiocephaly and craniofacial asymmetry. Surgical lengthening of the muscle is indicated for resistant cases or for those diagnosed after the age of one.

Conclusion

Head and neck masses in children are common and can be congenital or acquired. A thorough evaluation of the child is essential before formulating a management plan. Surgical treatment is the rule for congenital masses and relies on extensive knowledge of head and neck anatomy.

References

1. Guarisco JL. Congenital head and neck masses in infants and children part I. Ear Nose Throat J 1991;70:40–47.
2. Guarisco JL. Congenital head and neck masses in infants and children part II. Ear Nose Throat J 1991;70:75–82.
3. Foley DS, Fallat ME. Thyroglossal duct and other congenital midline cervical anomalies. Semin Pediatr Surg 2006;15:70–75.
4. Telander RL, Deane SA. Thyroglossal and branchial cleft cysts and sinuses. Surg Clin North Am 1977;57: 779–791.
5. Gupta P, Maddalozzo J. Preoperative sonography in presumed thyroglossal duct cysts. Arch Otolaryngol Head Neck Surg 2001;127(2):200–202.
6. Lim-Dunham JE, Feinstein KA, Yousefzadeh DK, et al. Sonographic demonstration of normal thyroid gland excludes ectopic thyroid in patients with thyroglossal duct cyst. Am J Roentgenol 1995;164(6):1489–1491.
7. Sistrunk WE. The surgical treatment of cysts of the thyroglossal tract. Ann Surg 1920;71:121–122.
8. Chandler JR, Mitchell B. Branchial cleft cysts, sinuses, and fistulas. Otol Clin North Am 1981;14:175–201.
9. Acierno S, Walhausen J. Congenital cervical cysts, sinuses and fistulae. Otolaryngol Clin North Am 2007;40:161–176.
10. Work WP. Newer concepts of first branchial cleft defects. Laryngoscope 1972;82:1581–1593.
11. McRaeRG, LeeKJ, GoertzenE. First branchial cleft anomalies and the facial nerve. Otol Head Neck Surg 1983;91: 197–202.
12. Sandborn WD, Shafer AD. A branchial cleft cyst of fourth pouch origin. J Pediatr Surg 1972;7(1):82.

13. Smith RJ, Burke DK, Sato Y, et al. OK-432 therapy for lymphangiomas in infants and children. Arch Otolaryngol Head Neck Surg 1996;122:1195–1199.
14. de Serres LM, Sie KC, Richardson MA. Lymphatic malformations of the head and neck. A proposal for staging. Arch Otolaryngol Head Neck Surg 1995;121:577–582.
15. Brock ME, Smith RJH, Parey SE, et al. Lymphangioma. An otolaryngologic perspective. Int J Pediatr Otorhinolaryngol 1987;14:133.
16. Orvidas LJ, Kasperbauer JL. Pediatric lymphangiomas of the head and neck. Ann Otol Rhinol Laryngol 2000; 109:411.
17. Emran MA, Josee D, Laberge L, et al. Alcoholic solution of zein (ethibloc) sclerotherapy for treatment of lymphangiomas in children. J Pediatr Surg 2006;41:975–979.
18. Ogita S, Tsuto T, Nakamura K, et al. OK-432 therapy in 64 patients with lymphangiomas. J Pediatr Surg 1994;29: 784–785.
19. Okazaki T, Iwatani S, Yanai T, Hiroyuki K, et al. Treatment of lymphangioma in children: our experience of 128 cases. J Pediatr Surg 2007;42:386–389.
20. Strome M, Eraklis A. Thymic cysts in the neck. Laryngoscope 1977;87:1645–1649.
21. Khariwala SS, Nicollas R, Triglia JM, Garabedian EN, Marianowski R, Van Den Abbeele T, April M, Ward R, Koltai PJ. Cervical presentations of thymic anomalies in children. Int J Pediatr Otorhinolaryngol 2004;68(7):909–914.
22. Do TT. Congenital muscular torticollis: current concepts and review of treatment. Curr Opin Pediatr 2006; 18(1):26–29.

Pediatric Stridor

David J. Brown

Key Points

- The first priority in evaluating a child with stridor is to determine if there is respiratory compromise.
- The history is an important component when evaluating stridor and can direct the clinician to the site of lesion and help with the differential diagnosis.
- Patients with dysphagia and failure to thrive should have a swallowing evaluation.
- Laryngomalacia is the most common cause of stridor.
- The incidence of subglottic stenosis has decreased over the past four decades.
- Children with airway symptoms out of proportion to their clinical exam findings and children without a firm diagnosis after the history, physical examination, and radiologic evaluation should undergo a direct laryngoscopy and bronchoscopy.

Keywords: Stridor • Neonate • Infant • Airway • Congenital • Laryngomalacia

Definition

Stridor is the abnormal sound produced by air passing through an airway lumen of decreased caliber. The production of stridor is related to the Venturi effect – as air passes through a constricted lumen, the air speed increases while the pressure decreases. This results in a vacuum, airway soft tissue fluttering and ultimately, the audible sound termed stridor. Stridor may be inspiratory, expiratory, or biphasic. Inspiratory stridor correlates clinically with lesions of the supraglottis and glottis. Expiratory stridor is associated with anomalies of the subglottis, trachea, and bronchi. Biphasic stridor can be heard from glottic and subglottic pathologies.

D.J. Brown
Division of Pediatric Otolaryngology, Children's Hospital of Wisconsin, Department of Otolaryngology – Head and Neck Surgery, Medical College of Wisconsin, Milwaukee, WI, USA
e-mail: djbrown@mcw.edu

Evaluation

The history is a key component in evaluating the child with stridor and can often direct the clinician to the location of the lesion as well as the differential diagnosis. The history should begin with the child's birth. The clinician should inquire about the child's birth weight, mode of delivery (vaginal vs. caesarian section), extraction difficulties, cyanosis, respiratory distress, and the need for endotracheal intubation. For those infants who had endotracheal intubation, the duration of intubation, size of the endotracheal tube, and number of intubations give the clinician an idea of how much potential trauma the airway has sustained.

Associated signs and symptoms can localize the airway lesion. Choking with feeding suggests a supraglottic or glottic pathology. A weak cry or hoarseness can point to glottic etiologies such as vocal fold paralysis or laryngeal webs. Positional changes should be noted, such as decreased stridor while prone in infants with laryngomalacia. The clinician should ask about actions that exacerbate the stridor such as agitation and crying which amplify stridor in laryngomalacia. Cutaneous vascular malformations such as hemangiomas or lymphatic malformations should alert the examiner to potential airway vascular lesions.

R.B. Mitchell and K.D. Pereira (eds.), *Pediatric Otolaryngology for the Clinician*,
DOI: 10.1007/978-1-60327-127-1_18, © Humana Press, a part of Springer Science + Business Media, LLC 2009

The past medical and surgical histories are also useful in the evaluation. A viral prodrome with fever suggests an infectious etiology. Neurologic conditions can affect aerodigestive tract tone and coordination. Syndromic features are sometimes associated with airway anomalies such as the midline abnormalities in Opitz syndrome which include a posterior laryngeal cleft. Complex cardiac anomalies often present with airway anomalies. Recurrent aspiration pneumonias suggest an abnormal conduit between the airway and digestive tracts as seen in vocal fold paralysis, posterior laryngeal clefts, and tracheoesophageal fistulas. A history of cardiopulmonary or intracranial surgery can result in an injury to the vagus or recurrent laryngeal nerves. A maternal history of vaginal condylomata should raise suspicion of airway papillomas.

Since breathing and swallowing are highly coordinated events of the aerodigestive tract that can be disrupted by airway lesions, a feeding history should be obtained. Newborns and infants should gain weight appropriately and the clinician should be concerned if the child falls off his growth curve. Children with failure to thrive or respiratory distress with feeding should have a swallowing evaluation. Some children with stridor may need a feeding tube if their underlying aerodigestive anomaly significantly affects their growth and development.

Physical Examination

When examining a child with stridor, the first priority is to determine if the child is in acute distress by assessing for cyanosis, tachypnea, drooling, retractions (supraclavicular, intercostal, and substernal), and unusual breathing positions (tripod posture). Patients in acute distress may require an airway evaluation and intervention in a controlled setting such as the operating room. Children who are not in acute distress can be evaluated in the clinic. The general appearance should be observed including signs of cyanosis, respiratory rate, and retractions. The voice quality should be assessed for hoarseness, weakness, and aphonia. Stridor should be characterized by its phase (inspiratory, expiratory, or biphasic), pitch (high or low), and intensity level (load or soft). A barking cough should be noted if present. Auscultation of the neck and chest with a stethoscope is helpful for localizing the lesion and hearing subtle airway sounds. The remaining head and neck examination should be completed with emphasis on cranial nerve deficits, craniofacial and syndromic features, tracheal deviation, and neck masses. The skin should be examined for vascular malformations such as hemangiomas and lymphatic malformations.

A flexible fiberoptic laryngopharyngoscopy (FFL) should be performed if the child is not in acute distress. FFL is useful for evaluating the upper airway from the nose to the glottis and sometimes gives a view of the subglottis. Patency of the choanae should be noted as well as adenoid hypertrophy, vallecular cysts, supraglottic collapse, vocal fold mobility, and lesions of the larynx.

Children with respiratory compromise requiring airway stabilization, those with symptoms that are out of proportion to their clinical findings, and those without a diagnosis after the history, physical examination, and radiologic evaluation should undergo evaluation by direct laryngoscopy and rigid bronchoscopy under general anesthesia.

Radiologic Evaluation

The radiologic evaluation can support and supplement findings found on history and physical examination. High kilovolt anterior-posterior (AP) and lateral neck films and chest X-rays (CXRs) can identify subglottic narrowing, tracheal deviation, and abnormal lung ventilation. Airway fluoroscopy can demonstrate collapse of the supraglottis, tracheal narrowing from tracheomalacia, and airway narrowing from vascular compression. A barium esophagram can identify compression by vascular anomalies and a tracheoesophageal fistula. Computed tomography (CT) and magnetic resonance imaging (MRI) of the brain can identify entities associated with increased intracranial pressure (Arnold-Chiari malformation, myelomeningocele, and hydrocephalus) and therefore compression of the vagus nerve. CT and MRI of the neck and chest can be helpful in identifying tumors and vascular anomalies.

Differential Diagnosis

Laryngeal

Laryngomalacia is the most common cause of infantile stridor and represents over 75% of the cases *(1, 2)*. The stridor in laryngomalacia is inspiratory and caused by collapse of the epiglottis and arytenoid mucosa. The quality of the stridor can be high-pitched and musical or a low-pitched, coarse, and fluttering sound. The stridor may be initiated or exacerbated by agitation, feeding, or while lying in the supine position.

The etiology of laryngomalacia has yet to be elucidated, but a common theory is that the larynx is floppy secondary to neurologic immaturity *(3)*. Gastroesophageal reflux disease (GERD) is highly associated with laryngomalacia and is also thought to be secondary to neurologic immaturity *(3,4)*. Matthews et al. found that of 24 infants diagnosed with laryngomalacia who had 24-h double-probe pH monitoring, 92% had three episodes of pharyngeal reflux and 100% had at least one episode *(5)*.

The diagnosis of laryngomalacia is made by FFL. The infant's inspiratory stridor should correlate with collapse of the epiglottis or arytenoid mucosa. In addition to supraglottic collapse, signs of GERD (laryngeal edema, erythema, and pooling of gastric refluxate) should be noted. Although well-controlled data are lacking to support the treatment of GERD in patients with laryngomalacia, its empiric treatment has been advocated.

High-kilovolt AP and lateral neck films are usually obtained to evaluate for secondary airway lesions. Secondary airway lesions can be found in over 10% of patients, especially if there is associated cyanosis *(6)*. Airway fluoroscopy may show supraglottic collapse and may also be useful in identifying secondary airway lesions.

Laryngomalacia is self-limited and resolves within 1–2 years in more than 90% of infants *(1)*. Findings that warrant further evaluation with direct laryngoscopy, bronchoscopy, and possibly supraglottoplasty include: stridor inconsistent with the FFL findings, abnormal neck films, concern for a secondary lesion, respiratory distress, cyanosis, and failure to thrive *(7, 8)*. During the airway endoscopy, secondary lesions should be sought. For cases of primary laryngomalacia with respiratory distress or failure to thrive, a supraglottoplasty can be performed. This procedure has many variations and techniques. For supraglottic collapse, the aryepiglottic folds can be lysed. For stridor secondary to redundant arytenoid mucosa, the lateral arytenoid mucosa can be trimmed while sparing the medial arytenoid mucosa to decrease the risk of interarytenoid scarring. The supraglottoplasty can be performed using a CO_2 laser, the microdebrider, or sinus instruments (Fig. 1). In the past, a tracheostomy was performed for severe cases of laryngomalacia, but since the development of endoscopic supraglottoplasty techniques, tracheostomy is rarely needed.

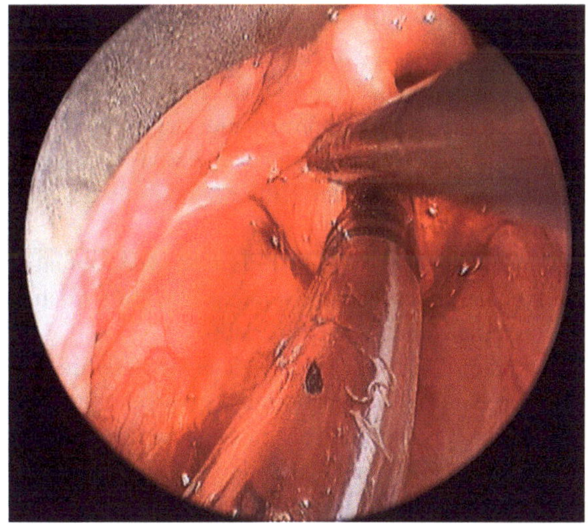

Fig. 1 Supraglottoplasty using sinus instruments. The left aryepiglottic fold is being compressed and incised with a through-cutting forcep

Vocal fold paralysis is the second most common cause of stridor in neonates and comprises 10% of congenital laryngeal anomalies *(9)*. Vocal fold paralysis may be congenital or acquired. Congenital forms of vocal fold paralysis can be inherited as an autosomal dominant, autosomal recessive, or X-link-associated trait or associated with congenital abnormalities of the central nervous or cardiovascular systems *(10)*. Central nervous system anomalies such as Arnold-Chiari malformations, hydrocephalus, and myelomeningocele put pressure on the vagus nerve from increased intracranial pressure which can result in bilateral vocal fold paralysis. Congenital cardiovascular anomalies can put pressure on the recurrent laryngeal nerve resulting in a unilateral vocal fold paralysis. Trauma to the recurrent laryngeal nerve from a traumatic childbirth delivery or from cardiothoracic surgery leads to vocal fold paralysis that may be temporary or permanent.

The remaining etiologies of vocal fold paralysis include tumors of the neck and mediastinum and idiopathic causes.

The most common presentation of infants with vocal fold paralysis is stridor and a weak cry. Some children may also present with respiratory distress and recurrent aspiration.

The diagnosis is made by FFL in an awake infant or by direct laryngoscopy of the infant with mild sedation but no topical anesthesia or paralytics.

The radiologic evaluation is determined by the history and clinical findings. In infants with choking during feeding, a modified barium swallow may confirm aspiration. A CXR can be useful to evaluate for aspiration pneumonia. For infants with bilateral vocal fold paralysis, MRI can determine if there are central nervous system lesions.

Suspected tumors and cardiovascular anomalies of the neck and chest can be evaluated by CT or MRI.

The first priority for patients with vocal fold paralysis is to have a stable airway. Some infants with respiratory distress will require a tracheostomy while others require close monitoring. The second priority is to ensure adequate nutrition without airway compromise. Some patients may require thickened feeds, a temporary nasogastric tube, or a surgical feeding tube.

Congenital laryngeal webs occur secondary to incomplete resorption of the laryngeal lumen epithelium during embryologic development. Infants present with stridor, a weak cry, hoarseness, respiratory distress, or aphonia. Most congenital laryngeal webs are anterior because the resorption proceeds in a dorsal to ventral direction (Fig. 2). Laryngeal webs are associated with cardiac and 22q11 anomalies *(11)*. Laryngeal webs can also be acquired secondary to vocal fold trauma from laryngeal surgery or endotracheal intubation (Fig. 3). The diagnosis is made by FFL or direct laryngoscopy. Thin webs can be managed by endoscopic lysis with or without mitomycin-C *(12)*. Thicker webs and those who fail endoscopic lysis are managed with open laryngofissure and placement of a laryngeal keel or stent.

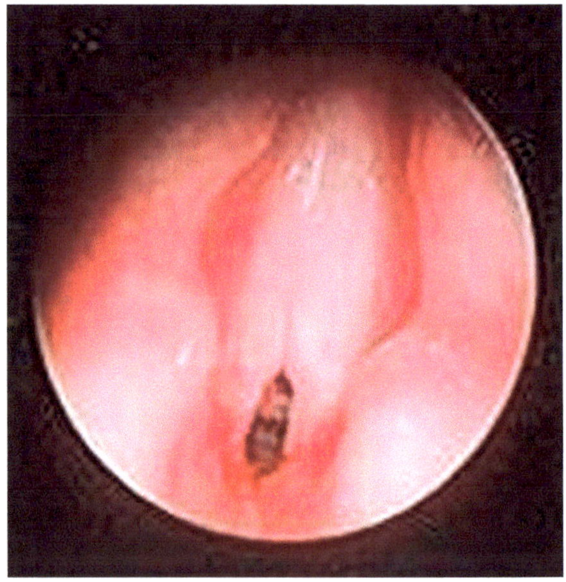

Fig. 2 Near complete anterior glottic web

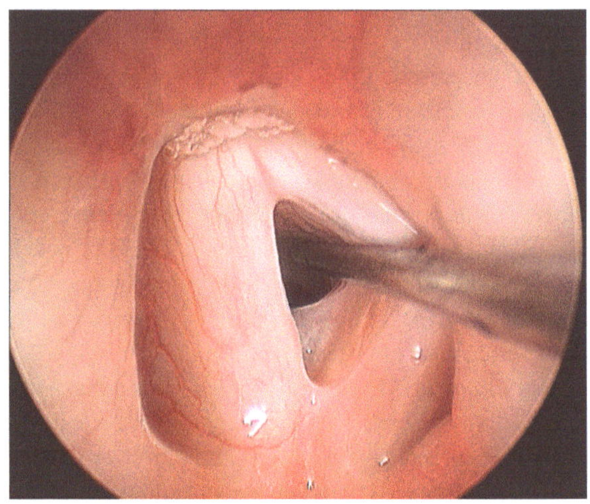

Fig. 3 Posterior glottic web. The probe is retracting the right true vocal fold laterally to demonstrate the posterior glottic web

Laryngeal cysts are mucous retention cysts that present with stridor, respiratory distress, cyanosis, dysphagia, and failure to thrive. De Santo et al. defined two types of laryngeal cysts, saccular and ductal *(13)*. *Saccular cysts* are submucosal cysts caused by mucous accumulation within the laryngeal saccule. They are differentiated from laryngoceles by being fluid-filled and by not having a communication with the laryngeal lumen. Saccular cysts are further divided into lateral and anterior subtypes. The lateral saccular cyst presents as a mass distorting the lateral epiglottis, aryepiglottic fold, false vocal fold, and ventricle. Extension of a large lateral saccular cyst through the thyrohyoid membrane can present as a lateral neck mass. Anterior saccular cysts present as protrusions through the anterior ventricle that overlay the true vocal fold. CT and MRI of the neck can define the extent of the cyst. Saccular cysts are managed surgically by endoscopic techniques or external approaches depending on the cyst size and location.

Ductal cysts arise from fluid accumulation secondary to obstructed submucosal glands. The most common type of the ductal cyst is the vallecular cyst which can cause significant retroflexion of the epiglottis, supraglottic airway obstruction, stridor, and cyanosis (Fig. 4).

Vallecular cysts can be diagnosed by FFL, direct laryngoscopy, or a modified barium swallow study. They are difficult to see on plain film radiographs, but can be identified on CT or MRI. The management of vallecular cysts is surgical. Marsupialization of the cyst and removal of the mucosal lining can be performed with a CO_2 laser, cold knife, or a microdebrider. After removal of the vallecular cyst, most children have resolution of their symptoms within days.

Posterior laryngeal clefts are uncommon congenital anomalies caused by incomplete formation of the septum between the esophagus and the larynx and/or trachea. They present with stridor, choking, aspiration, chronic cough, and failure to thrive. The incidence of posterior laryngeal clefts is less than 0.1% ***(13)***. As many as one in three posterior laryngeal clefts are associated with tracheoesophageal fistulas ***(14,15)***, Genetics may play a role in the etiology since an autosomal dominant inheritance pattern has been observed in addition to being associated with midline anomaly syndromes such as Optiz G and Pallister-Hall syndromes ***(16–19)***.

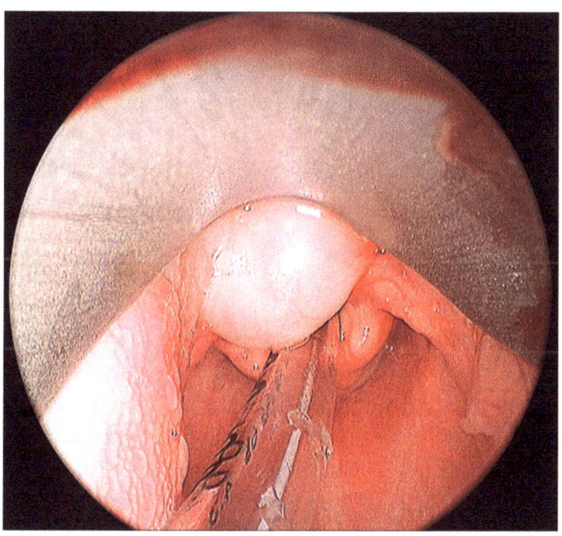

Fig. 4 Vallecular cyst partially obstructing visualization of the larynx

The Benjamin-Inglis classification system describes four types of posterior laryngeal clefts: Type 1 clefts are interarytenoid and lie above the level of the true vocal folds, Type 2 clefts extend below the true vocal folds and partially through the cricoid cartilage, Type 3 clefts extend into the extrathoracic trachea, and Type 4 clefts extend into the intrathoracic trachea ***(20)***.

The diagnosis of posterior laryngeal clefts can be challenging, especially in the less severe, Type 1 clefts. Chien et al. found Type 1 posterior laryngeal clefts in 1 of 13 patients presenting to their institution with symptoms of chronic cough or aspiration over a 3-year period ***(21)***. Therefore, a Type 1 cleft should be part of the differential diagnosis for children with chronic cough and aspiration. These children should be evaluated for aspiration with a modified barium swallow or a functional endoscopic evaluation of swallowing study. Direct laryngoscopy and bronchoscopy should be performed. Bimanual palpation and probing of interarytenoid area confirms the diagnosis. For larger clefts, redundant esophageal mucosa may be seen prolapsing through the posterior cleft and into the laryngeal lumen. The bronchoscopy will indentify the distal extent of the cleft and the presence of other airway anomalies such as a tracheoesophageal fistula.

The management of posterior laryngeal clefts depends on the extent of the cleft. The treatment for Type 1 clefts is evolving. Chien et al. recommend that Type 1 clefts have a trial of nonsurgical management first with a proton pump inhibitor to treat GERD, upright feedings, and thickened of feedings ***(21)***. Those children who fail conservative treatment should have surgical repair. Types 1 and 2 posterior laryngeal clefts can be repaired endoscopically. Open procedures should be performed on those with Type 3 and 4 clefts and those who fail endoscopic management. Open surgical techniques include repair through a laryngofissure, a lateral pharyngotomy, and a thoracotomy (for Type 4 clefts).

Subglottic

Subglottic stenosis (SGS) is defined as subglottic narrowing of less than 4 mm in a term infant and less than 3 mm in the premature infant (Fig. 5) ***(22)***. Children with SGS present with stridor (inspiratory or biphasic) and may have a barking cough. The stenosis can be

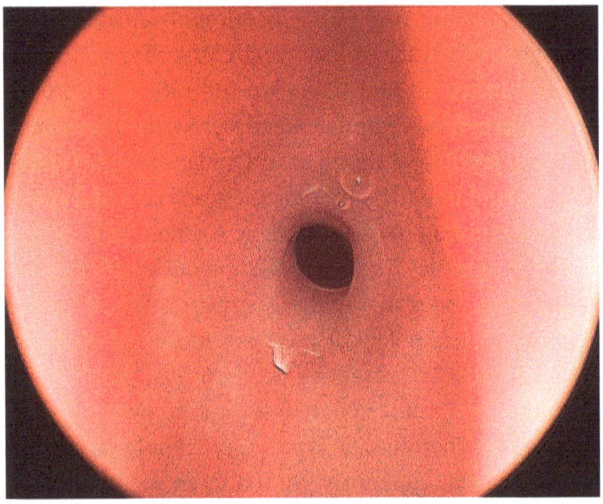

Fig. 5 Myer-Cotton Type 3 subglottic stenosis

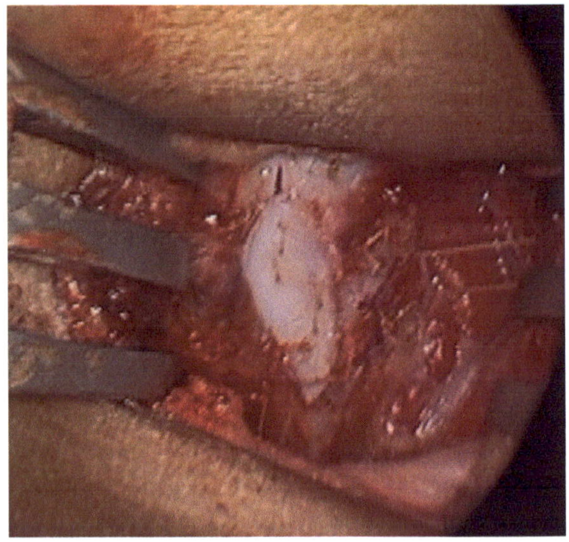

Fig. 6 Thyroid ala cartilage anterior graft for subglottic stenosis

congenital or acquired from endotracheal intubation. Congenital subglottic stenosis is generally less severe and easier to manage than acquired subglottic stenosis. The incidence of SGS has been decreasing because of improved airway management in the neonatal intensive care unit and especially the use of appropriately sized endotracheal tubes made of less traumatic materials. In the 1970s, the incidence was as high as 8% of intubated infants but a 2001 review by Walner et al. suggests that the incidence is now less than 2% *(23)*.

If the child is not intubated, FFL can be performed. In isolated SGS there will be a normal supraglottic examination. Occasionally, subglottic narrowing can be seen below the true vocal folds. High KV airway films may show narrowing of the subglottic airway.

The definitive evaluation of SGS is with direct laryngoscopy and bronchoscopy. SGS is confirmed in a child without a leak <30-cm H_2O while using an age-appropriate endotracheal tube. The Myer-Cotton SGS grading system is the most common system used and is as follows: Type 1 – less or equal to 50% stenosis, Type 2 – 51–70% stenosis, Type 3 – 71–99% stenosis, and Type 4 – complete stenosis *(24)*.

The surgical management of subglottic stenosis depends on the extent of stenosis, age of the child, and comorbid conditions. Neonates who have subglottic stenosis and multiple failed extubations may require a tracheostomy. Cotton and Seid described an alternative to tracheostomy for some neonates, the anterior cricoid split *(25)*. The anterior cricoid split is indicated in the neonate who has failed multiple extubations, weighs more than 1,500 g, has an oxygen requirement of less than 35%, no heart failure, and does not require mechanical ventilation. The procedure consists of a vertical incision extending from the second tracheal cartilage, through the anterior cricoid ring, and up to the lower half of the thyroid cartilage. The airway is then stented with an ETT for one week. To decrease the failure rate and complications related to postoperative self extubation, Forte et al. advocated using thyroid ala cartilage to augment and support the anterior cricoid split airway (Fig. 6) *(26)*. Other surgical options for subglottic stenosis include balloon dilation, laryngotracheal reconstruction, and cricotracheal reconstruction *(27, 28)*.

Subglottic hemangiomas are vascular tumors secondary to endothelial proliferation and present clinically with biphasic stridor within the first 3–6 months of life. One half of infants with subglottic hemangiomas have cutaneous hemangiomas. Lateral neck films may show asymmetric subglottic narrowing of the airway. The diagnosis is confirmed by direct laryngoscopy and bronchoscopy. The subglottic hemangioma is often located in the posterior lateral quadrant with the left side being more common than the right. Circumferential subglottic hemangiomas may also be seen. The hemangioma may appear blue or red and is soft to palpation. After confirming the diagnosis, some recommend MRI of the neck and chest to evaluate the extent of the disease *(29)*. There are many treatment options for subglottic hemangiomas. For children with minimal symptoms and no airway obstruction, watchful waiting is an option. Medical management includes corticosteroids (systemic or intralesional), interferon, and vincristine. Potential side effects of corticosteroids include growth abnormalities and cushingoid changes while interferon and vincristine have potential neurotoxic effects. Lasers have been used to remove hemangiomas but there is a risk of subglottic stenosis. Open excision with laryngotracheoplasty and cartilage graft to augment the airway is one of the surgical approaches used. Another management option is to perform a tracheostomy to secure the airway until the hemangioma resolves either spontaneously or with the assistance of medical therapy.

Subglottic cysts are mucous retention cysts that cause biphasic stridor and respiratory distress (Fig. 7). The cysts have been characterized as congenital or acquired. Congenital cysts are thought to cause respiratory distress in the newborn period requiring urgent ETT intubation. Acquired cysts are found in infants with a history of ETT intubation. Prematurity increases the risk for acquired subglottic cysts. Since the cysts cannot be identified other than by direct laryngoscopy in a stable infant, there is controversy as to whether the cysts can be congenital or are always acquired from ETT trauma. The cysts may be single or multiple and are thought to occur from ETT mucosal trauma, which leads to mucosal gland obstruction and mucous retention. The infant may be symptomatic with stridor immediately after extubation or not until months later.

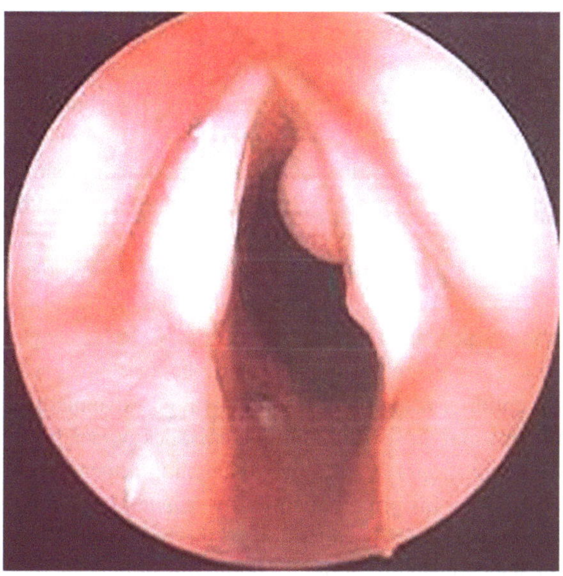

Fig. 7 Right subglottic cyst from prior endotracheal intubations

Subglottic cysts can be managed with laser or sharp dissection removal. They have a high recurrence rate (>40%) and therefore these patients should be followed closely and may require a surveillance direct laryngoscopy and bronchoscopy 3–6 months after the last excision ***(30)***.

Tracheal

Tracheomalacia is anterior-posterior collapse of the trachea that is secondary to weak tracheal cartilage or from external compression (Fig. 8). Children with tracheomalacia present with expiratory stridor, wheezing, and coughing. Conditions that affect the structural integrity of the trachea such as tracheoesophageal fistulae, esophageal anomalies, vascular rings and slings, and innominate artery anomalies can cause tracheomalacia. In addition to compressing the trachea, vascular anomalies can impinge on the esophagus and result in dysphagia. Tracheomalacia can present after surgery on the trachea as seen after tracheoesophageal fistulae repair or tracheostomy.

Lateral airway fluoroscopy shows dynamic collapse of the trachea. Esophagrams will demonstrate vascular anomalies as well as esophageal anomalies. MRI can be useful to evaluate the extent of vascular anomalies.

Bronchoscopy under general anesthesia with spontaneous breathing can demonstrate the anterior-posterior collapse. Flexible or rigid bronchoscopy can be

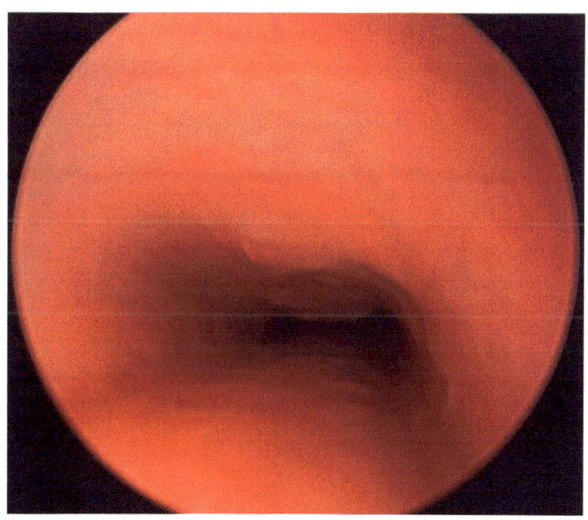

Fig. 8 Tracheomalacia with anterior-posterior collapse of the trachea

performed to diagnose tracheomalacia. However, the potential for rigid bronchoscopy to stent the airway and distort the findings leads some to prefer flexible bronchoscopy.

Tracheomalacia related to floppy tracheal cartilage will often resolve spontaneously in 2–3 years as the child and the tracheal airway grow. Infants who are symptomatic with respiratory distress may require continuous positive airway pressure. The treatment of tracheomalacia secondary to external compression depends on the offending anomaly. After repairing the compressing anomaly, treatment options include airway stents, cartilage grafting, aortopexy, and tracheostomy.

Congenital tracheal stenosis occurs when tracheal cartilages form a complete ring instead of the usual inverted U shape (Fig. 9). This rare congenital anomaly is associated with pulmonary slings and other cardiovascular anomalies. These patients present with biphasic stridor, cough, and dyspnea on exertion. High KV neck and chest films may pick up the abnormally small tracheal lumen. CT, 3D CT, and MRI are more useful because they can determine the stenotic length, bronchial involvement, and the presence of associated vascular anomalies. Bronchoscopy confirms the presence of complete tracheal rings and their length. The airway evaluation should be performed with minimal mucosal trauma using small (<2 mm) rigid or flexible scopes. The management depends on the child's symptoms, the length of stenosis, and the location of the stenosis. Some children with complete tracheal rings have minimal symptoms and can be managed conservatively with nonoperative observation. Rutter et al. estimate that 1 in 10 children with complete tracheal rings can be managed without surgery ***(31)***. For symptomatic children, tracheal resection with end-to-end anastomosis can be done for short-segment stenosis. Long-segment stenosis is best managed by performing a slide tracheoplasty ***(32)***. This procedure is often performed while the child is on cardiopulmonary bypass, especially if there is distal tracheal stenosis or if the infant's cardiovascular anomalies are being repaired at the same time.

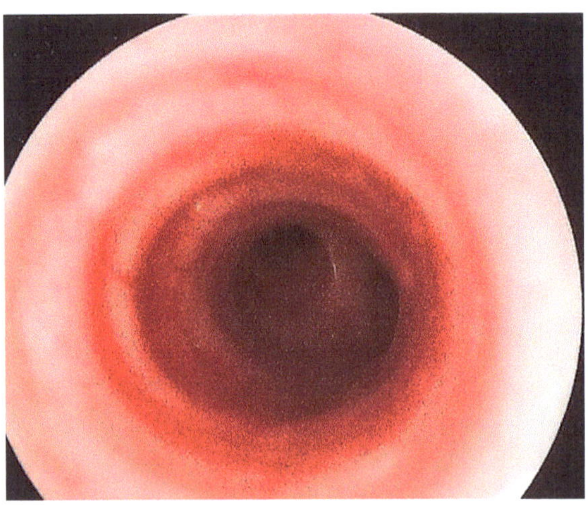

Fig. 9 Complete tracheal rings with a circular appearance

Infectious

Croup, or viral laryngotracheobronchitis, is a viral infection which commonly affects children from 6 to 36 months of age. Croup is the most common cause of acute upper airway obstruction in children under 6 years and has an annual incidence of 3% ***(33)***. Parainfluenza viruses account for up to 75% of croup cases with respiratory syncytial virus, adenovirus, and influenza A and B viruses also contributing to the etiology. These patients often have a viral prodrome that is followed by a barking cough, with or without biphasic stridor and hoarseness. The diagnosis is made from the history and physical exam with classical findings on plain X-ray films of the neck. The classic croup AP neck film shows a subglottic steeple sign. Mild cases of croup can be treated with close observation and humidified air as needed. Moderate to severe cases are treated with humidified air, corticosteroids, and racemic epinephrine. The use of dexamethasone has decreased the rate of hospitalization for croup but more severe cases continue to require hospital admission with close observation ***(34)***. Endotracheal intubation may be required in up to 2% of children but should be avoided if possible because of the risk of subglottic stenosis ***(35)***. The endotracheal tube should be removed when the child has defervesced and there is an appropriate leak around the endotracheal tube. Rigid airway endoscopy to evaluate for subglottic stenosis is reserved for children who do not respond to aggressive medical therapy and those with multiple episodes of croup.

Acute epiglottitis is a life-threatening upper airway obstruction historically caused by *Haemophilus influenzae* type B (HiB) infection of the epiglottis. Since the widespread use of the *Haemophilus influenzae* type B vaccine began in the 1980s, the incidence of this severe infection has fortunately decreased dramatically *(36, 37)*. Acute epiglottitis affects children from 3 to 6 years of age with a rapid onset of fever, stridor, and a toxic appearance. Additionally, the clinical findings of tachypnea, respiratory distress, drooling, and a tripod breathing posture should be considered suspicious for acute epiglottitis. Children who are in acute distress should not be agitated by performing procedures such as fiberoptic laryngoscopy or intravenous line access. If there is respiratory distress and a high index of suspicion, radiologic evaluation is not necessary. If lateral neck films are obtained, the epiglottis will be enlarged and have a "thumb" sign. The ideal management of epiglottitis requires a team effort with experienced specialists from anesthesiology, otolaryngology, and nursing in the operating room. Since this is an airway emergency, the bronchoscopy and tracheostomy equipment should be available. Muscle relaxants should be avoided because the child's respiratory effort is crucial for oxygenation and ventilation through the edematous larynx. Inhalation anesthesia will allow the child to spontaneously breathe but may take longer than usual since the laryngeal lumen is narrowed. Once the child is anesthetized, direct laryngoscopy and intubation should be performed. If there is difficulty securing the airway with the endotracheal tube, the bronchoscope can be used for airway visualization and ventilation. In cases with airway instability, a tracheostomy may be necessary. The epiglottis has a "cherry red" appearance and should be cultured for appropriate antibiotic coverage. After 2–3 days of IV antibiotics, direct laryngoscopy can determine if the epiglottic edema and erythema has resolved enough for extubation.

Bacterial tracheitis is emerging as a more common infectious cause of pediatric respiratory failure since corticosteroids are being used more commonly to manage croup and the HiB vaccine has decreased the incidence of acute epiglottitis. In their series of infectious causes of airway obstruction between 1997 and 2006, Hopkins et al. report that bacterial tracheitis was three times more likely to progress to severe respiratory distress than both croup and epiglottis combined *(38)*. Bacterial tracheitis is most commonly caused by *Staphylococcus aureus* as well as group A Streptococcus and *Haemophilus influenza.* The child may present with a viral prodrome, a croup-like cough, stridor, and fever. The chest X-ray may show a steeple sign similar to that found in croup.

Bronchoscopy confirms the diagnosis with the presence of diffuse inflammation and pseudomembranes extending from the true vocal folds to the trachea and possibly to the mainstem bronchi. Debriding the airway can assist with recovery and may have to be repeated. Cultures should be obtained during the bronchoscopy and IV antibiotics should be initiated to treat the common bacteria associated with tracheitis.

Recurrent respiratory papillomatosis (RRP) consists of benign papillomas of the airway and is caused by human papilloma virus (HPV) subtypes 6 and 11 (Fig. 10). The incidence of RRP in US children is about 4 per 100,000 *(39)*. Most cases of RRP are contracted when the child passes through the birth canal but there have been reports of RRP in children born by caesarian section. Children with RRP commonly present with stridor and hoarseness between 2 and 5 years of age. More aggressive forms of RRP, with high mortality, have been reported in infants diagnosed at less than 6 months of age. For example, Loyo et al. reported a neonate born by caesarian section with aggressive RRP *(40, 41)*.

Because of papilloma regrowth, these patients require multiple airway evaluations and debulkings to give them an adequate airway and to improve voice quality. During the airway evaluation, biopsies should be obtained for HPV subtyping and malignancy evaluation. The carbon dioxide laser was once the primary technique for papilloma removal, but recently the microdebrider has surpassed the carbon dioxide laser and is used by more than half of the pediatric otolaryngologists surveyed from the American Society of Pediatric Otolaryngology (ASPO) *(42)*.

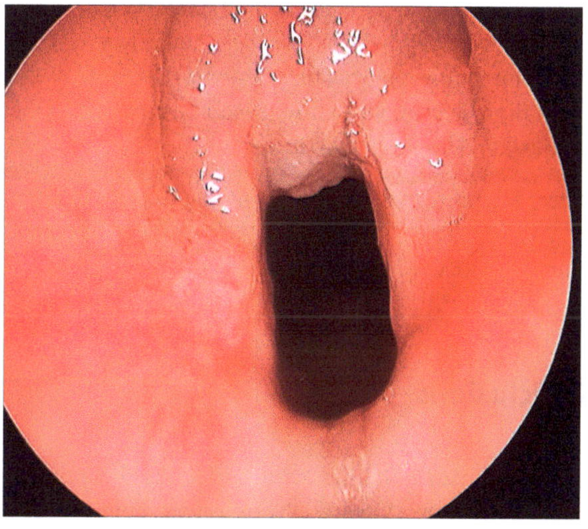

Fig. 10 Laryngeal papillomas of the anterior true vocal folds and anterior commisure

Because of the aggressive nature of this disease, the inability for complete surgical excision, and the morbidity associated with repeated operations, adjuvant therapies have been tried for RRP. The most promising adjuvant therapy is the antiviral cidofovir, a cytosine nucleotide analog. Other therapies include photodynamic therapy, interferon, and methotrexate. A survey of ASPO members found that more than 60% report clinical improvement with intralesional cidofovir ***(42)***. Adjuvant therapies were initially used for more severe cases and those with distal spread, but cidofovir is now being used for less aggressive disease ***(43)***.

Although benefit has been reported with intralesional cidofovir, there is a concern for long-term malignant transformation potential. Broekema and Dikkers reviewed 31 publications to assess the toxicity of cidofovir. They found that the malignant potential in the cidofovir-treated group was similar to the non-treated group (2.7% vs. 2.3%) but highlighted the need for long-term data ***(44)***. In an effort to balance the benefits and risks of cidofovir, the RRP Task Force have the following recommendations ***(43)***:

- Cidofovir should be offered to patients with moderate to severe disease who have failed other surgical and nonsurgical therapies and still require more than three debulkings per year.
- Mild forms of RRP with less morbidity should not be considered for cidofovir until the long-term sequelae are better understood.
- Informed consent should be obtained for cidofovir injections. The parents should be counseled on the risk of nephrotoxicity and the unknown risk of future malignant transformation.
- Malignant transformation should be reported to the FDA and the RRP task force.

There are presently vaccines available to prevent HPV in young women. Time will tell how these vaccines alter the course of pediatric RRP.

Conclusions

When evaluating children with stridor, the first priority is to determine if there is respiratory compromise. Obtaining a strong history is important in evaluating pediatric stridor and can direct the subsequent work-up. Most patients with stridor are evaluated by FFL, direct laryngoscopy, and bronchoscopy. The management of stridor is determined by the diagnosis and severity of symptoms and may include watchful waiting, medical treatment, and surgery.

References

1. Holinger LD. Etiology of stridor in the neonate, infant and child. The Annals of Otology, Rhinology, and Laryngology 1980;89(5 Pt 1):397–400.
2. Cotton RT, Reilly JS. Congenital malformations of the larynx. In: Bluestone CD, Stool SE, eds. Pediatric Otolaryngology. Vol 2. Philadelphia: W.B. Saunders; 1983:1300–1.
3. Belmont JR, Grundfast K. Congenital laryngeal stridor (laryngomalacia): etiologic factors and associated disorders. The Annals of Otology, Rhinology, and Laryngology 1984;93(5 Pt 1):430–7.
4. Roger G, Denoyelle F, Triglia JM, Garabedian EN. Severe laryngomalacia: surgical indications and results in 115 patients. The Laryngoscope 1995;105(10):1111–7.
5. Matthews BL, Little JP, McGuirt WF, Jr., Koufman JA. Reflux in infants with laryngomalacia: results of 24-hour double-probe pH monitoring. Otolaryngology and Head and Neck Surgery 1999;120(6):860–4.
6. Friedman EM, Vastola AP, McGill TJ, Healy GB. Chronic pediatric stridor: etiology and outcome. The Laryngoscope 1990;100(3):277–80.
7. Mancuso RF, Choi SS, Zalzal GH, Grundfast KM. Laryngomalacia. The search for the second lesion. Archives of Otolaryngology–Head & Neck Surgery 1996;122(3):302–6.
8. Olney DR, Greinwald JH, Jr., Smith RJ, Bauman NM. Laryngomalacia and its treatment. The Laryngoscope 1999; 109(11):1770–5.
9. Holinger PH, Brown WT. Congenital webs, cysts, laryngoceles and other anomalies of the larynx. The Annals of Otology, Rhinology, and Laryngology 1967;76(4): 744–52.
10. Tarin TT, Martinez JA, Shapiro NL. Familial bilateral abductor vocal cord paralysis. International Journal of Pediatric Otorhinolaryngology 2005;69(12):1693–6.
11. Fokstuen S, Bottani A, Medeiros PF, Antonarakis SE, Stoll C, Schinzel A. Laryngeal atresia type III (glottic web) with 22q11.2 microdeletion: report of three patients. American Journal of Medical Genetics 1997;70(2):130–3.
12. Unal M. The successful management of congenital laryngeal web with endoscopic lysis and topical mitomycin-C. International Journal of Pediatric Otorhinolaryngology 2004;68(2):231–5.
13. DeSanto LW, Devine KD, Weiland LH. Cysts of the larynx—classification. The Laryngoscope 1970;80(1):145–76.
14. Cohen SR. Cleft larynx A report of seven cases. The Annals of Otology, Rhinology, and Laryngology 1975;84(6):747–56.
15. Evans KL, Courteney-Harris R, Bailey CM, Evans JN, Parsons DS. Management of posterior laryngeal and laryngotracheoesophageal clefts. Archives of Otolaryngology–Head & Neck Surgery 1995;121(12):1380–5.

16. Phelan PD, Stocks JG, Williams HE, Danks DM. Familial occurrence of congenital laryngeal clefts. Archives of Disease in Childhood 1973;48(4):275–8.
17. Cote GB, Katsantoni A, Papadakou-Lagoyanni S, et al. The G syndrome of dysphagia, ocular hypertelorism and hypospadias. Clinical Genetics 1981;19(6):473–8.
18. Hall JG, Pallister PD, Clarren SK, et al. Congenital hypothalamic hamartoblastoma, hypopituitarism, imperforate anus and postaxial polydactyly – a new syndrome? Part I: clinical, causal, and pathogenetic considerations. American Journal of Medical Genetics 1980;7(1):47–74.
19. Ondrey F, Griffith A, Van Waes C, et al. Asymptomatic laryngeal malformations are common in patients with Pallister-Hall syndrome. American Journal of Medical Genetics 2000;94(1):64–7.
20. Benjamin B, Inglis A. Minor congenital laryngeal clefts: diagnosis and classification. The Annals of Otology, Rhinology, and Laryngology 1989;98(6):417–20.
21. Chien W, Ashland J, Haver K, Hardy SC, Curren P, Hartnick CJ. Type 1 laryngeal cleft: establishing a functional diagnostic and management algorithm. International Journal of Pediatric Otorhinolaryngology 2006;70(12):2073–9.
22. Willging JP, Cotton RT. Subglottic stenosis in the pediatric patient. In: Myer CM, Cotton RT, Shott SR, eds. The Pediatric Airway. Philadelphia: JB Lippincott; 1995:111–32.
23. Walner DL, Loewen MS, Kimura RE. Neonatal subglottic stenosis – incidence and trends. The Laryngoscope 2001; 111(1):48–51.
24. Myer CM, 3rd, O'Connor DM, Cotton RT. Proposed grading system for subglottic stenosis based on endotracheal tube sizes. The Annals of Otology, Rhinology, and Laryngology 1994;103(4 Pt 1):319–23.
25. Cotton RT, Seid AB. Management of the extubation problem in the premature child. Anterior cricoid split as an alternative to tracheotomy. The Annals of Otology, Rhinology, and Laryngology 1980;89(6 Pt 1):508–11.
26. Forte V, Chang MB, Papsin BC. Thyroid ala cartilage reconstruction in neonatal subglottic stenosis as a replacement for the anterior cricoid split. International Journal of Pediatric Otorhinolaryngology 2001;59(3):181–6.
27. Durden F, Sobol SE. Balloon laryngoplasty as a primary treatment for subglottic stenosis. Archives of Otolaryngology–Head & Neck Surgery 2007;133(8):772–5.
28. Hartley BE, Rutter MJ, Cotton RT. Cricotracheal resection as a primary procedure for laryngotracheal stenosis in children. International Journal of Pediatric Otorhinolaryngology 2000;54(2–3):133–6.
29. Rahbar R, Nicollas R, Roger G, et al. The biology and management of subglottic hemangioma: past, present, future. The Laryngoscope 2004;114(11):1880–91.
30. Lim J, Hellier W, Harcourt J, Leighton S, Albert D. Subglottic cysts: the Great Ormond Street experience. International Journal of Pediatric Otorhinolaryngology 2003;67(5):461–5.
31. Rutter MJ, Willging JP, Cotton RT. Nonoperative management of complete tracheal rings. Archives of Otolaryngology–Head & Neck Surgery 2004;130(4):450–2.
32. Grillo HC. Slide tracheoplasty for long-segment congenital tracheal stenosis. The Annals of Thoracic Surgery 1994;58(3):613–9 discussion 9–21.
33. Denny FW, Murphy TF, Clyde WA, Jr., Collier AM, Henderson FW. Croup: an 11-year study in a pediatric practice. Pediatrics 1983;71(6):871–6.
34. Johnson DW, Jacobson S, Edney PC, Hadfield P, Mundy ME, Schuh S. A comparison of nebulized budesonide, intramuscular dexamethasone, and placebo for moderately severe croup. The New England Journal of Medicine 1998; 339(8):498–503.
35. Kairys SW, Olmstead EM, O'Connor GT. Steroid treatment of laryngotracheitis: a meta-analysis of the evidence from randomized trials. Pediatrics 1989;83(5):683–93.
36. Broadhurst LE, Erickson RL, Kelley PW. Decreases in invasive Haemophilus influenzae diseases in US Army children, 1984 through 1991. JAMA 1993;269(2):227–31.
37. Mayo-Smith MF, Spinale JW, Donskey CJ, Yukawa M, Li RH, Schiffman FJ. Acute epiglottitis. An 18-year experience in Rhode Island. Chest 1995;108(6):1640–7.
38. Hopkins A, Lahiri T, Salerno R, Heath B. Changing epidemiology of life-threatening upper airway infections: the reemergence of bacterial tracheitis. Pediatrics 2006;118(4):1418–21.
39. Derkay CS. Task force on recurrent respiratory papillomas. A preliminary report. Archives of Otolaryngology–Head & Neck Surgery 1995;121(12):1386–91.
40. Chipps BE, McClurg FL, Jr., Freidman EM, Adams GL. Respiratory papillomas: presentation before six months. Pediatric Pulmonology 1990;9(2):125–30.
41. Loyo M, Pai SI, Netto GJ, Tunkel DE. Aggressive recurrent respiratory papillomatosis in a neonate. International Journal of Pediatric Otorhinolaryngology 2008;72(6):917–20.
42. Schraff S, Derkay CS, Burke B, Lawson L. American Society of Pediatric Otolaryngology members' experience with recurrent respiratory papillomatosis and the use of adjuvant therapy. Archives of Otolaryngology–Head & Neck Surgery 2004;130(9):1039–42.
43. Derkay C. Cidofovir for recurrent respiratory papillomatosis (RRP): a re-assessment of risks. International Journal of Pediatric Otorhinolaryngology 2005;69(11): 1465–7.
44. Broekema FI, Dikkers FG. Side-effects of cidofovir in the treatment of recurrent respiratory papillomatosis. European Archives of Otorhinolaryngology 2008;265(8):871–9.

Inflammatory Disorders of the Pediatric Airway

Alessandro de Alarcon and Charles M. Myer III

Key Points

- Inflammatory disorders of the pediatric airway compromise a distinct group of diseases that can present with acute and chronic airway compromise.
- Acute causes of inflammation include croup, epiglottitis, and membranous laryngotracheobronchitis.
- Chronic causes of inflammation include GERD and eosinophilic esophagitis.
- Diagnosis is based on clinical presentation, diagnostic studies, and endoscopy.
- Management is based on the specific disorder and the degree of airway distress.
- Acute causes of inflammation are often self-limited but can be life threatening.
- Chronic causes of inflammation can mimic some acute causes of obstruction and resolution of symptoms is based on appropriate diagnosis of the disorder and its treatment.

Keywords: Croup • Epiglottitis • Laryngotracheobronchitis • Gastroesophageal reflux • Eosinophilic esophagitis

A. de Alarcon
Division of Pediatric Otolaryngology – Head and Neck Surgery, Cincinnati Children's Medical Center, Cincinnati, OH USA

C.M. Myer III (✉)
Department of Otolaryngology – Head and Neck Surgery, University of Cincinnati College of Medicine, Pediatric Otolaryngology – Head and Neck Surgery, Cincinnati Children's Medical Center, Cincinnati, OH, USA
e-mail: Charles.Myer@cchmc.org

Introduction

Inflammatory disorders of the pediatric airway encompass an array of pathologic processes affecting the laryngotracheal complex. The major illnesses that cause inflammation within the airway can present with varying degrees of airway distress and can lead to major airway compromise, and in some cases, if untreated, death. It is of paramount importance that the clinician has an algorithm for the evaluation and management of children who present with acute airway compromise. Once the airway has been stabilized, the most likely underlying etiology should be considered and the appropriate treatment initiated.

It is beyond the scope of this chapter to describe all etiologies of pediatric airway obstruction and these are summarized in Table 1. The differential can be narrowed further based on the evaluation of the child, paying particular attention to clinical signs and symptoms (Table 2). Management of the acutely decompensating child mandates safety first and often involves cooperation from multiple specialists such as emergency medicine physicians, anesthesiologists, critical care physicians, pediatricians, and otolaryngologists.

Once a child is stable, the etiology of airway obstruction can be explored further. History and physical examination, as well as directed studies can help in the evaluation of these children. Inflammatory processes of the airway can be separated into those that are acute in nature and those that are chronic. It is important to recognize that some children with a chronic inflammatory process can present acutely with symptoms that may masquerade as a different disease process.

R.B. Mitchell and K.D. Pereira (eds.), *Pediatric Otolaryngology for the Clinician*,
DOI: 10.1007/978-1-60327-127-1_19, © Humana Press, a part of Springer Science + Business Media, LLC 2009

Table 1 Differential diagnosis of airway obstruction in children

Location	Congenital	Inflammatory	Neoplastic	Traumatic	Idiopathic
Nose/ Nasopharynx	Choanal atresia/Stenosis	Rhinitis	Juvenile angiofibroma	Nasal fracture	
	Pyriform aperture stenosis	Adenoid hypertrophy	Granulomatous disease	Septal fracture	
	Encephalocele	Retropharygeal abscess	Malignancy	Septal hematoma	
	Dermoid				
	Glioma				
	Craniofacial anomaly				
Oropharynx/ Hypopharynx	Glossoptosis	Tonsillar hypertrophy	Hemangioma		
	Lingual thyroid	Retropharygeal abscess	Lymphangioma		
	Dermoid	Cellullitis	Granulomatous disease		
	Vallecular cyst		Malignancy		
	Cricopharyngeal achalasia				
	CNS disease (hypotonia)				
Supraglottic	Laryngomalacia	Epiglottitis	Hemangioma		
	Laryngocele	Angioneurotic edema	Lymphangioma		
	Cyst	Abscess	Papilloma		
			Granulomatous disease		
			Malignancy		
Glottic	Web	Laryngitis	Hemangioma	Hematoma	
	Atresia	Spasm	Lymphangioma	Fracture	
	Cleft	Tuberculosis	Papilloma	Stenosis	
	Stenosis	GERD	Granulomatous disease	Foreign body	
	Vocal cord paralysis	Eosinophilic esophagitis	Malignancy		
Subglottic	Stenosis	Laryngotracheobronchitis (viral)	Hemangioma	Chondritis	
	Cyst	Laryngotracheobronchitis (bacterial)	Papilloma	Stenosis	
		Eosinophilic esophagitis	Malignancy	Fracture	
				Foreign body	
Tracheobronchial	Stenosis	Tracheitis (viral)	Thyroid	Stenosis	
	Complete rings	Tracheitis (bacterial)	Mediastinal tumors	Foreign body	
	Tracheomalacia		Malignancy		
	Vascular ring				
	Tracheoesophageal fistula				
	Reduplication of the trachea				
	Reduplication of the esophagus				
	Goiter				
Pulmonary	Hiatal hernia	Pneumonitis	Malignancy		
	Diaphragmatic hernia	Pneumonia			
	Pulmonary cyst	Toxic			
		Cystic fibrosis			

Evaluation

The evaluation of children with inflammatory processes of the airway should begin with a complete history and physical examination. Ancillary tests are helpful in establishing the diagnosis as well as eliminating other etiologies of obstruction. Airway films, flexible nasolaryngoscopy, and blood work have important roles when major causes of inflammatory airway disorders are considered and will be further discussed later in the chapter.

Table 2 Signs and symptoms of airway obstruction

Location	Voice	Airway noise	Retractions	Feeding	Cough
Oropharygeal	Muffled	Coarse/Stertor	Late	Drooling, jaw forward, poor feeding	None
Supraglottic	Muffled	Inspiratory	Late	Jaw forward, poor feeding	None
Glottic	Hoarse to aphonic	Biphasic	Present	Normal until late and severe	None
Subglottic	Normal	Biphasic	Present	Normal until late and severe	Barking
Tracheobronchial	Normal	Extrathoracic-biphasic Intrathoracic-expiratory washing machine	Late	Normal until late and severe Poor feeding early with extrinsic esophageal pressure	Brassy

Acute Inflammatory Disorders

The three main entities that are most common in children with acute airway obstruction secondary to an inflammatory process are viral laryngotracheobronchitis, membranous laryngotracheobronchitis, and epiglottitis *(1)*. An algorithm for the evaluation of acute airway disorders is presented in Fig. 1.

Croup

Acute laryngotracheobronchitis (LTB), or croup, is a viral upper respiratory infection that is most commonly caused by parainfluenza virus types I and II. Other upper respiratory viruses are sometimes implicated in this process such as respiratory syncitial virus (RSV) and influenza virus types A and B. Mycoplasma pneumoniae can cause LTB in the older child. The age of presentation is typically between 6 months and 3 years of age, with a peak incidence at age 2 *(2, 3)*. LTB commonly occurs during the late fall and early winter season: transmission is by direct contact. The incubation time is dependent on the particular virus and can range from 2 to 6 days. However, infected children can shed viral particles for up to 2 weeks following the acute episode. Children that are hospitalized for LTB should be placed in contact isolation and strict hand-washing protocols should be used to prevent nosocomial spread of infection, especially with RSV, which can be lethal if spread to children with congenital heart disease, chronic pulmonary disease, or immunodeficient patients.

The hallmarks of presentation are an upper respiratory infection for 1–3 days, low grade fevers, hoarseness, and a barking cough. A complete white blood cell count is often normal and is used to differentiate from bacterial causes such as epiglottitis and membranous laryngotracheobronchitis. The diagnosis should be suspected by the history and examination. Plain films will confirm the diagnosis by demonstrating hypopharyngeal overdistention as well as variable degrees of subglottic narrowing which is symmetric with a wider air column noted on expiration when compared to inspiration, thickened and irregular vocal cords and normal configuration of the epiglottis and aryepiglottic folds (Fig. 2). Flexible laryngoscopy often demonstrates normal supraglottic structures with variable degrees of erythema. The subglottis is often seen below the cords and may be edematous and erythematous.

Management is based on the degree of respiratory embarrassment of the child. Mild cases can be followed as outpatients while those with more severe obstruction, underlying medical issues, or severe distress should be placed under close observation. Medical management includes humidified air, racemic epinephrine, and steroids *(4)*. Rarely patients will need more definitive securement of the airway, i.e., intubation. The risk of subglottic stenosis in this setting is low (less than 3%); however, every precaution should be taken to prevent potential injury (for example, using appropriate-sized endotracheal tubes, shorter intubation times, and nasotracheal intubation). Rigid microlaryngoscopy and bronchoscopy should be reserved for those that fail medical management or extubation (to identify a cause of failure).

Children who present with recurrent croup should be evaluated for other pathology at a time when the airway is not acutely inflamed. Subglottic stenosis, gastroesophageal reflux disease (GERD), and eosinophilic esophagitis should be considered in the differential of these children.

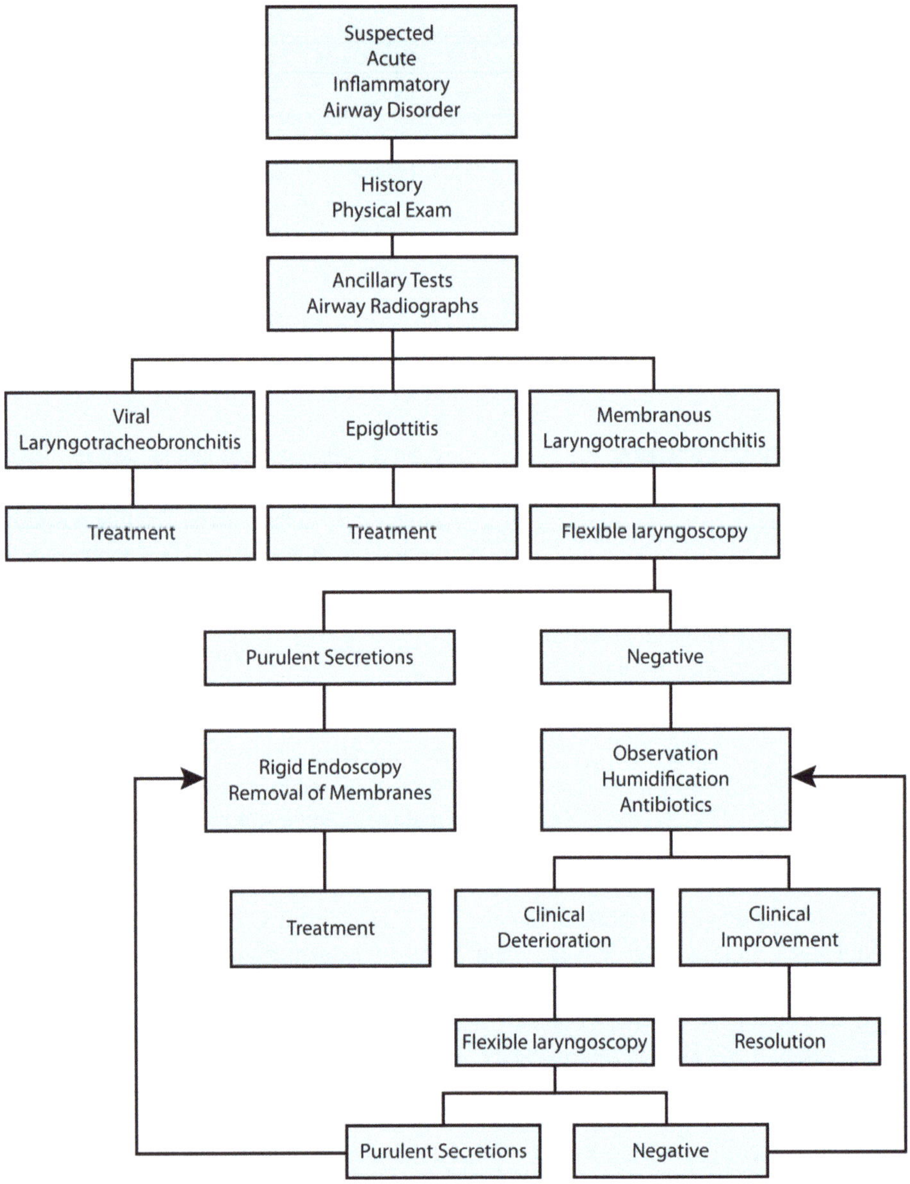

Fig. 1 Management algorithm for acute inflammatory airway disorders

Membranous Laryngotracheobronchitis

Membranous laryngotracheobronchitis (MLTB) is a condition which can overlap with LTB but with potentially more severe consequences. The illness has been called membranous croup as well as bacterial tracheitis. The age range affected is much broader than in LTB and tends to be an older population with an average age of 5 years but includes those in their teens *(5–7)*. The disease is believed to be secondary to a bacterial superinfection of an existing viral upper respiratory infection. The most commonly implicated organisms are *Staphylococcus aureus* and *Haemophilus influenza*, although other pathogens such as *Moraxella catarrhalis*, *Streptococcus pneumoniae* and, in rare

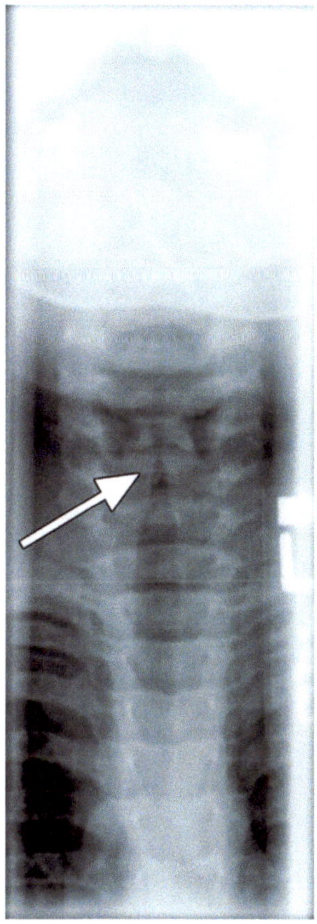

Fig. 2 Viral laryngotracheobronchitis. Frontal view X-ray. *Arrow* indicates classic "steeple" sign

cases, *Pseudomonas aeruginosa* have been identified in MLTB *(8,9)*.

The presentation again can be variable and can overlap with LTB. However, there are some distinct clinical characteristics that can differentiate a child with MLTB. These children usually appear more toxic than those with LTB. Additional indicators of severe MLTB are hoarseness (bordering on aphonia). Children often will not vocalize because of pain and the physical presence of membranes. Tenderness in the laryngotracheal complex which is out of portion to what would be expected can be a subtle clue. In the stable child, airway films and flexible nasolaryngoscopy may confirm a suspected diagnosis. Airway films often show shaggy exudates on the tracheal wall while endoscopy will demonstrate the thick purulent secretions in the airway (Fig. 3a,b).

MLTB requires operative management with microlaryngoscopy, rigid bronchoscopy, and removal of the offending membranes *(6, 7)*. Blood cultures and cultures of the membranes themselves should be performed. Endotracheal intubation may be needed after removing the membranes and this should be a decision made by the clinician based on the severity of the illness. Postdebridement management is essential in these patients. Intubated children will need frequent scheduled suctioning to prevent plugging. Humidification is important as secretions often persist for 3–5 days and it prevents the secondary accumulation of thickened membranes and crusts. Broad spectrum antibiotics should be used initially with more focused coverage when culture results return. There is no standard length of administration of antibiotics or observation in the hospital. However, conservative treatment should be employed to prevent potentially life-threatening events or recurrence.

Epiglottitis

The incidence of epiglottitis as an illness has all but disappeared since the implementation of the *H. influenza B* vaccine. Nontypable *H. influenza* has become a rare cause of epiglottitis *(10–12)*. In those who forego immunization or who come from other countries, one may see more cases of epiglottitis. The potential severity of this condition mandates that the clinician recognizes this entity, its hallmarks, and the treatment *(13)*.

In children with epiglottitis, there is a lack of a characteristic prodrome of a viral upper respiratory infection like that seen in LTB and MLTB. A common complaint is a rapidly progressive sore throat. As the infection progresses, the child becomes more toxic, lethargic, and with increasing symptoms of airway obstruction. These symptoms often begin 4–8 h after the initial sore throat. Tachypnea is common and the child will often sit in the "tripod" position, assuming an upright position with the neck extended and the arms providing support to maximize the size of the supraglottic airway. As the supraglottic edema progresses and tissues prolapse into the airway, the obstruction and stridor worsen. The voice will become muffled and drooling ensues. Lateral airway films will demonstrate the characteristic thumb sign of a thickened epiglottis (Fig. 4).

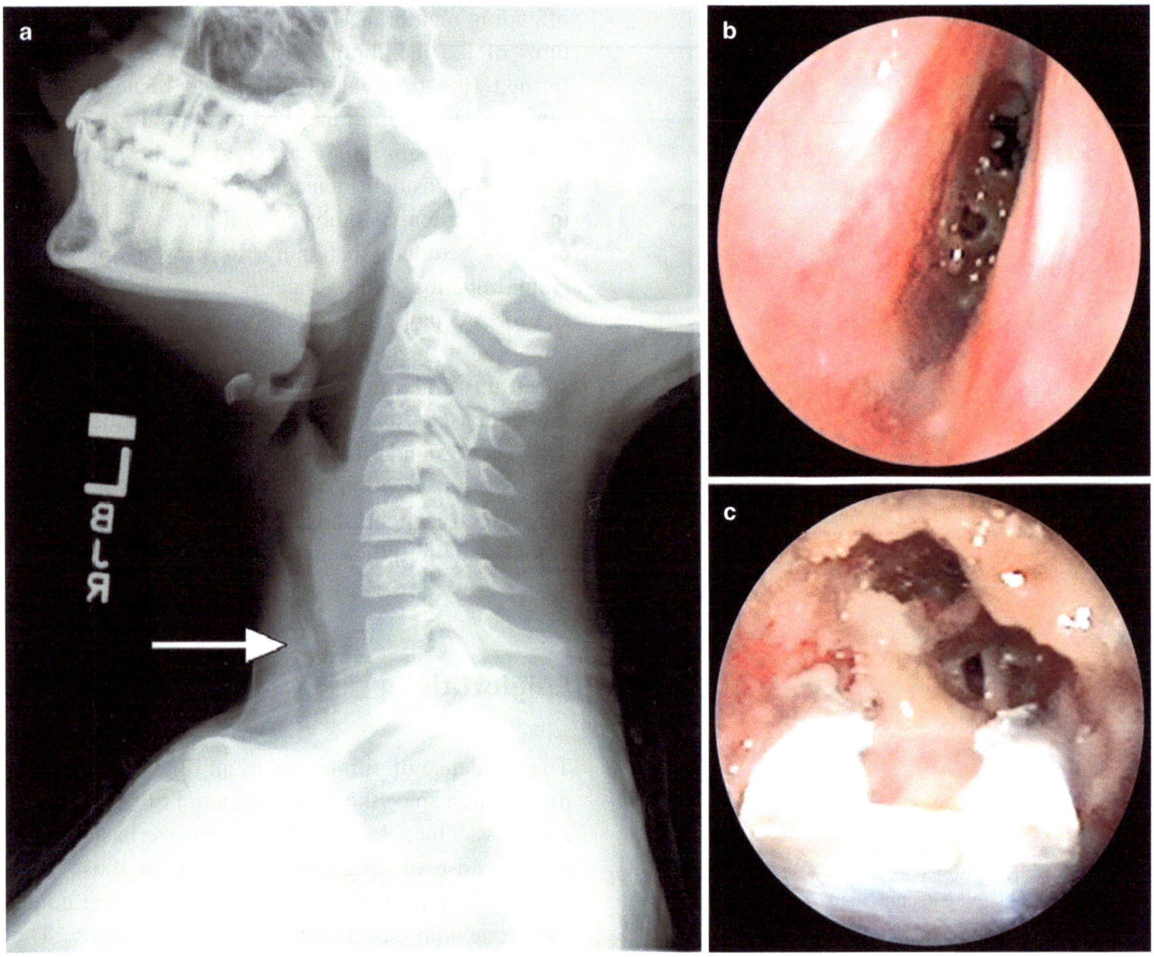

Fig. 3 (**a**) Membranous laryngotracheobronchitis. Lateral view X-ray. *Arrow* indicates the shaggy exudate on the anterior tracheal wall. (**b**) Membranous laryngotracheobronchitis. Endoscopic view of membranes occluding the subglottic lumen

If epiglottitis is suspected, the child should be under constant observation and placed in a setting where intubation can be performed readily and safely. Evaluation should be performed with the child breathing spontaneously. Endoscopic evaluation will reveal erythema and edema of the supraglottic structures (Fig. 5). Following diagnosis, nasotracheal intubation should be performed. If this is not successful, a ventilating bronchoscope should be used to secure the airway. Should this also fail, tracheotomy should be performed. Extubation is usually possible after 48 h and is guided by the ability to see the normal supraglottic structures with resolution of inflammation. Aerobic and anaerobic cultures should be taken to help direct appropriate antibiotic therapy and broad spectrum antibiotics should be used with a spectrum including *H. influenza* until culture results return.

Chronic Inflammatory Disorders

Children who have chronic inflammation of the laryngotracheal complex can mimic other acute airway disease processes. These disorders often can be distinguished based on the chronicity of the symptoms or, more commonly, the recurrence of symptoms (Fig. 6). Children with recurring symptoms should be evaluated for other pathology such as an underlying mild subglottic stenosis *(14,15)*.

Evaluation

Children with chronic airway inflammation are evaluated in a similar manner to those with acute inflammation. In these children, there may not be hallmark

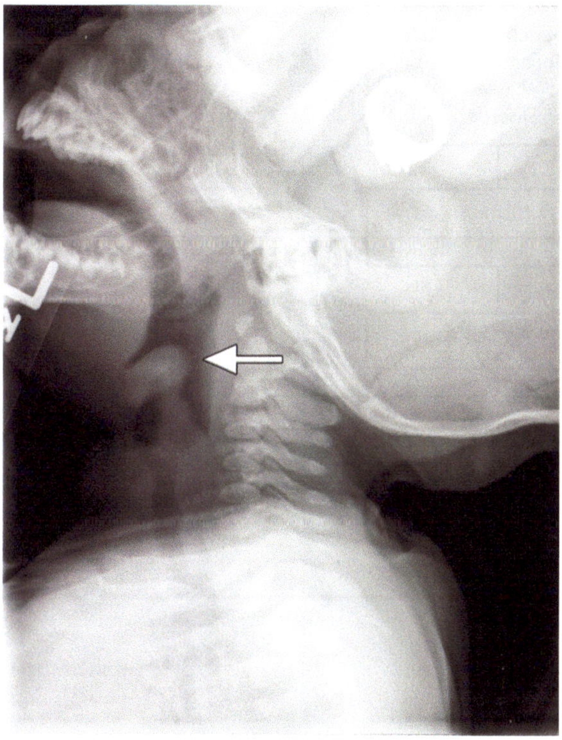

Fig. 4 Epiglottitis. Lateral view X-ray. *Arrow* indicates swollen epiglottis

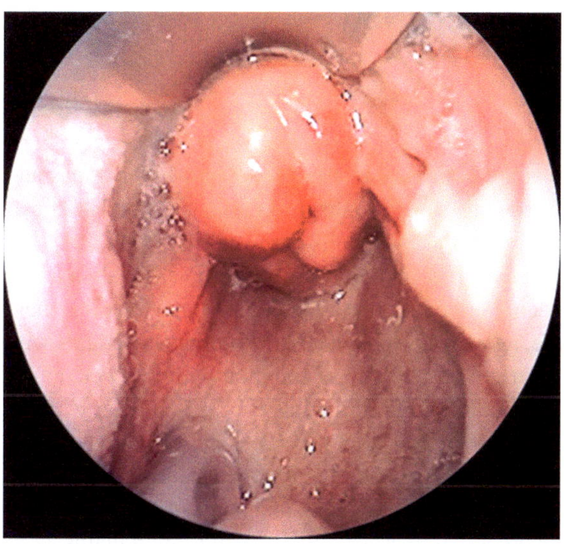

Fig. 5 Epiglottitis. Endoscopic view demonstrating inflamed and edematous epiglottis

signs or symptoms that will help identify the specific disorder. There are often clues from the history, physical exam, and lastly from the diagnostics preformed.

Like children with acute symptoms, airway films are obtained as part of the evaluation. They are often normal or with very little pathology that might explain the disease.

In these children, endoscopic evaluation in the operating room is often the modality that provides the key information that identifies the underlying etiology. Unlike those with an acute presentation, it is often best to bring these children for evaluation when they are less symptomatic or clinically well. Microlaryngoscopy, rigid bronchoscopy, and esophagoscopy are performed to evaluate for congenital, inflammatory, neoplastic, or traumatic disorders. Adjuncts that can help identify a potential etiology are flexible bronchoscopy and placement of an impedance probe or dual pH probe. These procedures often are performed in conjunction with pulmonologists and gastroenterologists. Once these evaluations are completed, a team approach can be useful in developing a treatment strategy. Two of the more common etiologies that can cause chronic inflammation of the airway are GERD and eosinophilic esophagitis (EE) ***(16–21)***.

Reflux-Associated Laryngitis

Reflux has been implicated as a frequently unrecognized cause of airway symptoms and pathology. Diagnosis is often difficult because the signs and symptoms can be subtle and nonspecific. Laryngeal findings such as arytenoid edema, erythema, pachydermia, and pseudosulcus vocalis all have been implicated as indicators of reflux. Impedance probe results, BAL washings showing lipid-laden macrophages, and esophageal biopsies showing chronic reflux esophagitis can help make the diagnosis.

Many of these children can be treated empirically with proton pump inhibitors and H_2 blockers in an effort to eliminate reflux as a possible etiology. Behavioral modification to decrease the symptoms associated with reflux include: completing the last meal two hours prior to bedtime, limiting caffeine intake, and modifying the diet to foods that do not stimulate acid secretion. The vast majority will see improvement with resolution of symptoms. If medical management fails, surgical management such as a Nissen fundoplication can be pursued ***(21)***.

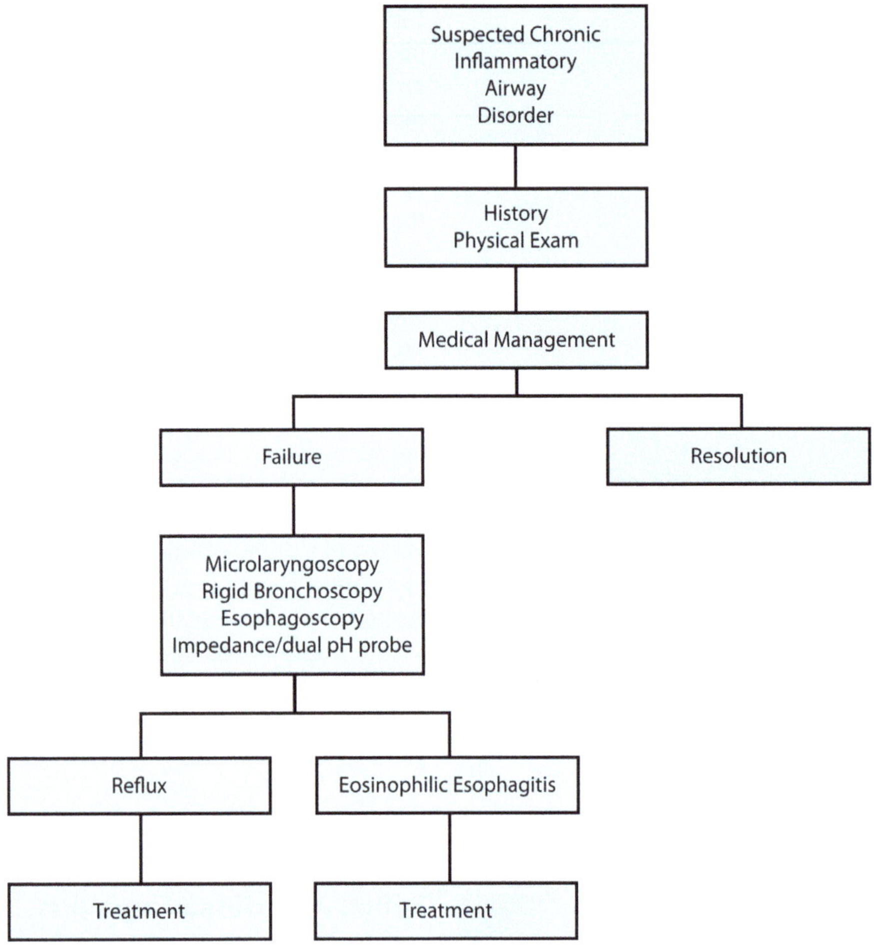

Fig. 6 Management algorithm for chronic inflammatory airway disorders

Eosinophilic Esophagitis

Eosinophilic esophagitis (EE) is an inflammatory disease with a predominately eosinophilic infiltrate within the esophagus that is unresponsive to acid suppression therapy. Although many of the symptoms of disease are associated with the esophagus, including dysphagia, choking and vomiting, and food impaction, airway symptoms are not uncommon and can be the initial presentation and the predominant problem *(19)*. Children will often have a history of allergy, in particular to foods, which may give a clue to the diagnosis.

Diagnosis is made by esophagoscopy and biopsy. Biopsies will show an eosinophilic infiltrate typically numbering greater than 24 eosinophils per high-powered field. The esophagus can appear normal on endoscopy. However, there are some characteristic findings that are indicative of EE, including white plaques and furrowing of the esophagus in mild cases and trachealization of the esophagus in severe cases (Fig. 7).

Laryngeal findings can be variable. Erythema and edema mimicking reflux are common. However, there are, again, some characteristic findings in patients with recurrent croup that are common with EE. Vocal nodules and blunting of the false vocal fold/anterior commisure region are common. There may be an associated mild grade I or grade II subglottic stenosis *(16)*.

Management involves treatment of the underlying disorders. Topically applied steroids are a mainstay of treatment, utilizing a "bad" inhaler technique with swallowing of the inhaled medication form of steroid inhalers. Diet modification and allergy testing also play a role *(22)*. These patients will need follow-up esophagoscopy to monitor disease and should be referred to a specialist who treats EE.

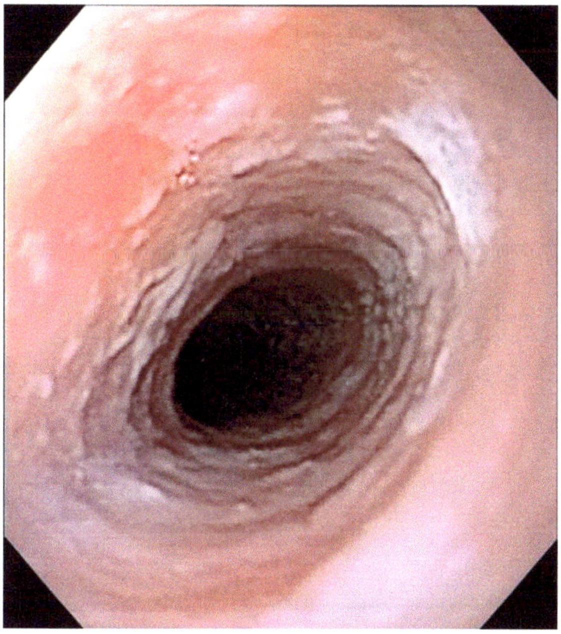

Fig. 7 Eosinophilic esophagitis. Endoscopic view during EGD with classic trachealization of the esophagus

Conclusion

Inflammatory disorders of the airway encompass diseases which can affect the airway in the acute and the chronic setting. Management of the airway is of paramount importance to the safety of the patient in the acute setting. A solid understanding of the more common acute etiologies and their hallmark signs and symptoms will ensure proper diagnosis and management. Chronic inflammatory processes can mimic some acute inflammatory diseases. Gastroesophageal reflux disease and eosinophilic esophagitis should always be kept in mind in this setting as they are treatable causes of airway inflammation.

References

1. Stroud RH, Friedman NR. An update on inflammatory disorders of the pediatric airway: epiglottitis, croup, and tracheitis. Am J Otolaryngol 2001;22:268–75.
2. Myer CM, 3rd., Holmes DK. Management of croup. Am J Dis Child 1990;144:267.
3. Myer CM, 3rd.. Inflammatory diseases of the pediatric airway. In: Cotton R, Myer IC, eds. Practical Pediatric Otolaryngology (1st edition). Philadelphia: Lippincott-Raven Publishers; 1999:547–59.
4. Bjornson CL, Johnson DW. Croup. Lancet 2008;371:329–39.
5. Salamone FN, Bobbitt DB, Myer CM, Rutter MJ, Greinwald JH, Jr. Bacterial tracheitis reexamined: is there a less severe manifestation? Otolaryngol Head Neck Surg 2004;131:871–6.
6. Gallagher PG, Myer CM, 3rd.. An approach to the diagnosis and treatment of membranous laryngotracheobronchitis in infants and children. Pediatr Emerg Care 1991;7:337–42.
7. Eckel HE, Widemann B, Damm M, Roth B. Airway endoscopy in the diagnosis and treatment of bacterial tracheitis in children. Int J Pediatr Otorhinolaryngol 1993;27:147–57.
8. Gold SM, Shott SR, Myer CM, 3rd. Radiological case of the month. Membranous laryngotracheobronchitis. Arch Pediatr Adolesc Med 1996;150:97–8.
9. Brook I. Aerobic and anaerobic microbiology of bacterial tracheitis in children. Clin Infect Dis 1995;20(Suppl 2):S222–3.
10. Gonzalez Valdepena H, Wald ER, Rose E, Ungkanont K, Casselbrant ML. Epiglottitis and Haemophilus influenzae immunization: the Pittsburgh experience – a five-year review. Pediatrics 1995;96:424–7.
11. Shah RK, Roberson DW, Jones DT. Epiglottitis in the Hemophilus influenzae type B vaccine era: changing trends. Laryngoscope 2004;114:557–60.
12. Guldfred LA, Lyhne D, Becker BC. Acute epiglottitis: epidemiology, clinical presentation, management and outcome. J Laryngol Otol 2007;25:1–6.
13. Verghese ST, Hannallah RS. Pediatric otolaryngologic emergencies. Anesthesiol Clin North Am 2001;19: 237–56, vi.
14. Kwong K, Hoa M, Coticchia JM. Recurrent croup presentation, diagnosis, and management. Am J Otolaryngol 2007;28:401–7.
15. Zalzal GH. Stridor and airway compromise. Pediatr Clin North Am 1989;36:1389–402.
16. Thompson DM, Orvidas LJ. Otorhinolaryngologic manifestations of eosinophilic esophagitis. Gastrointest Endosc Clin N Am 2008;18:91–8, ix.
17. Thompson DM, Arora AS, Romero Y, Dauer EH. Eosinophilic esophagitis: its role in aerodigestive tract disorders. Otolaryngol Clin North Am 2006;39:205–21.
18. Dauer EH, Freese DK, El-Youssef M, Thompson DM. Clinical characteristics of eosinophilic esophagitis in children. Ann Otol Rhinol Laryngol 2005;114:827–33.
19. Dauer EH, Ponikau JU, Smyrk TC, Murray JA, Thompson DM. Airway manifestations of pediatric eosinophilic esophagitis: a clinical and histopathologic report of an emerging association. Ann Otol Rhinol Laryngol 2006;115: 507–17.
20. Yellon RF, Goldberg H. Update on gastroesophageal reflux disease in pediatric airway disorders. Am J Med 2001;111(Suppl 8A):78S–84S.
21. Suskind DL, Zeringue GP, 3rd., Kluka EA, Udall J, Liu DC. Gastroesophageal reflux and pediatric otolaryngologic disease: the role of antireflux surgery. Arch Otolaryngol Head Neck Surg 2001;127:511–4.
22. Furuta GT, Liacouras CA, Collins MH, et al. Eosinophilic esophagitis in children and adults: a systematic review and consensus recommendations for diagnosis and treatment. Gastroenterology 2007;133:1342–63.

Tracheostomy in Children

Emily F. Rudnick and Ron B. Mitchell

Key Points

- Children needing a tracheostomy are more likely to be less than one year of age.
- Tracheostomy is indicated in children for one of three reasons:
  - Prolonged ventilator dependence (usually due to lung disease of prematurity)
  - Upper airway obstruction (including congenital, acquired, and craniofacial etiologies)
  - Increased need for pulmonary toilet (underlying neurological disease)
- Management of a tracheostomy in a child requires an interdisciplinary team of medical professionals who can assist with postoperative care, education, and therapy for the child and his or her family.
- Tracheostomy-related deaths have decreased in incidence, but still occur in up to 4% of children most commonly due to mucous plugging or accidental decannulation.
- Long-term complications of tracheostomy include tracheostomal granulation and persistent tracheocutaneous fistula after decannulation.

Keywords: tracheotomy • tracheostomy • ventilator dependence • neonatal tracheostomy

E.F. Rudnick (✉)
Division of Pediatric Otolaryngology, Department of Otolaryngology – Head and Neck Surgery, Johns Hopkins University School of Medicine, Baltimore, MD, USA
e-mail: erudnic2@jhmi.edu

R.B. Mitchell
Division of Pediatric Otolaryngology, Department of Otolaryngology – Head & Neck Surgery, Cardinal Glennon Children's Medical Center, Saint Louis University School of Medicine, St. Louis, MO, USA

Introduction

Tracheotomy is a complex procedure that has been performed on children since the seventeenth century. Historically, tracheotomy was performed to quickly relieve upper airway obstruction due to infectious processes such as diphtheria, epiglottitis, or croup. With the advent of improved neonatal care in recent decades, tracheostomy is now most commonly indicated in premature infants who require prolonged ventilatory support or because of failure of extubation secondary to congenital or acquired airway abnormalities. Another evolving indication for tracheotomy is control of pulmonary toilet in neurologically impaired children. Compared to in adults, tracheostomy in children is associated with significantly greater morbidity and mortality. However, complications have decreased significantly in recent years. In addition to complications related to the surgical procedure itself, children who undergo tracheostomy may experience prolonged difficulties with deglutition, speech, and general development. Therefore, the decision to perform tracheostomy should involve an interdisciplinary team of medical professionals who can assist with postoperative care, education, and therapy for the child and his or her family.

Definitions

Tracheotomy: Greek, meaning "to cut the trachea." *Tracheotomy* refers to the surgical procedure itself.

Tracheostomy: Greek, meaning "to furnish the trachea with an opening." *Tracheostomy* refers to the physical hole in the trachea (or the tube placed through it).

R.B. Mitchell and K.D. Pereira (eds.), *Pediatric Otolaryngology for the Clinician,*
DOI: 10.1007/978-1-60327-127-1_20, © Humana Press, a part of Springer Science + Business Media, LLC 2009

Demographics

The majority of tracheotomies are performed in children less than one year of age *(1)*. The incidence of tracheostomy among infants admitted to a NICU is 0.5–3% and declining in comparison to number of hospital admissions per year. Less than 30% of neonates who require prolonged mechanical ventilation will undergo tracheostomy.

Indications

Prolonged ventilatory support is the most common modern indication for tracheostomy in the pediatric population. Significant advances in neonatal care have dramatically increased survival rates of premature infants. Infants are now born younger and sustained for longer periods even with severe bronchopulmonary dysplasia and other comorbidities of prematurity. An important component of these advances is management of the airway in premature infants. The development of the polyvinyl chloride endotracheal tube has reduced intubation trauma and has made prolonged intubation the standard of care for premature infants requiring ventilatory support. These patients may be intubated for several months before tracheostomy is considered. The trend, however, is toward fewer days of intubation and ventilation with early extubation. Tracheostomy is usually recommended when safe extubation is not possible because of multiple failed attempts complicated by chronic lung disease or upper airway obstruction.

Upper airway obstruction is another common indication for tracheostomy in children. The main causes of upper airway obstruction in children that require tracheostomy for airway maintenance are:

- *Subglottic stenosis:* Subglottic stenosis is most often a result of prolonged endotracheal tube intubation. The endotracheal tube may cause ischemia and pressure necrosis of the tracheal mucosa and cartilages that results in circumferential stenosis at the level of the cricoid ring. A tracheostomy is often the first line of therapy allowing the child time to wean from the ventilator, leave the ICU, and later be considered for airway expansion surgery and decannulation.
- *Tracheomalacia:* Tracheomalacia is characterized by a collapse of the posterior membranous wall of the trachea during expiration which may cause significant or complete obstruction of the tracheal lumen. In tracheomalacia, the ratio of cartilaginous to membranous posterior wall is significantly smaller than in the normal trachea. While this condition in an otherwise healthy baby may resolve in 18–24 months, children with severe tracheomalacia may require mechanical positive pressure ventilation through a tracheostomy tube to sustain them. In the past, severe laryngomalacia, which is characterized by inward collapse of laryngeal structures on inspiration due to a delay in maturation of laryngeal structures, was managed with a tracheostomy. This has become less common, as successful endoscopic management of laryngomalacia has become more common.
- *Craniofacial syndromes*: Children born with syndromes that cause abnormal development of the craniofacial skeleton often display severe airway obstruction due to structural abnormalities of the maxilla, mandible, and palate that lead to crowding of the nasopharynx and oropharynx. This results in a complex clinical picture that may vary over time. In *Treacher-Collins* syndrome (mandibulofacial dysostosis), children may require tracheostomy due to significant micrognathia. In *Pierre-Robin* sequence, the upper airway obstruction is due to glossoptosis and micrognathia. Children with *Apert's* syndrome have a hypoplastic maxilla, pyriform aperture or choanal stenosis, and resultant naso/oropharyngeal crowding. Other craniofacial syndromes known to cause airway obstruction that may require tracheostomy include *Beckwith-Wiedemann* syndrome, *Crouzon* syndrome, *Pfeiffer* syndrome, and the *CHARGE* association.
- *Neoplasms:* Benign neoplasms such as respiratory papillomas, lymphangiomas, or subglottic hemangiomas occasionally cause severe upper airway obstruction requiring tracheostomy. Malignant tumors are far more rare causes of upper airway obstruction in pediatric patients.

Neurological condition requiring pulmonary toilet: A minority of patients who are neurologically impaired require tracheostomy to assist with ventilation, prevent chronic aspiration, or facilitate pulmonary toilet. Children who undergo tracheostomy for purposes of pulmonary toilet and neurological impairment are generally slightly older and have experienced multiple hospital admissions for upper respiratory infections and pneumonia. Most of these children are fed via a gastrostomy tube to reduce the frequency of aspiration. Common neurological conditions in children requiring tracheostomy include cerebral palsy, encephalopathy, myasthenia gravis, and traumatic brain injury.

Surgical Procedure

Tracheotomy is best performed in the operating room over an endotracheal tube. A rigid bronchoscope should be available for control of the airway and ventilation if needed.

The patient is positioned on a shoulder roll to optimize extension and exposure. The cricoid and hyoid cartilages are identified and marked preoperatively. A small incision is made in the skin just below the level of the cricoid cartilage. Subcutaneous fat is removed using electrocautery. The midline avascular muscular raphe is bluntly divided, and dissection is continued until the anterior tracheal wall is identified. Occasionally the isthmus of the thyroid gland obscures the tracheal wall. The isthmus may be either carefully elevated and divided using Electrocautery, or undermined and retracted superiorly. When the trachea is well visualized, a cricoid hook may be placed to carefully elevate the trachea into the field of view. Silk or polypropylene "stay" sutures are placed through the tracheal cartilages on either side of the planned vertical incision in the trachea. These sutures will facilitate tracheostomy tube change or replacement in the setting of an accidental decannulation. Using an 11-blade scalpel, a vertical incision is made through the 2nd and 3rd tracheal rings. The endotracheal tube is slowly retracted under direct visualization, and the tracheostomy tube is carefully inserted and connected to the ventilatory circuit. A chest X-ray is obtained postoperatively to confirm tube placement and proper lung expansion. In order to allow the tracheocutaneous fistula to mature, the child is usually observed for one week postoperatively. Observation in an intensive care unit is recommended in case of accidental decannulation and need for emergency airway access. The tracheostomy tube is changed on postoperative day 7 at which time the stay sutures are removed.

Tubes

Tracheostomy tube (Fig. 1) choice is dependent on the age and weight of the child as well as the indication for tracheostomy. In general, the tube with the smallest lumen that will maintain adequate ventilation is indicated in order to minimize mucosal trauma. Standard tracheostomy tube diameters and lengths for age are depicted in Table 1. Important principles to consider when choosing the appropriate tube include ***(2)***:

Inner diameter: Tubes are numbered according to the inner diameter (ID) of the tube in millimeters (mm). A premature infant may require a 3.0-mm ID tube, whereas a term infant should accommodate a 3.5-mm ID tube.

Length: Tubes are manufactured in neonatal, pediatric, pediatric long, and adjustable lengths. The distal tip of the tracheostomy tube should lie 7–20 mm proximal to the tracheal carina. This distance can be adequately measured by a plain chest radiograph.

Presence of cuff: Tracheostomy tubes are either cuffed or uncuffed. Cuffed tubes may be valuable in maintaining mechanical ventilation without significant air leak, or in assisting with control of aspiration and pulmonary toilet. Children with tracheostomy for relief of upper airway obstruction in general do not require cuffed tubes.

Caps and valves: Depending on the severity of ventilation requirements, children may be able to tolerate a speech valve or cap to assist with phonation and daytime activities. A Passy-Muir speech valve is a one-way valve that allows inspiration through the tracheostomy tube lumen but forces air out through the vocal cords allowing for production of sound and speech. Tracheostomy tube caps do not allow air to enter the lumen of the tube and should be worn only when the tracheostomy is in place to assist with daytime air exchange and phonation, or when decannulation is being considered. Children should be closely monitored during capping trials.

Complications

Tracheostomy complications are quite common and may occur up to 70% of the time ***(3)***. The incidence of tracheostomy-related mortality is reported to be up to 4% and is usually due to mucous plugging or accidental decannulation. Complications may occur during the operation, in the immediate postoperative period, and weeks, months, or years after tracheotomy in the delayed postoperative period. Important complications to consider include:

Hemorrhage: Careful surgical technique may prevent significant bleeding intraoperatively. Bleeding from the tracheostomy site postoperatively may stem from the raw mucosal surface of the fistula or from

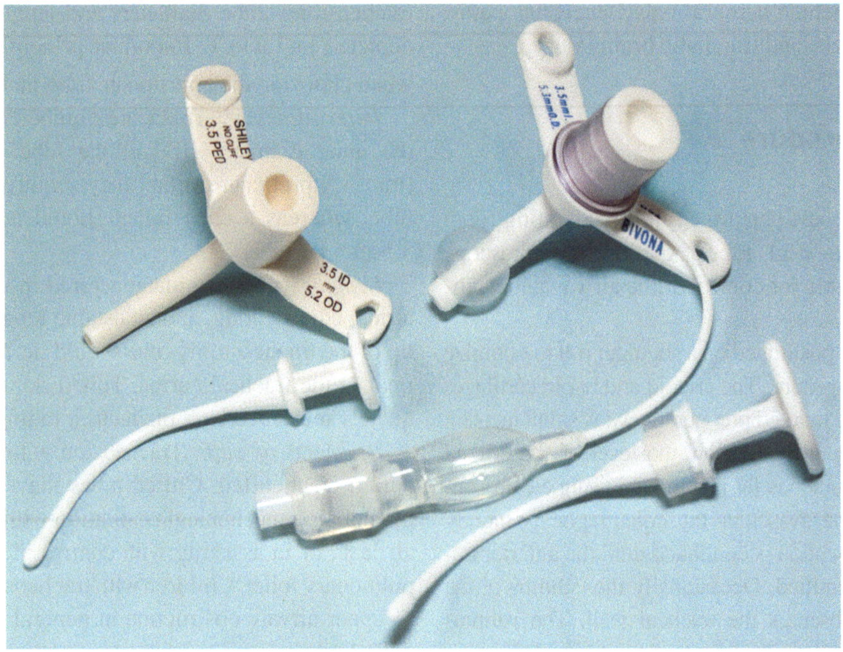

Fig. 1 Tracheostomy tubes and obturators. A cuffless 3.5 Shiley PED tube with obturator (*left*) and a cuffed Bivona 3.5 NEO tube with obturator (*right*)

Table 1 Common tracheostomy tube brands and size appropriate for age

		Shiley		Bivona		Portex	
Age	Suggested ID for age	ID	Length	ID	Length	ID	Length
Premature							
<1 kg	2.5	2.5 (neo)		2.5 (neo)	30		
				2.5 (peds)	38		
1–2.5 kg	3.0	3.0 (neo)	30	3.0 (neo)	32	3.0	36
			39	3.0 (peds)	39		
Neo to 6 months	3.0–3.5	3.5 (neo)	32	3.5 (neo)	34	3.5	40
		3.5 (peds)	40	3.5 (peds)	40		
6 months to 1 year	3.5–4.0	4.0 (neo)	34	4.0 (neo)	36	4.0	44
		4.0 (peds)	41	4.0 (peds)	41		
1 year to 2 years	4.0–4.5	4.5	42	4.5	42	4.5	48
>3 years	(Age in years + 16)/4	5.0	44	5.0	44	5.0	50
		5.5	46	5.5	46	5.5	52
		4 adult					
		6 adult					

ID Inner diameter in millimeters

Length Length of tube shaft in millimeters

Shiley (Shiley laboratories, Irvine, CA) tracheostomy tubes come as cuffless or cuffed (TTS-tight to shaft), fenestrated. An adjustable-length Shiley tube is also available measuring up to 80 mm in length

Bivona (Bivona Corporation, Gary, IN) tracheostomy tubes come cuffless or cuffed

Portex (Portex corporation) tracheostomy tubes are all cuffed and are longer than Shiley or Bivona tubes

granulation tissue. Over time, it is possible for the side or tip of the tracheostomy tube to erode into the innominate artery. This erosion which is often fatal can produce massive hemorrhage requiring emergency tamponade and surgical repair via median sternotomy.

Infection: Tracheostomy-related infections may be caused by stomal skin breakdown or celullitis. Tracheitis may occur episodically and is worse in the winters. Infections are managed expectantly with antibiotics, humidification, and wound care.

Stomal granulation: Granulation tissue is contact-induced inflammatory tissue that may develop in and around the tracheocutaneous tract. It will often bleed on manipulation, and excessive tissue may make tube changes more difficult. Granulation may be observed, cauterized at the bedside, or excised. It will frequently recur.

Tracheal suprastomal granulation or stenosis: Tracheostomy tubes may also irritate the mucosa within the tracheal lumen. Frequently, granulation develops in the suprastomal area or in the mucosa surrounding the tip of the tracheostomy tube. Tracheal stenosis may develop if the tube is placed too close to the cricoid cartilage or if the tip or cuff causes pressure necrosis on the tracheal mucosa and cartilage. These anatomical changes often require surgical removal or reconstruction, particularly if decannulation is anticipated.

Tracheocutaneous fistula: Following decannulation, a fistula may persist between the tracheal lumen and skin at the former site of the tracheostomy tube. This fistula can produce persistent drainage, skin irritation, and limit sound and speech production. It may occur up to 40% of the time. Correction is with surgical excision of the fistula.

Accidental decannulation: Accidental decannulation may occur at any stage following tracheostomy tube placement. Decannulation may be due to a small tube size, short tube length, or excessive patient motion in the setting of an immature tract. Particular care should be taken in attempting to reinsert a tracheostomy tube as a false passage may be created and subsequent ventilation may produce a pneumomediastinum and subcutaneous emphysema that obscures the airway. Decannulation can be an emergency and may lead to death.

Tracheostomy tube plugging: Mucous plugging of the tracheostomy tube may be severe and can lead to respiratory arrest and death. Plugging may be prevented with careful suctioning, humidification, and cleaning of the tube as well as with routine tube changes.

Additional Considerations

Speech: Children with tracheostomies who do not have significant airway stenosis should be encouraged to temporarily occlude their tube to create sound. Early intervention with a speech therapist is important in developing the most effective way of verbal communication for the individual patient.

Swallowing: Presence of a tracheostomy may produce significant difficulties with deglutition. Aspiration has been noted in a significant number of patients with tracheostomy due to loss of the normal laryngeal reflex. Pressure or interruption of the strap musculature may also contribute to swallowing difficulties, along with presence of an indwelling tube exerting pressure on the esophageal wall. Thickening liquids and swallow therapy may help in preventing aspiration.

Decannulation: Decannulation is often feasible in children with tracheostomy when their underlying problem has resolved. Large series evaluating tracheostomy patients report that up to 60% of patients are ultimately decannulated ***(4)***. Children who underwent tracheotomy as neonates for prolonged ventilation are the most likely patients to be successfully decannulated when they are older and have been off the ventilator for a significant period of time. Frequently, surgical intervention is required prior to decannulation to address tracheostomy-induced granulation, suprastomal collapse, or tracheal stenosis. Decannulation should always be performed in a controlled setting after monitored capping trials and a detailed endoscopic evaluation of the airway in the operating room. Children are routinely observed overnight following decannulation.

References

1. Carron JD, Derkay CS, Strope GL, et al. Pediatric tracheotomies: changing indications and outcomes. Laryngoscope 2000; 110(7):1099–1104.
2. Cochrane LA, Bailey CM. Surgical aspects of tracheostomy in children. Paediatr Respir Rev 2006; 7(3):169–174.
3. Wetmore RF, Marsh RR, Thompson ME, et al. Pediatric tracheostomy: a changing procedure. Ann Otol Rhinol Laryngol 1999; 108(7 Pt 1):695–699.
4. Sidman JD, Jaguan A, Couser RJ. Tracheotomy and decannulation rates in a level 3 neonatal intensive care unit: a 12-year study. Laryngoscope 2006; 116(1):136–139.

Cleft Lip and Palate

Kathleen Wasylik and James Sidman

Key Points

- Cleft lip and palate is a common birth defect, and is the most common congenital defect of the head and neck.
- More than 300 syndromes are known to be associated with orofacial clefting but cleft palate is more likely to be syndromic than cleft lip ± palate.
- There are many issues that result from a cleft lip and palate. These include feeding problems, speech difficulties, otologic issues, midface growth impairment, cleft lip nasal deformities, and dental problems. A multidisciplinary team approach is mandatory.
- Often patients with a cleft palate have velopharyngeal insufficiency, requiring either a pharyngeal flap or a sphincter pharyngoplasty.
- Many of the unilateral and bilateral cleft lip patients will also require at least one revision surgery to deal with the commonly associated cleft lip nasal deformities.

Keywords: Cleft lip • Cleft palate • Velopharyngeal insufficiency

Introduction

Cleft lip and palate is a common birth defect that can be isolated or part of a syndrome. As a newborn, palatal clefts can cause difficulties with feeding and failure to thrive, requiring special attention and alternative feeding methods. Clefts of the lip are repaired very early in life, and may only require a single surgery. Later issues that arise with isolated cleft lips are generally related to the associated nasal deformities. Cleft palates can be more complicated and are almost always associated with eustachian tube dysfunction, palatal incompetence, and speech problems. Additionally, patients with cleft palates experience midface growth deficiency often requiring orthognathic surgical intervention. Patients with cleft lips often require a secondary rhinoplasty later in adolescence (Fig. 1).

Facial clefting can be divided into either cleft palate or cleft lip with or without palate. Cleft lips can be unilateral or bilateral. The cleft can be incomplete or complete, depending on whether the cleft extends superiorly into the nasal sill and involves a complete interruption of the orbicularis oris muscle. There is also a phenotypic spectrum of the incomplete cleft lip. The most minor form of incomplete cleft lip is termed microform, which is a lack of fusion of the orbicularis muscle with an overlying intact skin. The superior portion of the incomplete cleft lip can either contain normal orbicularis oris muscle or only a fibrous attachment, termed the Simonart's band.

Cleft palates associated with cleft lips can involve either the primary or secondary palate. The palate is divided into primary and secondary based on its location relative to the incisive foramen. The primary is located anteriorly and the secondary is located posteriorly. When it involves the primary palate, it extends from the incisive foramen anteriorly through the maxillary alveolus. Clefting of the secondary palate is the result of the failure of the palatine processes to fuse in the midline. The vomer, however, can be fused to

J. Sidman, M.D., (✉)
Department of Otolaryngology, University of Minnesota, Children's Hospitals and Clinics, Minneapolis, MN, USA
e-mail: sidma001@umn.edu

K. Wasylik
Pediatric Otolaryngology Head and Neck Surgery Associates, St. Petersburg, FL, USA

R.B. Mitchell and K.D. Pereira (eds.), *Pediatric Otolaryngology for the Clinician*,
DOI: 10.1007/978-1-60327-127-1_21, © Humana Press, a part of Springer Science + Business Media, LLC 2009

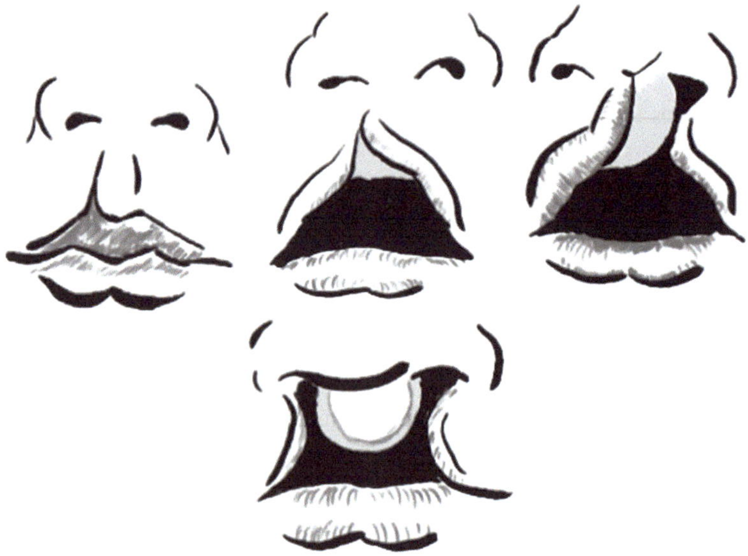

Fig. 1 Spectrum of lip clefting. *Left–right*, microform cleft lip, incomplete unilateral cleft lip, complete unilateral cleft lip, and complete bilateral cleft lip. *Reproduced with permission from Timothy Lander M.D*

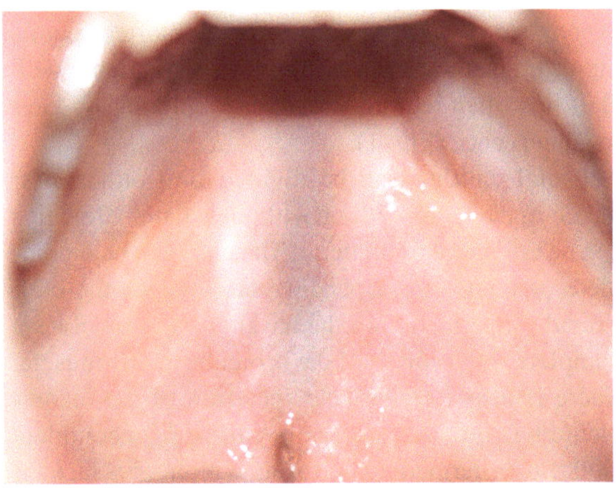

Fig. 2 A submucous cleft palate, with the typical zona pellucida secondary to the muscular dehiscence

either side *(1)*. A cleft lip can be associated with either primary or secondary cleft palates. A cleft in the primary palate can occur with a cleft lip, but embryologically it is impossible for a notched maxillary alveolus to be present in an isolated fashion.

It is best not to describe the cleft palate as unilateral or bilateral, but whether it involves the hard palate in addition to the soft palate, and whether or not the vomer is fused to one side or another. A submucous cleft palate indicates a muscular dehiscence in the soft palate despite an overlying intact mucosal envelope, and can often go undetected (Fig. 2).

Epidemiology

Clefting of the lip and/or palate is one of the most common congenital defects, and is the most common to occur in the head and neck. Its incidence ranges from 1:300 to 1:1,200 *(2)*. A cleft lip with or without a cleft palate is considered to be a distinct epidemiological and embryologic entity from an isolated cleft palate *(3)*. Cleft lip is associated with a palatal cleft in two thirds of cases *(3)*.

The incidence of cleft lip with or without cleft palate varies significantly by racial group. The highest incidence occurs in children with an Asian or Native American background, approaching 1:500 births. That incidence is 1:1,000 births in the Caucasian population and 1:2,500 in those with an African descent *(3)*. However, the incidence of isolated cleft palate is about 1:1,500–2,000 births with no racial variability *(3)*. Isolated cleft palate is less common than cleft lip with or without palate *(1)*. Unilateral cleft lip with or without palate is twice as common as bilateral cleft lip with or without palate and for reasons that are unclear, the unilateral cleft lip more commonly affects the left side. It also tends to occur more frequently in males *(1)*.

Anatomy

The principal muscle of the lip is the orbicularis oris, which interdigitates with other muscles of expression of the mid and lower face. In a complete cleft lip, this muscle parallels the margins of the cleft and inserts on the alar base laterally and the columellar base medially. These abnormal insertions result in an abnormal rotation of the premaxilla outward, while the unopposed lateral segment is retrodisplaced (Figs. 3 and 4).

The septum becomes displaced into the noncleft side, due to both muscular tension as well as lack of bony support. This deviation of the septum results in a shortening of the columella and a flattening of the ipsilateral lateral crus (Figs. 5 and 6).

The lip has a shortened philtum, and the peak of Cupid's bow is rotated. Incomplete cleft lips will have a similar arrangement, except that it is possible for the superior fibers of the orbicularis oris sphincter to be intact. Often even the incomplete cleft lip has a complete dehiscence of the muscular sling, and only the soft tissue known as Simonart's band is present. The microform lip is usually a minor muscular dehiscence with vermillion notching, although the overlying soft tissue envelope is entirely intact *(3)*. Microform cleft

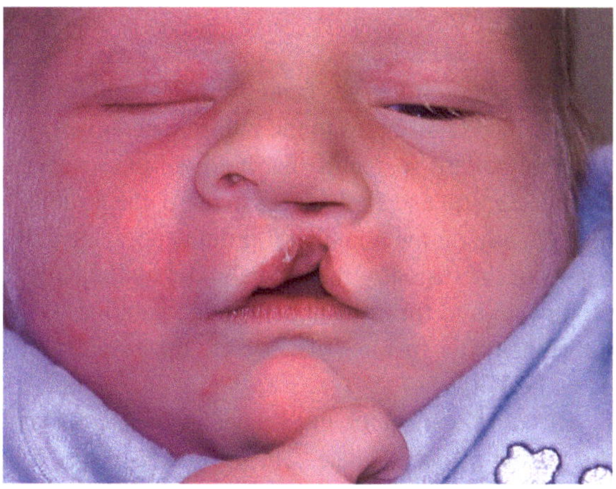

Fig. 3 An incomplete unilateral cleft lip

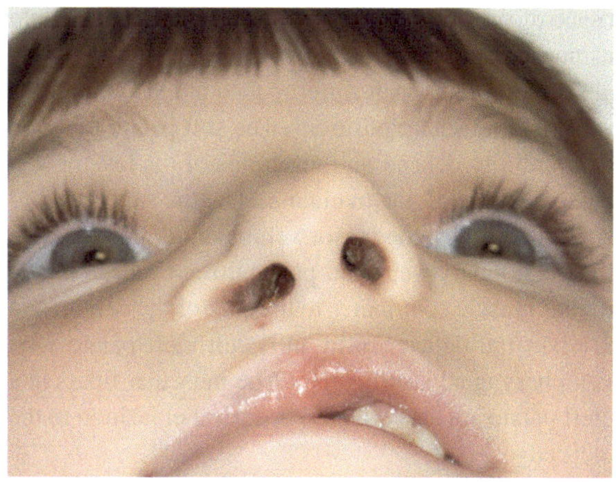

Fig. 5 The typical cleft lip nasal deformity associated with a unilateral cleft lip. Note the ipsilateral collapsed ala

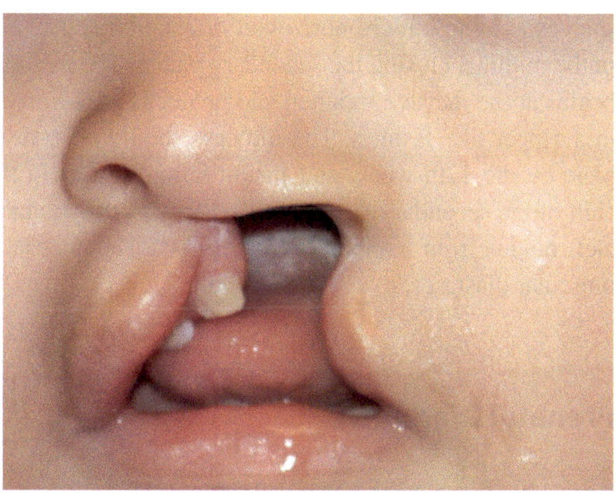

Fig. 4 A complete unilateral cleft lip

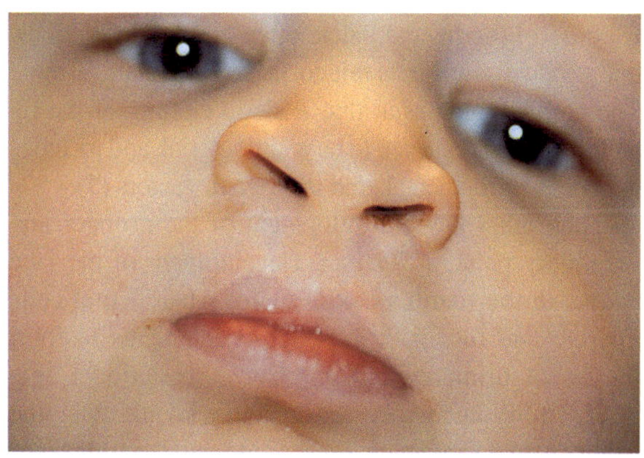

Fig. 6 The typical cleft lip nasal deformity associated with a bilateral cleft lip. Note the markedly shortened columella, and the flared ala

lip is often recognized by the associated flattened lower lateral cartilage of the nose.

The bilateral cleft lip has similar anatomical tendencies, with the orbicularis fibers arranged parallel to the cleft and inserting on the lateral ala. The prolabium has no muscular fibers. It is flattened and has no philtral markings. The unopposed midface will result in an unrestrained forward growth of the vomer and nasal septum. This can result in significant protrusion of the premaxilla. The columella is very short and has no bony support. Like the unilateral lip, the alae have a flattened lateral crura. The projected vomer and premaxilla can result in a locked-out premaxilla after the lip repair, where the lateral palatal shelves have collapsed medially behind the premaxilla, so that after repair of the soft tissue of the lip, the premaxilla is unable to recede into its normal anatomical position *(4)*.

The problems with a cleft palate are also due to its abnormal muscular positions. The soft palate function and mobility depend on the actions of the levator veli palatine muscles, the uvula muscles, the superior constrictor muscles, the tensor veli palatine muscles, and the palatopharyngeus and palatoglossus muscles. The uvular muscle contributes to the bulk of the velum, and is often the deficiency in an occult cleft palate with velopharyngeal insufficiency. The muscular fibers in a cleft palate are also oriented in a parallel fashion to the cleft edges.

Embryology

Clefting of the lip and palate often clusters in families, but is usually not transmitted in a Mendelian fashion. The embryologic insult that leads to clefting of the lip and/or palate is believed to be multifactorial, and includes genetic, environmental, and teratogenic factors *(5)*.

The embryologic development of the primary and secondary palate is distinct. Development of the face begins in the fourth week in utero, when neural cells migrate and fuse with mesodermal elements to form the facial primordium. At 35 days gestational age, three embryonic processes become identifiable: the frontonasal prominence, the paired medial nasal prominences, and the maxillary prominences *(6)*. The frontonasal prominence is the central segment of the face that primarily develops into the forehead, supraorbital ridges, nose, philtrum, and primary palate. The paired medial nasal prominences form the intermaxillary segment, which contributes to the philtrum and gives rise to the maxillary segments that hold the incisor teeth. During the fifth and sixth weeks in utero, the proliferative growth of the maxillary prominences medially results in the fusion of the medial nasal and maxillary prominences to form the upper lip and anterior alveolus. When this fusion fails, a cleft lip and alveolus occur *(7)* (Fig. 7).

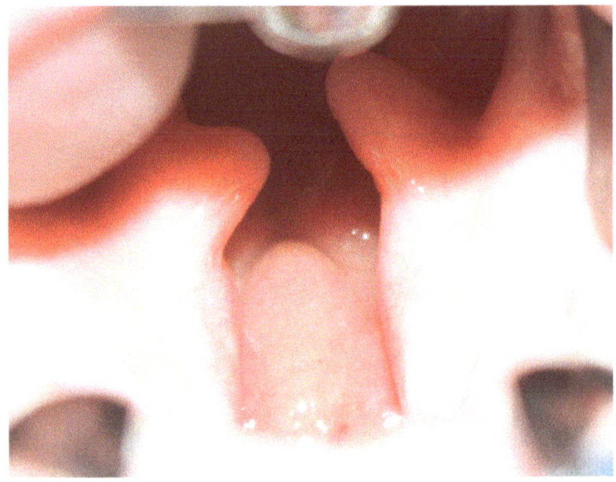

Fig. 7 A surgical perspective of a cleft palate involving both the hard and soft palate, with the vomer present in the midline

The development of the secondary palate follows that of the primary palate. The secondary palate is a result of the fusion of the paired outgrowths of the maxillary prominences. These prominences, termed palatal shelves, are evident during the sixth week of development as vertically oriented growths on either side of the tongue. By the following week in utero, the palatal shelves assume a more horizontal orientation and fuse in the midline, closing the secondary palate. The fusion begins at the incisive foramen and proceeds posteriorly in a zipper-like fashion. This process should be complete by the 12th week, and fusion failure results in a cleft of the secondary palate. The severity of the palatal cleft ranges from a submucous cleft, or a submucosal muscular diastases, to a complete cleft *(3)*.

Prenatal Diagnosis

The ultrasound diagnosis of facial clefting was first reported over 20 years ago *(8, 9)*. It is highly sensitive in diagnosing a cleft lip, but has variable success in diagnosing a cleft palate in utero. Although the midline structures are fused by 8 weeks, imaging is not reliably achieved until week 15 because of head positioning and the relatively small size of the face in comparison to the tranducer. Generally, although the specificity of prenatal diagnosis by ultrasound is high, the sensitivity is low. This can be attributed to an unfavorable position of the fetus, the skill of the sonographer, or lack of emphasis on this diagnosis *(8)*. The isolated cleft palate is particularly difficult to identify prenatally because of the acoustic shadow of the facial bones *(8)*. Recent advances in ultrasound allow for three-dimensional images, which can illustrate facial abnormalities with increased clarity.

Associated Syndromes

Over 30% of infants born with a cleft lip and palate (and over 50% of those with cleft palate) have other associated malformations. The central nervous system and skeletal system are the most commonly involved systems *(10)*. More than 300 syndromes are known to be associated with orofacial clefting. A careful craniofacial and skeletal exam at birth should reveal clues to any associated syndromes. For example, down-slanting lateral canthi may indicate Treacher Collins syndrome. Auricular abnormalities may reveal a hemifacial microsomia. Lip pits are often indicative of the autosomal dominant transmission of Van Der Woude's syndrome. Paralysis of cranial nerves six and seven is the hallmark of Mobius syndrome. Digital malformations can include Nager syndrome or Otopalataldigital syndrome. Micrognathia and glossoptosis in addition to the cleft palate defines Pierre Robin Sequence. Finally, the syndrome most commonly associated with Pierre Robin Sequence is Stickler syndrome, a progressive condition affecting collagen, which can be identified with ophthalmologic examination and genetic testing.

The most common associated chromosomal abnormality is a deletion of the long arm of the 22q11, which occurs in 90% of those diagnosed with velocardiofacial syndrome (VCF). Almost 10% of children with a cleft palate (but without a cleft lip) will be diagnosed with VCF *(11)*. Children with velocardiofacial syndrome can have long-term learning disabilities, as well as psychosocial issues. DiGeorge syndrome also involves abnormalities in the same chromosomal region, which can in turn have associated immunological deficiencies. Any conotruncal abnormalities should prompt the physician to investigate the possibility of VCF or DiGeorge syndrome. Trisomy 13 and 18 are also chromosomal abnormalities commonly associated with a cleft palate *(10)*.

Feeding Issues

One of the greatest initial challenges of a newborn with a cleft palate is difficulty with feeding. Because of the cleft in the palate, the infant is unable to create a seal and generate an adequate suck. Affected children are unable to generate negative pressures, and this feeding difficulty can lead to failure to thrive. In order to avoid this, alternative feeding methods are undertaken. Parents need to be taught to use special squeeze bottles, such as the Haberman or Pigeon bottle, that eliminate the need to generate negative pressure by the infants *(12)*. These bottles also reduce air ingestion allowing for the overall improvement of digestion. A newborn with a cleft should be able to ingest 3 ounces within 20–30 min. Having a cleft palate prohibits the ability to breast feed, except under very unusual circumstances *(3)*. Infants with isolated cleft lips do not experience these difficulties with feeding, and can be breast- or bottle-fed.

Otologic Issues

The presence of middle ear effusions in children with cleft palate is universal *(13)*. The underlying etiology of otitis media with effusion is the abnormal palatal musculature, and in particular, altered tensor veli palatini function leading to eustachian tube dysfunction *(2)*. Instead of its normal insertion along the posterior edge of the hard palate and the palatal aponeurosis, the tensor muscle inserts along the bony edges of the cleft *(3)*. Additional abnormalities include diastases of the uvular muscle as well as an interruption of the levator sling. Because of this eustachian tube dysfunction, children with cleft palates will almost uniformly have serous otitis media at some time in early childhood and require insertion of tympanostomy tubes *(13)*.

Many syndromes that occur with clefts are also associated with sensorineural hearing loss including Stickler, Van der Woude, Waardenbergs, and Klippel-Feil syndromes. Auditory brainstem evaluations are often a necessary step in the diagnostic evaluation of these children.

It has been suggested in the past that surgical repair of cleft palate will normalize eustachian tube function *(14, 15)* but it has not been proven. Ultimately, children's eustachian tube function normalizes by the time they are 5 or 6 years of age in 75–94% of patients but may require lifelong otologic examinations *(16– 18)*.

Speech Issues

Earlier repair of the cleft palate is associated with better speech development. The speech difficulties in association with cleft palate are twofold. Hypernasality and nasal air escape from velopharyngeal insufficiency can result from inadequate length or poor movement of the palate. This will often lead to unintelligibility. As a result of this unintelligibility, there are often secondarily learned compensatory responses, such as glottal stops, pharyngeal fricatives, and consonant substitutions.

If intense speech therapy fails, there are two surgical options for velopharyngeal insufficiency. A sphincter pharyngoplasty is indicated when there is deficient movement of the lateral walls of the pharynx, or when there is a combined deficiency of the lateral walls and palate. The sphincter, which is characterized by a central port, is created by rotating superiorly based posterior tonsillar pillars and suturing them to the posterior pharyngeal wall as high as possible, just below the inferior aspect of the adenoid pad. The resulting sphincter is considered to be dynamic *(19)*. The alternative is a pharyngeal flap, which rotates a superiorly based myomucosal flap from the posterior pharyngeal wall, and insetting it into the palate, obliterating most of the nasopharyngeal passage. Two lateral ports for nasal airflow are incorporated *(20)*. This surgical technique is particularly helpful for short palates. The pharyngeal flap is at much higher risk for precipitating obstructive sleep apnea. It is felt the dynamic sphincter pharyngoplasty confers better speech results *(21, 22)*.

Presurgical Maxillary Orthopedics

Nasoalveolar molding devices (NAM) are utilized to reduce the severity of the initial cleft lip deformity, and are designed to optimize the repair by altering the bony and soft tissue components. Some devices address the alveolus, lip, and the nose. The goals of the NAM are to mold the lip segments so that they are in contact at rest (Figs. 8 and 9).

In a bilateral cleft lip, the presurgical orthopedics can gently retract the premaxilla until it is in contact with the lateral alveolar segments, achieving a normal dental arch, ideally preventing the maxilla from becoming locked out. The primary lip repair is then generally delayed a couple of months until it is felt that the cleft

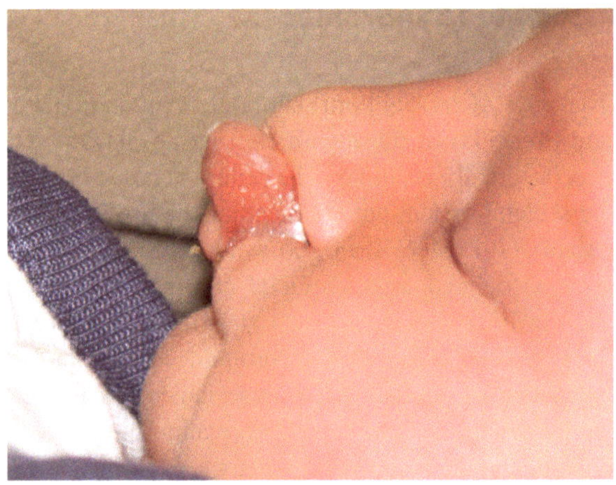

Fig. 8 A bilateral cleft lip with premaxilla protrusion

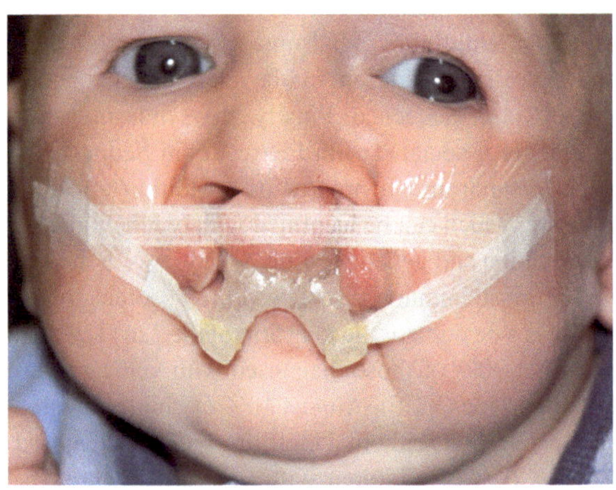

Fig. 9 The nasoalveolar molding device used prior to repair of the bilateral cleft lip

can be closed without significant tension. Complications of the presurgical orthopedics are related to irritation, ulceration, and intolerance of the device *(23)*.

Surgical Intervention

Both cleft lips and palates need to be surgically repaired. The timing of repair can be debated, but generally cleft lips are repaired between 8 and 12 weeks, and the palate is repaired between 9 and 12 months. Commonly quoted criteria for the initial lip repair would follow the "rule of 10s," indicating the infant must be 10 weeks old, weigh 10 pounds, and have a hemoglobin of 10 g/dL. This, however, is considered antiquated with modern anesthesia, and is only applicable in Third-World countries. Bone grafts to repair alveolar notching and incisive foramen fistulae are undertaken when the child is 5 or 6 years of age, before the eruption of permanent dentition *(24)*. Definitive rhinoplasty is performed when the female child reaches 14 years of age, and when the male child is between 15 and 16 years of age to allow for completion of facial growth. Occasionally, should social pressures necessitate it, the rhinoplasty may be done at an earlier age, with the understanding that as bone grafts are performed, and facial growth occurs, the overlying soft tissue envelope will change, altering the outward appearance.

Most commonly, all palatal interventions are performed in a single-staged fashion. There are, however, advocates of the two-stage palate repair. This involves closing the soft palate early, between 3 and 6 months of age, and delaying the repair of the hard palate until the child is several years old *(25)*. This would theoretically limit the effect of the hard palate repair on maxillary growth. It is suggested that the subperiosteal scarring impairs midfacial growth *(3)*. There are several studies, however, that have shown there is no significant difference in craniofacial morphology between kids that have their repair at 8 months versus 8 years *(3, 26)*. The real downfall of delaying palate surgery is an unacceptable compromise on speech, and so hard palate obturators must be used until surgical repair is undertaken.

The goals of the surgical intervention of the lip include providing adequate length of the lip, precise alignment of the vermillion border, and good muscular approximation of the orbicularis sphincter. The Millard rotation advancement repair is the workhorse of cleft lip surgery. It is designed such that the medial portion of the cleft side becomes the rotation flap, and allows for the downward rotation of the short lip. The advancement flap is designed from the lateral soft tissues, and is inset medially into the defect that results from the rotation of the medial lip. The triangular flap, also known as the Randall-Tennison repair, is an alternative method for cleft lip repair, and is often utilized for the complete unilateral cleft lip, especially when the defect is wide, but does not recreate the philtral column as naturally as the rotation-advancement flap.

The bilateral cleft lip is best approached with the Straight Line Closure of Veau, which allows for the creation of the appropriate philtral width out of the prolabium tissues. The orbicularis oris muscle is approximated at the inferior aspect of the prolabium *(27)*.

It is not unusual for cleft lip repairs to require revision surgery. Revision may range from minor vermillion adjustments to full take downs to gain additional lip length, or even a lip switch procedure for severely deficient soft tissue. These procedures usually occur as the patient is about to enter school to avoid social pressures.

The overall goals of repairing the palate include closing the cleft, providing sufficient length to the palate, as well as obtaining good muscle approximation to improve velopharyngeal function. The type of cleft involving the palate will generally dictate what type of closure is required. A cleft involving only the soft palate can be repaired with a Double Z-Plasty, which has several benefits, including nonopposing suture lines, as well as the potential lengthening of the palate *(28, 29)*. All clefts involving the hard and soft palate require a two-layer closure, with both nasal flaps and oral flaps. The von Langenbeck variation allows for laterally placed relaxing incisions, and the anterior oral mucosa is released off the hard palate as one unit. The Wardill-Kilner (V-Y) palatoplasty leaves the anterior oral mucosa down by connecting the lateral incisions to the incisions made for the nasal turn in flaps. This in theory also allows for a lengthening of the palate, but without a concurrent release of the nasal mucosa, it is unlikely there is any substantial gain in length. Finally, if the cleft of the hard palate is complete, the oral mucosa incision parallels the cleft margins, resulting in a two-flap palatoplasty. The incisive foramen fistula is unavoidable, and is generally repaired with an alveolar bone graft around 5 years of age, which allows for timely tooth eruption ***(30, 31)***.

There is much discussion about rhinoplasty at the time of the primary lip repair. Certainly, the nasal deformity is improved with the cleft lip repair. Because the growth of the facial skeleton changes the appearance of the overlying soft tissue so much, it is unrealistic to think that anything beyond minor modifications of the position of the ala and lower lateral cartilages is useful. Definitive rhinoplasties are best done upon the completion of the growth of the facial skeleton and any bone grafts that need to be done.

Conclusion

Cleft lips and palates are the most common congenital defect of the head and neck. There are many associated issues that can plague the child permanently. It is important to coordinate the care of the cleft patient using a multidisciplinary team approach.

References

1. Campbell S, Lees C, Moscoso G, Hall P. Ultrasound antenatal diagnosis of cleft palate by a new technique: the 3D reverse face view. Ultraound Obstet Gynecol 25:2005.
2. Goudy S, Lott D, Canady J. Conductive hearing loss and otopathology in cleft palate patients. Otolaryngol Head Neck Surg 134:2006.
3. Arosarena O. Cleft lip and palate. Otolaryngol Clin North Am 40:2007.
4. Mulliken J. Bilateral cleft lip. Clin Plast Surg 31:2004.
5. Eppley B. The spectrum of orofacial clefting. Plast Reconstr Surg 115(7):2005.
6. Jiang, R, Bush J, Lidral A. Development of the upper lip: morphogenetic and molecular mechanisms. Dev Dyn 235:2006.
7. Marazita M, Mooney M. Current concepts in the embryology and genetics of cleft lip and palate. Clin Plast Surg 31:2004.
8. Johnson N, Sandy J. Prenatal diagnosis of cleft lip and palate. Cleft Palate Craniofac J 40(2):2003.
9. Stoll C, Dott B, Alembik Y, Roth M. Evaluation of prenatal diagnosis of cleft lip/palate by fetal ultrasonographic examination. Ann Gene 43:2003.
10. Stoll C, Alembik Y, Dott B, Roth M.P. Associated malformations in cases with oral clefts. Cleft Palate Craniofac J 37:2000.
11. Goldber R, Motzkin B, Marion R, et al. Velocardiofacial syndrome: a review of 120 Patients. Am J Med Genet 45(3):1993.
12. Robin N, et al. The multidisciplinary evaluation and management of cleft lip and palate. South Med J 99(10): 2006.
13. Paradise J, Bluestone C, Felder H. The universality of otitis media in 50 infants with cleft palate. Pediatrics 44:1969.
14. Bluestone C, et al. Roentgenographic evaluation of eustachian tube function in infants with cleft and normal palates. Cleft Palate J 93:1972.
15. Braganza R. Closure of the soft palate for persistent otorrhea after placement of pressure equalization tubes in cleft palate infants. Cleft Palate Craniofac J 28:1991.
16. Gould H. Hearing loss and cleft palate: the perspective of time. Cleft Palate J 27:1990.
17. Moller P. Hearing, middle ear pressure, and otopathology in a cleft palate population. Acta Otolaryngol 92:1981.
18. Smith T. Recovery of eustachian tube function and hearing outcome in patients with cleft palate. Arch Otolaryngol 101:1975.
19. Sie K. Sphincter pharyngoplasty: speech outcome and complications. Laryngoscope108(8):1998.
20. de Serres L, Sie K. Results with sphincter pharyngoplasty and pharyngeal flap. Int J Pediatr Otorhinolaryngol 48:1999.
21. Smith B, Guyette T. Evaluation of cleft palate speech. Clin Plast Surg 31:2004.
22. Marsh J. The evaluation and management of velopharyngeal dysfunction. Clin Plast Surg 31:2004.
23. Grayson B, Maull D. Nasoalveolar molding for infants born with clefts of the lip, alveolus, and palate. Clin Plastic Surg 31:2004.
24. Daw J, Patel P. Management of alveolar clefts. Clin Plast Surg 31:2004.
25. Liao Y, Mars M. Hard palate repair timing and facial growth in cleft lip and palate: a systematic review. Cleft Palate Craniofac J 43(5):2006.
26. Rohrich R. Optimal timing of cleft palate closure. Plast Reconstr Surg 106(2):2000.
27. McCarthy J. Plastic surgery. Volume 4: Cleft Lip and Palate and Craniofacial Abnormalities. W.B. Saunders, Philadelphia. 1990.
28. Gage-White L. Furlow palatoplasty: double opposing Z-plasty. Facial Plast Surg 9:1993.
29. Furlow L. Cleft palate repair by double opposing Z-plasty. Plast Reconstr Surg 78:1986.
30. Bitter K. Repair of bilateral cleft lip, alveolus, and palate: follow up criteria and late results. J Craniomaxillofac Surg 29:2000.
31. Newlands L. Secondary alveolar bone grafting in cleft lip and palate patients. Br J Oral Maxillofac Surg 38:2000.

Cough

Samantha Anne and Robert F. Yellon

Key Points

- Cough is a normal reflex mechanism that is important in maintaining a sterile and unobstructed respiratory tract.
- It can also be a pathological symptom and a sign of many underlying disorders and abnormalities.
- Chronic cough is a common denominator of many illnesses and can lead to significant impairment in the quality of life of an individual.
- This chapter will describe the reflex mechanism of cough, the necessary workup needed when a child presents with chronic cough, provide a brief description of the most common diagnoses in the differential diagnosis, and recommend treatment options.

Keywords: Chronic cough • Laryngomalacia gastroesophageal reflux • Asthma • Bronchitis • Sinusitis • Allergy

Classification of Cough

As described in Landau's review *(1)*, cough can be classified by duration. Acute cough lasts less than 2 weeks. Most have cough attributed to viral infection, which resolves within 2 weeks in 70–80% of children. Protracted cough is usually a postviral cough and lasts 2–4 weeks. Chronic cough is defined as lasting more than 4 weeks and the differential diagnosis is extensive *(1–4)* (Table 1).

Pathophysiology/Mechanism of Cough

The cough reflex arc is intricate. The afferent pathway begins with peripheral receptors located along the airway mucosa between the ciliated pseudostratified epithelial cells. The highest concentration of the receptors is at the level of the larynx. Based on the specific location in the airway, these sensory nerve fibers are derived from trigeminal, glossopharyngeal, vagal, and phrenic nerves. Once the receptors are stimulated, the signal travels along the respective nerve to the cough center located in the medulla. The signals are then integrated and a coordinated effector signal is elicited. The most common nerve stimulated is the vagus. The signal then travels with the vagal nerve to the larynx and tracheobronchial tree and with the phrenic nerve to the expiratory and thoracic musculature to elicit the cough.

There are four phases in cough. It begins with the inspiratory phase during which there is deep inspiration and then glottic closure. This is followed by the contracture phase during which various expiratory muscles are stimulated and contract against a closed glottis. These muscle contractions lead to the compressive phase during which there is an elevation of pressures along the airway from the subglottis to the level of the alveoli. Finally, during the expiratory phase, the glottis opens and there is rapid expulsion of trapped air at high flow rates which causes propulsion of secretions and foreign material.

S. Anne and R.F. Yellon (✉)
Department of Otolaryngology, University of Pittsburgh School of Medicine, Division of Pediatric Otolaryngology, Children's Hospital of Pittsburgh, Pittsburgh, PA, USA
e-mail: Robert.Yellon@chp.edu

R.B. Mitchell and K.D. Pereira (eds.), *Pediatric Otolaryngology for the Clinician*,
DOI: 10.1007/978-1-60327-127-1_22, © Humana Press, a part of Springer Science + Business Media, LLC 2009

Table 1 Differential diagnosis

Congenital	Infectious
Larynx	Chronic bronchitis
Laryngomalacia	Chronic sinusitis
Laryngeal clefts	Pertussis
Vocal cord paralysis	Laryngotracheitis
Tracheobronchial tree	*Chlamydia*
Double aortic arch	Tuberculosis
Aberrant innominate artery	*Mycoplasma*
Esophagus	
Tracheoesophageal fistula	
Esophageal atresia	
Inflammatory	**Traumatic**
Cough-variant asthma	Fractures
Asthma	Foreign body
Allergy	Intubation
GERD	
Smoke exposure	
Systemic	**Neoplastic**
Primary ciliary dyskinesia	Laryngeal, tracheal
Cystic fibrosis	or bronchial tumors
Habit cough	

Workup of Cough

History

When a child presents with cough, a detailed history is essential. The time course of the cough is important. A sudden onset should be distinguished from a more chronic gradual development of cough. Sudden onset of cough may suggest foreign body aspiration. It is equally important to determine whether symptoms are diurnal or constant throughout the day. Night time symptoms may suggest laryngo-pharyngeal reflux. Early morning cough suggests asthma and late morning onset may represent cystic fibrosis. Seasonal changes in severity of symptoms may suggest allergies. Cough associated with vigorous activity suggests exercise-induced asthma.

The nature of the cough is also important. The cough may be dry or productive. If the cough is productive, the quality of sputum must be determined. Thick purulent cough suggests an infection, while clear sputum suggests an inflammatory cause. Bloody sputum may be secondary to bronchiectasis or cystic fibrosis. Also, the sound quality of the cough is important. A barky cough suggests tracheobronchitis while a whooping sound suggests pertussis.

Other important factors are signs of aspiration, immunization status, neonatal infections, medications used to alleviate symptoms, and allergy symptoms. A history of hoarseness, intubation, or trauma is also important to ascertain. Smoke exposure must be documented in the history. A pooled analysis of 12 cross-sectional studies involving more than 50,000 children demonstrated clearly that there is strong link between parental smoking and nocturnal cough, wheeze, and asthma *(5)*. In addition, more ominous associations with cough such as persistent fevers, failure to thrive, cyanotic episodes, and ongoing lethargy and limitation of activity are helpful in reaching a diagnosis.

Physical Examination

The overall appearance of the child can give clues to the diagnosis. Cachexia suggesting failure to thrive must be noted. The child's vital signs, height, and weight must be plotted on growth charts. Examination starts with the eyes, looking for allergic shiners (vascular congestion around eyes) and allergic conjunctivitis. Examination of the nose includes looking for the allergic salute, a transverse crease at the supratip region of the nose from repeated rubbing in an upward direction, polyps, boggy turbinates, clear rhinorrhea, or purulent secretions. Oral cavity and oropharyngeal examination may identify posterior drainage, which suggests sinus disease, with prominent lymphoid tissue, and cobblestoning of mucosa with. Examination of the neck is important to document masses or lymphadenopathy. Flexible laryngoscopy may be indicated to evaluate for laryngeal anomalies such as clefting, vocal cord paralysis, laryngitis, and tumors. Finally, auscultation of the lungs must be done to evaluate for crackles, wheezing, or adventitial sounds.

Labs/Radiography

Laboratory evaluation can include CBC with differential to evaluate for WBC elevation and a neutrophilic left shift. In addition, eosinophilic count is helpful to determine a possible allergic etiology of cough. Sputum culture for cytology, bacteria, and fungus is helpful. TB skin testing and sweat/genetic testing for cystic fibrosis may be indicated in specific cases. A nasal smear may be helpful to evaluate for elevated eosinophils seen in allergic rhinitis. Pulmonary function tests, to evaluate for chronic obstructive or restrictive disease and methacholine challenge testing for presence of asthma or reactive airway disease may be indicated.

Initial evaluation can include inspiratory and expiratory radiographic views of the chest to evaluate for foreign bodies, infiltrates, consolidations, and cavitations. Further focused exams include CT of the sinuses to evaluate for presence of sinusitis, barium swallow, pH probe and nuclear scintiscan for evaluation of aspiration and acid reflux disease.

Endoscopy

Further evaluation to confirm the diagnosis, or for additional clues to the diagnosis after preliminary evaluation, usually involves flexible endoscopy of the upper airway in the clinic or a more detailed examination in the operating room. Complete airway evaluation is helpful if airway anomalies, foreign bodies, or neoplasms are suspected. In addition, broncho-alveolar lavage can be obtained for cytology, cultures, and lipid-laden macrophages which may indicate gastro-esophageal reflux and aspiration. If concern for primary ciliary dyskinesia or other cililary dysmotility syndromes arises, a biopsy can be taken of the respiratory mucosa for evaluation under phase contrast and electron microscopy.

Differential Diagnosis

The differential diagnosis for cough is extensive and also varies depending on the age of the child. It is important to keep this in mind when assessing a child with persistent cough. One study has shown that over 60% of children with a cough that lasted more than 4 weeks in a specific practice were initially diagnosed with asthma. Many of these children were on asthma medications and more than 12% of them had significant steroid side effects. However, in many of these children, the diagnosis of asthma was incorrect as other causes of cough such as airway lesions, aspiration, and reflux were identified ***(6)***.

There are congenital, infectious, inflammatory, traumatic, neoplastic, and systemic causes for cough (Table 1). The following are the most common diagnoses followed by a brief discussion of each cause:

Congenital

Congenital causes of cough mainly revolve around impingement of the airway by anomalous vessels or abnormal development of the aero-digestive tract. Diagnosis is often made by endoscopy and additional information can be attained with radiographic studies such as a barium swallow and/or a nuclear scan for aspiration.

Congenital defects at the level of the larynx result in an abnormal suck-breathe-swallow reflex in the infant, but aspiration and cough occurs because of an inability to protect the airway. For example, laryngeal clefts can result in aspiration with feeding because of the defect in the posterior septum that separates the esophageal inlet from the airway. The child coughs to clear the airway of aspirated food contents. In addition, vocal cord paralysis can also result in an inability to protect the airway from aspiration that results in cough.

One of the most common diagnoses of laryngeal anomalies in infancy is laryngomalacia. Some of these infants present with cough because of coexisting gastroesophageal reflux ***(7)***. The child often presents with a very characteristic history of worsening stridor on position changes, after feeding, and with crying. Resolution without surgical intervention is normally seen by the age of 2 years.

Chondromalacia can involve the entire laryngo-tracheo-bronchial tree and is fairly common. In one study, 34% of bronchoscopic procedures revealed laryngo-tracheo-bronchial malacia. It is important to determine the site of the malacia. Laryngomalacia is associated with inspiratory stridor while tracheomalacia and bronchomalacia are associated with expiratory stridor. Cough, wheeze, stridor, and persistent or recurrent pneumonia are the most common symptoms and signs ***(8,9)***. Cartilage deficiency is evidenced as loss of rigidity or support in the airway. This leads to collapse during expiration and increases during periods of increased airflow such as crying or coughing. Normal healthy infants have maximal expiratory airway pressures of approximately 125 cmH_2O. Infants with tracheomalacia have closing pressures between −8 and −27 cmH_2O, which indicates that the trachea easily collapses with increased airflow such as during a crying episode ***(10)***. Diagnosis can be best determined with bronchoscopy or possibly with radiological findings on fluoroscopy CT, or MRI. Treatment can be conservative as in isolated laryngomalacia. Interventions such as CPAP, pexy procedures, stenting, resections, or reconstructions may be necessary based on the severity of the disorder *(11)*.

Congenital defects of the tracheo-bronchial tree include aberrant inominate artery, where the vessel causes anterior compression of the trachea. This presents as repeated episodes of croup and a barky cough that often resolves over time. Vascular rings may not only compress the trachea but also the esophagus causing cough symptoms and dysphagia. A rare cause of compression is caused by an anterior bridging bronchus. This anomaly arises when the right lower lung lobe is supplied by a bronchus originating from the left main bronchus that crosses the mediastinum. These anomalies usually present with respiratory distress but can lead to cough *(12)*.

Congenital esophageal anomalies can also present with cough. Tracheoesophageal fistulas and atresia present with increased secretion retention in the nasopharynx and oropharynx and frank aspiration especially during feeding. In addition, tracheomalacia often accompanies this anomaly, which also serves to exacerbate the cough.

Infectious

Infectious causes of cough are the most common and the most treatable. Chronic bronchitis often results in chronic nonproductive or slightly productive cough and usually follows an acute respiratory illness. Viral bronchitis often presents with cough which resolves over 7–10 days. Longer duration suggests bacterial infection, comorbidities such as cystic fibrosis, or the presence of foreign bodies. Bacterial superinfections are usually caused by *Streptococcus pneumoniae* or *Haemophilus influenzae*.

Chronic rhinosinusitis is the second most common cause of chronic cough in children. Cough often results from postnasal drainage irritating the laryngeal receptors. It has also been attributed to laryngeal edema causing obstructive symptoms. The first line of treatment is antimicrobials but persistent and recurrent infections may require surgery with adenoidectomy and/or functional endoscopic sinus surgery (FESS).

Pertussis, caused by *Bordetella pertussis*, a Gram-negative coccobacillus, is rare in industrialized countries because of immunizations that are widely administered. However, there are rare cases in which a child presents with paroxysmal cough, which is often followed by a "whoop." The cough is, often, forceful and occurs in rapid succession, which often results in the child being short of breath and cyanotic. In infants less than 2 months of age there is a high likelihood of a pertussis infection if the infant has a cough or choking associated with cyanosis *(13)*. A markedly high lymphocyte count, in addition, is a useful indicator of pertussis *(14)*. Pertussis is usually a self-limiting disease process that improves over a one-month period. Antimicrobials directed against *Bordetella pertussis* can be effective in reducing the severity of the disease when administered in the first 4 weeks of infection and can also help reduce the risk of transmission *(15)*.

Laryngotracheobronchitis, more commonly referred to as croup, is the most common form of upper airway obstruction leading to cough. Most children start with an upper respiratory infection for 1–3 days before developing signs of upper airway obstruction. The child at this point develops the characteristic "barking" cough, hoarseness, and inspiratory stridor. Symptoms are characteristically worse at night and recur for several days. Symptomatic treatment is often all that is needed and chronic symptoms are rare. Severe, refractory, or recurrent croup warrants further evaluation for possible reflux or a structural airway lesion.

Chlamydia trachomatis usually affects the urogenital tract but can cause respiratory infections in children when exposure occurs during delivery. Infection usually occurs at age 1–3 months and can present as opthalmia neonatorum, neonatal conjunctivitis, or neonatal pneumonia. Chlamydia pneumonia typically has a protracted course and has a characteristic associated staccato cough. There is usually no wheezing or elevated temperature. Treatment is with erythromycin for 14 days *(16)*. Pulmonary infection with *Mycoplasma pneumoniae* may also cause a protracted cough with the most common symptoms including cough and fever. It most commonly affects children aged 5–9 years and is treatable with macrolides *(17)*.

Inflammatory

Inflammatory causes of cough are very common in children. Diagnosis is difficult because of the lack of anatomic anomalies or infectious findings on endoscopies and/or laboratory studies. The most common diagnosis is cough-variant asthma. It presents as a nonproductive chronic cough without wheezing that is often worse with exertion and at night. In a single series of 176 children with chronic cough, almost 35% had a diagnosis of cough-variant asthma *(18)*. Cough-variant asthma is most likely secondary to bronchoconstriction and subsequent activation of bronchial stretch receptors or from mucosal irritation of peripheral sensory receptors. Increased bronchial sensitivity has been demonstrated in cough-variant asthma and in classic asthma as compared to controls. In cough-variant asthma, however, there was significantly lower bronchoconstriction in response to nonspecific airway stimuli than in classic asthma. The absence of wheezing in cough-variant asthma is explained by this decreased bronchoconstriction and by less constriction and deformation of the airways *(19)*. Because of the paucity of associated findings, children may undergo a prolonged and complicated diagnostic workup. The diagnosis is made with a bronchoconstrictor challenge test resulting in a positive response to bronchodilators.

Children with cough-variant asthma often progress to classic asthma with wheezing and dyspnea. A high percentage of eosinophils in the sputum of children with cough-variant asthma may be significantly associated with subsequent development of classic asthma *(20)*. An important distinction is whether the cough is really secondary to asthma or an unrelated disease process. Many times, a child can undergo multiple inappropriate treatments with corticosteroids for treatment of asthmatic cough when it actually has a different etiology. Diagnosis of asthma can be made with increased confidence when there is a cough, wheezing, dyspnea, and airway hyperresponsiveness with a positive bronchodilator challenge. A recent study by Hartl et al. *(21)* has shown that bronchoalveolar lavage from asthmatic children has increased chemokines, such as thymus and activation-regulated chemokine (TARC) or macrophage-derived chemokine (MDC), and specific chemokine receptors on lymphocytes which can differentiate monasthmatic children from nonasthmatic children with chronic cough. Treatment of asthma often includes the use of inhaled corticosteroids *(21)*.

Allergy is a common diagnosis among children with cough. Associated sneezing, clear rhinorrhea, watery eyes, allergic shiners, and allergic salute should alert a physician about allergy as a source of cough. Antihistamines and topical intranasal corticosteroids can help decrease postnasal drip which often instigates the cough.

Gastroesophageal reflux disease (GERD) is physiologic in many infants and children but can be pathological leading to failure to thrive, esophagitis, and respiratory disease. It has been shown to also cause chronic cough, independent of the presence of esophagitis *(22)*. This causal relationship between chronic respiratory symptoms and GERD was well demonstrated using scintigraphy in a study done by Ravelli et al. *(23)*. Pulmonary aspiration was demonstrated with scintigraphy in half of the children with chronic respiratory symptoms such as chronic cough *(23)*. Other symptoms include regurgitation, irritability, crying, and fussiness. Diagnosis can be made with nuclear scintiscan esophageal biopsies, manometry, a PH probe, and examination of bronchoalveolar lavage (BAL) fluid. Farrell et al. *(24)* showed that pepsin in BAL was a specific and sensitive method to diagnose reflux. All children with observed aspiration had pepsin in BAL samples as opposed to none in the control group. Significantly elevated pepsin levels were demonstrated in children with proximal reflux and chronic cough *(24)*. Treatment of chronic cough secondary to reflux includes thickening feeds, elevating the head of the bed, smaller feeds, and antireflux medications.

Trauma

Laryngeal trauma can result in cough. With fractures of the laryngeal framework or with blunt trauma, there can be inflammation and edema that serve as an obstruction and can trigger cough. In addition, iatrogenic trauma with intubation may cause mucosal injury or arytenoid dislocation and subsequent vocal cord immobility which can cause obstruction and cough. Diagnosis is determined from endoscopy after securing a precarious airway if present.

Foreign body aspiration must always be suspected in children with a new onset of cough even with a normal physical examination and radiologic studies. The history is crucial in these children. In a review of children who had aspirated foreign bodies, sudden onset of cough and choking was noted in over 70% and approximately 60% had dyspnea and wheezing *(25)*. Nuts and seeds are the most common items recovered *(25–27)*. The clinical triad of acute coughing/choking, wheezing, and unilateral diminished breath sounds has been shown to have a high specificity for the presence of a foreign body (98%). In the same series, 32% of children with prolonged cough or a pulmonary affliction lasting more than 2 weeks that were unresponsive to medical therapy had an airway foreign body *(25)*.

Systemic

Primary ciliary dyskinesia is an autosomal recessive disorder characterized by defective ciliary structure and function. Cough is one of the most frequent symptoms associated with this disorder and is more prevalent when compared to normal, healthy children *(28)*. Diagnosis is made with analysis of ciliary structure and beat frequency using electron microscopy. Kartagener syndrome is ciliary dyskinesia with situs inversus seen on chest radiography.

Cystic Fibrosis, an autosomal recessive disorder, is another systemic disease with chronic cough as a common symptom. It is the most common lethal inherited disease among Caucasians. The tenacious secretions that drive the cough can emanate from a sinus or pulmonary etiology and persist despite aggressive pulmonary treatments, sinus lavages, surgeries, and antimicrobials. The standard diagnostic test is the sweat test and genetic testing is available to confirm the diagnosis. Treatment is usually through a multidisciplinary team that includes gastroenterologists, pulmonologists, otolaryngologists, and others.

Habit cough is a chronic cough with no detectable organic, anatomic, or physiologic etiology. Its diagnosis is made by exclusion of other etiologies. It is a habitual barking cough that has been previously described as a psychogenic cough. It causes significant disturbance to the child and caregivers and affects functioning at school and at home. The cough usually starts after an upper respiratory illness and is described as brief, explosive expiration with a "honking" or barking quality. Suspicion arises when there is an unusual history, limitation of cough to wakefulness, and a normal physical examination. Management can be as simple as explaining the benign nature of the cough and making the child aware of the habit. It can also become quite complex and may require mental health interventions, family therapy, and even rehabilitation programs *(29,30)*. Some studies have shown benefit with biofeedback, cognitive coping, and even hypnosis *(31,32)*.

Treatment

Treatment of cough depends on the underlying cause. There are a few general principles which guide treatment. In general, infectious causes respond to culture-directed antibiotics or antifungals and inflammatory causes respond to resolution of the cause such as acid reflux or asthma. Avoiding environmental insults such as allergens and tobacco smoke may improve symptoms. Of course, with foreign bodies, removal of the offending material is curative.

While waiting for these therapeutic measures to work, comfort measures can be used such as central-acting antitussives or peripherally acting anesthetics. In addition, over-the-counter medications, such as lozenges and humidity may be helpful. Expectorants and mucolytics also help to thin secretions to ease expulsion on cough.

References

1. Landau LI. Acute and chronic cough. Paediatr Respir Rev 2006;7:64–76.
2. Bluestone CD, Stool SE, Alper CM, et al. eds. Pediatric Otolaryngology,. 4th edPhiladelphia: WB Saunders, 2003:1395–1405.
3. Holinger LD, Lusk RP, Green CG. Pediatric Laryngology and Bronchoesophagology. Philadelphia: Lippincott-Raven, 1997:253–263.
4. Cotton RT, Myer CM. Practical Pediatric Otolaryngology. Philadelphia: Lippincott Williams & Wilkins, 1998.
5. Pattenden S, Antova T, Neuberger M, Nikiforov B, De Sario M, Grize L, et al. Parental smoking and children's respiratory health: independent effects of prenatal and postnatal exposure. Tob Control 2006;15:294–301.
6. Thomson F, Masters IB, Chang AB. Persistent cough in children and the overuse of medications. J Paediatr Child Health 2002;38:578–581.
7. Yellon RF. The spectrum of reflux-associated otolaryngologic problems in infants and children. Am J Med 1997;103:125–129.
8. Masters IB, Chang AB, Patterson L, et al. Series of laryngomalacia, tracheomalacia, and bronchomalacia disorders and their associations with other conditions in children. Pediatr Pulmonol 2002;34:189–195.
9. Yalcin E, Dogru D, Ozcelik U, Kiper N, Aslan AT, Gozacan A. Tracheomalacia and bronchomalacia in 34 children:

clinical and radiologic profiles and associations with other diseases. Clin Pediatr 2005;44(9):777–781.
10. Okazaki J, Isono S, Hasegawa H, Sakai M, Nagase Y, Nishino T. Quantitative assessment of tracheal collapsibility in infants with tracheomalacia. Am J Respir Crit Care Med 2004;170:780–785.
11. Rohde M, Banner J. Respiratory tract malacia: possible cause of sudden death in infancy and early childhood. Acta Pediatr 2006;95:867–870.
12. Rishavy TJ, Goretsky MJ, Langenburg SE, Klein MD. Anterior bridging bronchus. Pediatr Pulmonol 2003;35: 70–72.
13. Mackey JE, Wojcik S, Long R, Callahan JM, Grant WD. Predicting pertussis in a pediatric emergency department population. Clin Pediatr 2007;46:437–440.
14. Fung KS, Yeung WL, Wong TW, So KW, Cheng AF. Pertussis--a re-emerging infection? J Infect 2004;48: 145–148.
15. Singh M, Lingappan K. Whooping cough: the current scene. Chest 2006;130:1547–1553.
16. Miller KE. Diagnosis and treatment of chlamydia trachomatis infection. Am Fam Physician 2006;73(8):1411–1416.
17. Othman N, Isaacs D, Kesson A. Mycoplasma pneumoniae infections in Australian children. J Paediatr Child Health 2005;41:671–676.
18. Fujimura M, Abo M, Ogawa H, et al. Importance of atopic cough, cough variant asthma and sinobronchial syndrome as causes of chronic cough in the Hokuriku area of Japan. Respirology 2005;10:201–207.
19. Mochizuki H, Arakawa H, Tokuyama K, Morikawa A. Bronchial sensitivity and bronchial reactivity in children with cough variant asthma. Chest 2005;128(4):2427–2434.
20. Kim CK, Kim JT, Kang H, Yoo Y, Koh YY. Sputum eosinophilia in cough-variant asthma as a predictor of the subsequent development of classic asthma. Clin Exp Allergy 2003;33:1409–1414.
21. Hartl D, Griese M, Nicolai T, Zissel G, Press C, Konstantopoulos N, et al. Pulmonary chemokines and their receptors differentiate children with asthma and chronic cough. J Allergy Clin Immunol 2005;115(4): 728–736.
22. Chang AB, Cox NC, Faoagali J, Cleghorn GJ, Beem C, Ee LC, et al. Cough and reflux esophagitis in children: their co-existence and airway cellularity. BMC Pediatr 2006;6:4.
23. Ravelli AM, Panarotto MB, Verdoni L, Consolati V, Bolognini S. Pulmonary aspiration shown by scintigraphy in gastroesophageal reflux-related respiratory disease. Chest 2006;130:1520–1526.
24. Farrell S, McMaster C, Gibson D, Shields MD, McCallion WA. Pepsin in bronchoalveolar lavage fluid: a specific and sensitive method of diagnosing gastro-oesophageal reflux-related pulmonary aspiration. J Pediatr Surg 2006;41: 289–293.
25. Chiu CY, Wong KS, Lai SH, Hsia SH, Wu CT. Factors predicting early diagnosis of foreign body aspiration in children. Pediatr Emerg Care 2005;21(3):161–164.
26. Eren S, Balci AE, Dikici B, Doblan M, Eren MN. Foreign body aspiration in children: experience of 1160 cases. Ann Trop Paediatr 2003;23:31–37.
27. Aydogan LB, Tuncer U, Soylu L, Kiroglu M, Ozsahinoglu C. Rigid bronchoscopy for the suspicion of foreign body in the airway. Int J Pediatr Otorhinolaryngol 2006;70: 823–828.
28. Zihlif N, Paraskakis E, Lex C, Van de Pohl LA, Bush A. Correlation between cough frequency and airway inflammation in children with primary ciliary dyskinesia. Pediatr Pulmonol 2005;39:551–557.
29. Fitzgerald DA, Kozlowska K. Habit cough: assessment and management. Paediatr Respir Rev 2006;7:21–25.
30. Faught J, Fitzgerald DA. Habit cough and effective therapy. J Paediatr Child Health 2004;40:399–400.
31. Labbe EE. Biofeedback and cognitive coping in the treatment of pediatric habit cough. Appl Psychophysiol Biofeedback 2006;31:167–172.
32. Anbar RD, Hall HR. Childhood habit cough treated with self-hypnosis. J Pediatr 2004;144:213–217.

Hoarseness in Children

Craig S. Derkay and Stephen M. Wold

Key Points

- Voice disturbances in children are very common and usually of a benign etiology.
- Articulation disorders are more commonly addressed by a pediatric speech pathologist. Dysphonias often require the expertise of a voice therapist.
- Laryngoscopy, whether flexible, rigid, or both, is considered the "gold standard" for making a correct diagnosis.
- A complete history is key in establishing the etiology of childhood voice disturbances.
- Associated medical conditions, particularly extraesophageal reflux disease and allergic rhinitis, need to be investigated and treated to achieve a successful outcome.

Keywords: Hoarseness • Dysphonia • Recurrent respiratory papillomas • Vocal nodules • Voice therapy • Extraesophageal reflux disease

The overall prevalence of voice disorders (dysphonias) in children has been reported to be between 6 and 9%, but may be as high as 20% in some pediatric populations *(1,2)*. These may be broadly categorized in terms of their causes (congenital vs. acquired) or whether the condition is organic (anatomic or neurologic abnormality) versus functional (behavioral or psychogenic). Hoarseness, or the disturbance of clear vocal sound by local changes of the vocal folds, is the most common presenting sign and symptom of the patient with an underlying voice disorder. With the exception of older children and adolescents, dysphonia is frequently addressed at the request of a parent or referring physician, since most younger children lack the awareness of their own vocal quality or the perception that an abnormality exists *(2)*. Fortunately, the vast majority of pediatric dysphonias are the result of a benign process. However, a thorough evaluation and diagnosis is paramount for optimal treatment planning as well as to rule out those causes which are potentially more harmful.

Diagnosis

A thorough history and physical examination is the basis for diagnosis. The *history* should include inquiries into the birth history, prior intubations or surgery, previous trauma, colic, respiratory or feeding difficulties, gastroesophageal reflux (GER), environmental allergy symptoms, and a description of the child's voice use. In addition, one needs to establish the duration and progression of the abnormal voice and assess whether or not there is an associated stridor or stertor.

The *physical examination* should particularly document the voice quality, presence of abnormal airway noises, signs of respiratory distress, and any syndromic or abnormal craniofacial features. An assessment of the larynx, commonly done in the office by *flexible fiberoptic endoscopy*, is an essential element of the work-up and is often considered the gold standard. Office endoscopy in children can, however, be difficult to perform successfully, frequently requiring the assistance of the parents and nursing staff. If airway or respiratory difficulties exist, or to avoid physical restraint of an uncooperative child, examination may be deferred to the operating room under a general anesthetic. Video monitoring and photo documentation

C.S. Derkay (✉) and S.M. Wold
Department of Otolaryngology Head and Neck Surgery, Eastern Virginia Medical School, Norfolk, VA, USA
e-mail: Craig.Derkay@CHKD.org

R.B. Mitchell and K.D. Pereira (eds.), *Pediatric Otolaryngology for the Clinician*,
DOI: 10.1007/978-1-60327-127-1_23, © Humana Press, a part of Springer Science + Business Media, LLC 2009

are helpful to counsel and educate the family as well as to follow clinical progression and assist the voice pathologist in treatment. Videostroboscopy is extremely useful for the evaluation of the vocal folds and their movement during phonation (demonstrated by the "mucosal wave"). However, a rather high degree of cooperation is required from the patient.

Classification

Dysphonia may be further characterized in a number of different ways, but among the more widely accepted voice assessment tools is the GRBAS scale, which scores vocal quality via Grade (degree of abnormality), Roughness, Breathiness, Asthenia (weakness), and Strain *(3)*. The application of a standardized scoring system or scale provides a useful tool for both following clinical progression as well as for communication between care providers.

Additional Studies

Further work-up may be subsequently required for some patients including a work-up for gastroesophageal reflux, direct laryngoscopy with bronchoscopy, broncho-alveolar lavage, videostroboscopy, audiometry, laryngeal electromyography (EMG), chest X-ray, lab studies (i.e., ANA, lyme titers), computed tomography (CT), or magnetic resonance imaging (MRI).

Differential Diagnosis

Several of the more common etiologies of hoarseness/dysphonia are included:

Vocal Nodules ("Screamer" or "Singer" Nodules) – The most common cause of chronic pediatric hoarseness (perhaps as much as 78%), vocal fold nodules are generally considered to result from vocal abuse or misuse and are a benign, self-limited condition, often regressing following puberty *(2)*. The nodules are frequently observed along the anterior third of the true vocal folds bilaterally, and may result in early contact or incomplete glottic closure with a resultant hoarse or breathy voice (Fig. 1).

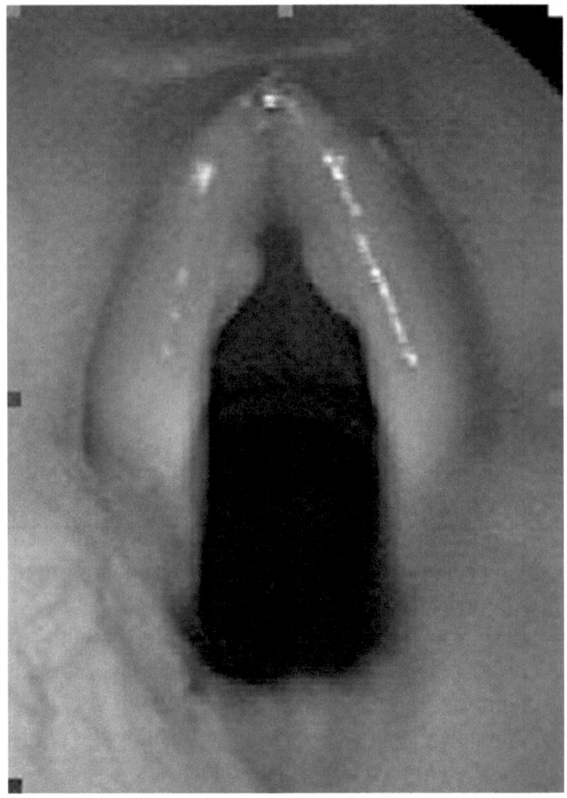

Fig. 1 Symmetric bilateral true vocal fold nodules

Recurrent Respiratory Papillomatosis (RRP) – The most common benign neoplastic cause of hoarseness, RRP can have a very aggressive, persistent, and refractory course. The process originates from the human papilloma virus (HPV) subtypes 6 and 11, transmitted most often in a vertical fashion from mother to fetus. Hoarseness is the most characteristic symptom of the disease when the larynx is affected and serves as the best indicator of recurrence. In some cases the disease may regress after puberty or be exacerbated by pregnancy. HPV subtyping may be helpful as HPV 16 and 18 have been shown to be associated with a more aggressive clinical course (Fig. 2).

Laryngomalacia – Typically presenting with neonatal stridor secondary to flaccidity or redundancy of the epiglottis and aryepiglottic folds, hoarseness is not a primary manifestation; however, may be present due to the common association with GER (Fig. 3).

Gastroesophageal Reflux – Extraesophageal reflux is an increasingly prevalent finding that may itself cause hoarseness from local posterior glottic edema and inflammation, but perhaps more importantly may contribute to

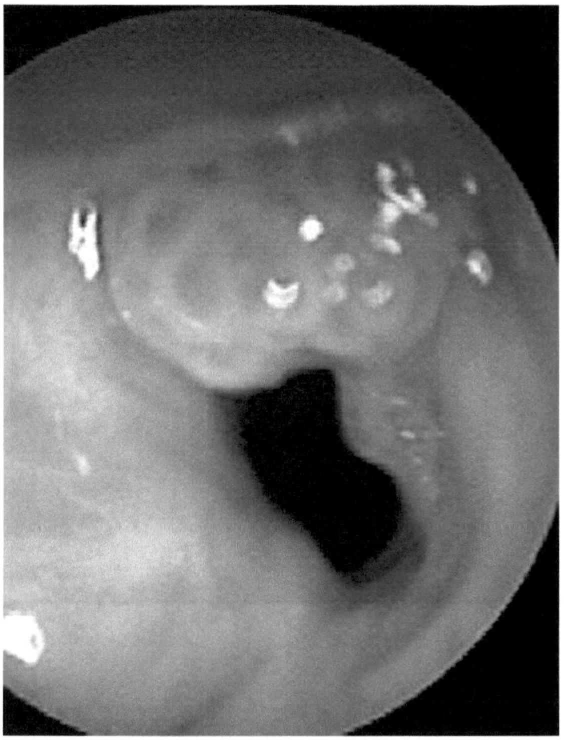

Fig. 2 Respiratory papilloma of the anterior commissure

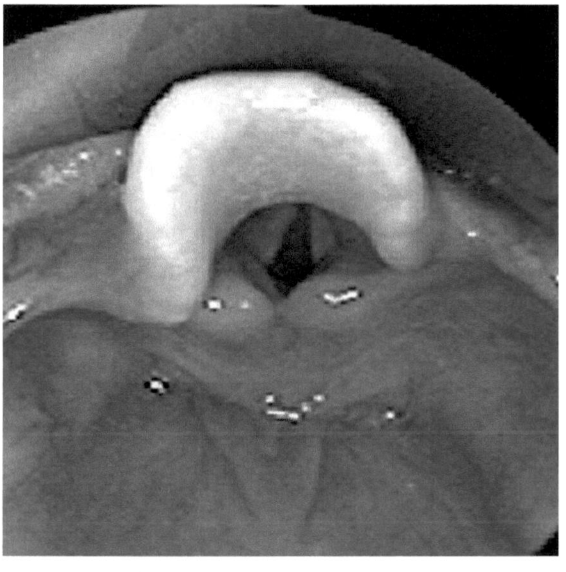

Fig. 3 Laryngomalacia evidenced by the shortened aryepiglottic folds and prolapsed arytenoids

or aggravate other laryngeal pathologies such as nodules, polyps, and laryngomalacia *(4)*. Radiographs, pH probe, multichannel intraluminal impedance, and empiric therapy

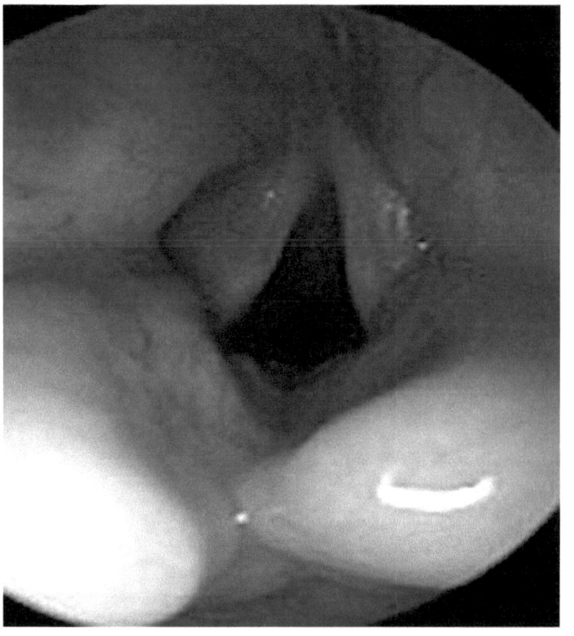

Fig. 4 Roughened, inflamed mucosa of the posterior glottis with edematous arytenoids

have all been suggested for the evaluation of GER; however, consensus is still lacking as to a standard for making the diagnosis (Fig. 4).

Vocal Fold Mobility Impairment (VFMI) – Abnormalities of vocal fold motion may result from both congenital and acquired causes, with unilateral VFMI occurring 4–5 times more frequently than bilateral. The most common etiologies in the pediatric population are idiopathic, followed by iatrogenic, neurologic, traumatic, and neoplastic *(5)*. The lesion may be at the level of the vocal folds themselves, as is the case with intubation injury and laryngeal fractures. It may also result from a recurrent laryngeal nerve injury or from a disorder of the central nervous system, as seen with the Arnold Chiari malformation, an uncommon cause of neonatal bilateral VFMI. Complications of some mediastinal and cardiothoracic procedures such as ligation of a patent ductus arteriosus may also result in recurrent laryngeal nerve injury, especially on the left where it takes a longer course through the chest. Neoplasms, which will be discussed later, may impair mobility at any level.

Laryngeal Webs/Laryngeal Cysts/Laryngoceles – Anatomic lesions of the larynx may result in respiratory difficulties, stridor, vocal "fullness," or hoarseness depending upon the specific location. These lesions

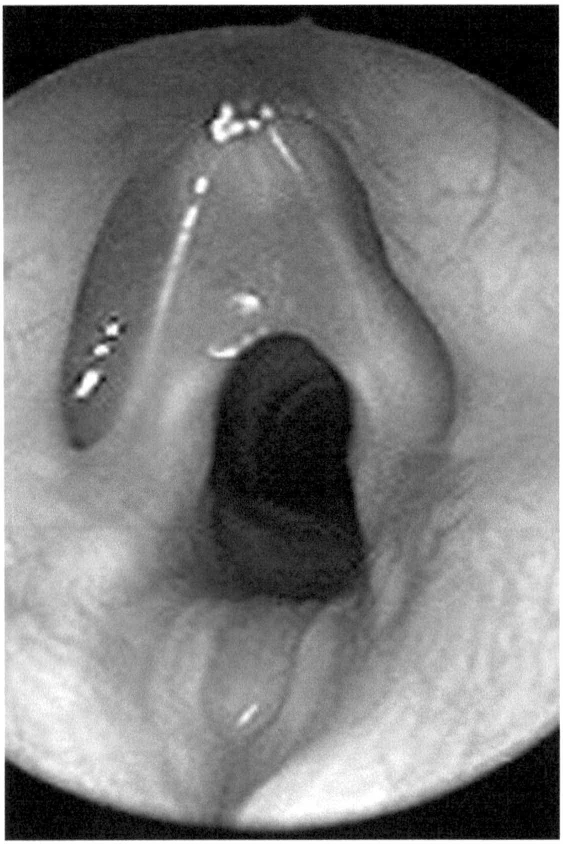

Fig. 5 Bilateral internal laryngoceles rooted within the laryngeal ventricles

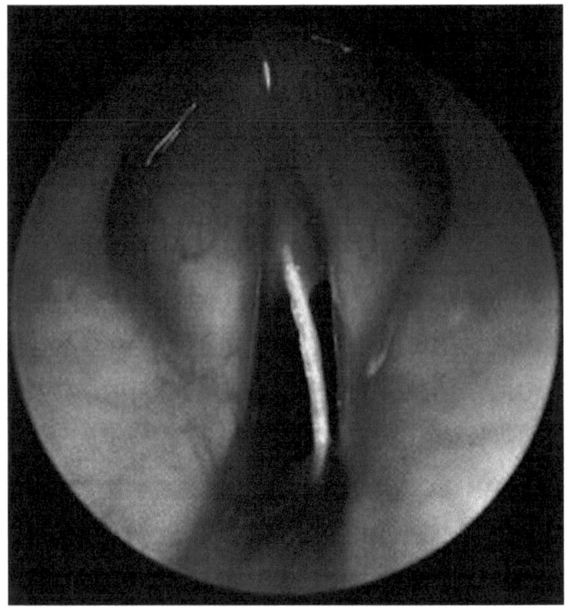

Fig. 6 Small fragment of a chicken bone lodged within the glottis

may result from developmental failure of airway recanalization, or may be acquired, most frequently from prior intubation (Fig.5).

Infection – Infectious laryngitis may result from inflammation caused by a number of viral, bacteria, and fungal agents. In children, the most common culprits of infectious laryngitis include *rhino, adeno*, and *parainfluenza* viruses. *Pneumococcus, haemophilus, candida, histoplasma, blastomyces*, and *mycobacteria* are seen much less frequently.

Foreign Body – Laryngeal foreign bodies are airway emergencies and require immediate intervention once suspected. Peanuts, grapes, popcorn, hot dogs, and sunflower seeds are most commonly aspirated in young children, while school supplies (i.e., pencil erasers) are more commonly aspirated in older children. Balloons can be particularly deadly because they tend to conform to the contours of the larynx (Fig. 6).

Allergic Rhinosinusitis (ARS) – Postnasal drainage is a common cause of persistent or recurrent hoarseness in children and is often associated with vocal resonance changes from nasal obstruction. True ARS is typically seen in children over 4 years of age and allergy testing may be warranted.

Subglottic Hemangioma – Hemangiomas are the most common pediatric head and neck neoplasms. They may cause hoarseness or other dysphonia depending upon their location. Symptoms are usually noted within the first 3–6 months of life during the proliferative phase and may be associated with biphasic stridor, respiratory distress, or cutaneous lesions (in as many as 50%). Small lesions may be self-limited and regress spontaneously over time.

Other Benign Neoplasms – Lymphatic malformations, hamartomas, neurofibromas, and myxomas may all cause vocal changes, though direct involvement of the larynx is rare, rendering hoarseness an uncommon finding.

Malignancy – Rhabdomyosarcoma, lymphoma, chondrosarcoma, fibrosarcoma, thyroid cancer, and squamous cell carcinoma may cause a variety of vocal changes through involvement of the larynx or the motor nerves that innervate the laryngeal muscles. Fortunately, malignant etiologies of hoarseness are rare in children.

Trauma – Intubation injury is the most common cause of traumatic hoarseness and may be due to placement of an improperly sized tube, traumatic intubation, uncontrolled GER, or prolonged intubation. Granulation and scarring often occur posteriorly and may ultimately cause webbing or stenosis. Other traumas include laryngeal fracture such as that seen in clothesline injuries, iatrogenic nerve injury as previously discussed, and foreign body aspiration. Taking a detailed history is particularly important in uncovering traumatic etiologies for hoarseness (Fig. 7).

Chronic Granulomatous Disease – Hoarseness secondary to vocal fold scarring, joint fixation, and airway stenosis may be seen with various systemic disorders such as sarcoidosis, Wegener's granulomatosis, and juvenile rheumatoid arthritis. In most cases, laryngeal involvement is not an isolated presentation, but rather in association with other organ system involvement. Radiographs and lab panels (ANA, RF, immune antibodies, etc.) are often useful to confirm the diagnosis.

Functional Dysphonias – Sometimes referred to as psychogenic or behavioral dysphonia, these patients present without any obvious organic lesion. It is thought that many of the conditions in this category stem from poor voice habits that are either learned or perhaps developed as a compensatory mechanism for other underlying disturbances (i.e., velopharyngeal insufficiency). In some patients, the dysphonia manifests consciously or subconsciously for the purpose of secondary gain. Diagnosis may be extremely challenging, and is typically made only after other etiologies have first been excluded. Without correction, however, these patients may in fact progress to develop true anatomic lesions, such as nodules, which perpetuate the symptoms.

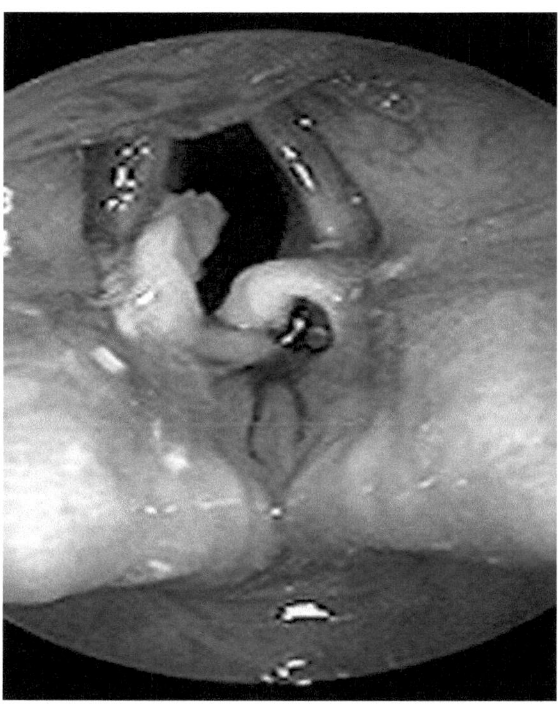

Fig. 7 Traumatic postintubation injury to the posterior vocal folds and arytenoids

Treatment

The hallmark of treatment for pediatric dysphonias is the institution of voice therapy. Of course, the success of therapy will depend greatly on the age of the child, his/her motivations for voice improvement, the cooperation and support of the family, and the skill of the therapist. Surgical correction of underlying anatomic abnormalities may also be necessary, depending upon the etiology, ranging from microlaryngoscopy techniques utilizing airway lasers and microdebriders to augmentation procedures for the correction of vocal fold mobility impairments. In addition to the noted modalities, maximal medical control of extraesophageal reflux utilizing proton pump inhibitors, histamine blockers, and dietary modification is often also advocated ***(1,3,5)***. Intralesional, topical, or systemic steroid therapy may also play a role in the resolution of some voice disorders, particularly in acute traumatic processes; however, experience in the pediatric population is largely anecdotal at this point.

Outcomes

Resolution of voice disturbance depends greatly on the underlying etiology. Children who have undergone airway reconstruction or who have developed scarring of the anterior commissure from prolonged periods of intubation or from repeated surgeries to remove laryngeal papillomas will not achieve successful voice outcomes. Children with vocal nodules who modify their behavior and resolve their underlying medical conditions are likely to normalize their voice. It should be noted that vocal improvement does not necessarily indicate that the underlying process has also been resolved and therefore follow-up and prophylactic care should be maintained ***(6)***. Compliance with treatment regimens is a large factor in the overall success of therapy. As previously noted, most young children lack the self-awareness of any voice disturbance, thus speech therapy is largely focused on behavior modification, whereas older kids may be more motivated to focus upon the voice itself. The concept of a multidisciplinary voice clinic serves as a promising model for optimizing voice and vocal care in the pediatric patient; however, these clinics are in their infancy and not widely available. Finally, although microlaryngeal techniques are commonly utilized in adults, they are not always applicable in children; hence, further experience, research, and instrument adaptation are required.

References

1. Requena R, Derkay CS, Darrow DH. Voice disorders in children: benign or serious? *J Respir Dis*. 1998;19(11):973–991.
2. Trani M, Ghidini A, Berganini G, Presutti. Voice therapy in pediatric functional dysphonia a prospective study. *Int J Pediatr Otorhinolaryngol*. 2007;71:379–384.
3. Ettema SL, Tolejano CJ, Thielke RJ, Toohil RJ, Merati AL. Perceptual voice analysis of patients with subglottic stenosis. *Otolaryngol Head Neck Surg*. 2006;135:730–735.
4. Koufman JA. The Otolaryngologic manifestations of gastroesophageal reflux disease (GERD): a clinical investigation of 225 patients using ambulatory 24-hour pH monitoring and an experimental investigation of the role of acid and pepsin in the development of laryngeal injury. *Laryngoscope*. 1991;101(4 Pt 2 Suppl 53):1–78.
5. Ishman SL, Halum SL, Patel NJ, Kerschner JE, Merati AL. Management of vocal paralysis: a comparison of adult and pediatric practices. *Otolaryngol Head Neck Surg*. 2006;135:590–594.
6. SM, Garrett CG. Utility of voice therapy in the management of vocal fold polyps and cysts. *Otolaryngol Head Neck Surg*. 2007;136:742–746.

Adenotonsillar Disease

David H. Darrow and Nathan A. Kludt

Key Points

- Tonsils and adenoid are important sources of J-chain bearing B-cell precursors that can eventually bind secretory IgA.
- Although most tonsillitis in children is viral, Group A streptococcal disease is the most common treatable disorder. Treatment is useful primarily in the prevention of sequelae. Tonsillectomy, however, may reduce the frequency of Group A streptococcal disease in selected individuals with recurrent disease.
- Acute infection with Epstein–Barr virus (infectious mononucleosis) usually occurs in older children and adolescents. Most individuals, acquire antibodies to the Epstein–Barr virus.
- Chronic infection of the adenoid may result in persistent nasal discharge as well as frequent or chronic otitis media.
- Lymphoma is the primary cause of neoplastic disease in the tonsils and adenoid and may arise primarily or as a result of a post-transplantation lymphoproliferative disorder.

Keywords: Pharyngitis • Tonsillitis • Streptococcus • Epstein–Barr virus • Adenoiditis • Tonsillectomy • Adenoidectomy • Tonsil lymphoma • Post-transplantation lymphoproliferative disorder

Adenotonsillar disease in children occurs as a result of infection, inflammation, or malignancy. Infection of the tonsils and adenoid is common in children due to exposure to upper respiratory infections of other children facilitated by day care and family settings. Conversely, malignancy of these tissues is exceedingly rare. Hyperplasia of the tonsils and adenoid leading to sleep-disordered breathing (SDB) is reviewed as a separate chapter in this textbook.

Waldeyer's ring is composed of the palatine tonsils bilaterally, the adenoid and tubal tonsils in the nasopharynx, and the lingual tonsil at the tongue base. These tissues are important in the development of regional immunity in children. Lymphoid follicles stimulated by antigen give rise to expansion of B-cell clones, induction of J-chain production, and differentiation of B-cells into memory cells and plasma cells associated with J-chain expression. Because J-chain is an essential component of secretory IgA, tonsils and adenoid may be an important source of B-cells for effector sites in the mucosa of the upper respiratory tract. However, there is no evidence that removal of the tonsils and/or adenoid increases the risk of immunomodulated disease *(1)*.

Infectious and Inflammatory Diseases of the Tonsils

Pharyngotonsillitis is a general term used to describe diffuse inflammation of the structures of the oropharynx, including the tonsils. The disorder presents with symptoms of odynophagia with objective signs of inflammation. Pharyngotonsillitis may be classified based on duration of symptoms as acute, subacute, or chronic, with most children presenting acutely. Alternatively, pharyngitis may also be characterized as nasopharyngitis, in which common symptoms include rhinorrhea, nasal congestion, sneezing, and cough.

D.H. Darrow (✉)
Departments of Otolaryngology – Head and Neck Surgery and Pediatrics, Children's Hospital of the King's Daughters, Eastern Virginia Medical School, Norfolk, VA, USA
e-mail: David.Darrow@chkd.org

N.A. Kludt
Surgical resident, University of California, Davis, CA, USA

R.B. Mitchell and K.D. Pereira (eds.), *Pediatric Otolaryngology for the Clinician*,
DOI: 10.1007/978-1-60327-127-1_24, © Humana Press, a part of Springer Science + Business Media, LLC 2009

Adenoviruses, influenza viruses, parainfluenza viruses, and enteroviruses are the most common etiologic agents. Nasopharyngitis of viral etiology may also cause a concomitant pharyngotonsillitis. The infection is most commonly acute and self-limited, with symptoms resolving within 10 days. Inflammation limited to the adenoid pad (adenoiditis) is difficult to diagnose in the primary care setting due to the inaccessibility of this tissue to direct visualization.

The etiologic agents responsible for pharyngotonsillitis are far more diverse than those of nasopharyngitis. Group A beta-hemolytic *Streptococcus*, adenoviruses, influenza viruses, parainfluenza viruses, enteroviruses, Epstein–Barr virus, and *Mycoplasma* account for over 90% of these infections *(2)*. Treatment of these illnesses varies depending on the etiology, and therefore throat culture for treatable bacterial etiologies is usually indicated. As in nasopharyngitis, most viral pharyngotonsillitis require no specific therapy. In the remainder of this chapter, we address other causes of pharyngotonsillitis, which may require more aggressive diagnosis and treatment.

Group A Beta-Hemolytic and Other Streptococci

The Group A beta-hemolytic streptococcus (GABHS) is the most common bacterium associated with pharyngotonsillitis in children. In the 60 years since the advent of antibiotics, most pharyngeal infections by GABHS have been benign, self-limited, and uncomplicated. In fact, most children improve symptomatically without any medical intervention. However, a small number of affected individuals continue to develop severe renal and cardiac complications following GABHS infection. In addition, there is evidence that early antibiotic therapy may be useful in treating the symptoms of GABHS. As a result, appropriate diagnosis and treatment of these infections is imperative.

The incidence of GABHS pharyngitis has not been estimated on the basis of population-based data *(3)*. Nevertheless, "strep throat" is well recognized as a common disease among children and adolescents. The incidence peaks during the winter and spring seasons, and is more common in cooler, temperate climates. Risk factors for GABHS pharyngitis include: close interpersonal contact in schools, military quarters, dormitories, and families with several children.

Transmission of GABHS is believed to occur through droplet spread. As a result, individuals are most infectious early in the course of the disease. The inoculum size and the virulence of the infecting strain are likely to be important factors in transmission. The incubation period is usually between 1 and 4 days. Following initiation of antimicrobial therapy, children may return to school within 36–48 h *(4)*. The role of individuals colonized with GABHS in the spread of the disease is uncertain, although data suggest that carriers rarely spread the disease to close contacts *(4)*.

The streptococci are Gram-positive, catalase-negative cocci characterized by their growth in long chains or pairs in culture. These organisms are traditionally classified into 18 groups with letter designations (Lancefield groups) on the basis of the antigenic carbohydrate component of their cell walls. While the Group A beta-hemolytic streptococcus is isolated from most patients with streptococcal pharyngitis, Group C, G, and B streptococci may also occasionally cause this disorder. Further subclassification of streptococci is made based on their ability to lyse sheep red blood cells in culture; the beta-hemolytic strains cause hemolysis associated with a clear zone surrounding their colonies, while alpha-hemolytic strains cause partial hemolysis and gamma-hemolytic strains cause no hemolysis. The primary determinant of streptococcal pathogenicity is an antigenically distinct protein known as the M protein. GABHS are capable of elaborating at least 20 extracellular substances that affect host tissue. Serologic detection of antibodies to these streptococcal antigens may provide evidence of previous streptococcal infection. The most commonly performed test is the Antistreptolysin O (ASO) titer.

Signs and symptoms of GABHS pharyngotonsillitis vary from mild sore throat and malaise (30–50% of cases) to high fever, nausea and vomiting, and dehydration (10%) *(4)*. The disorder is acute in onset, usually characterized by high fever, odynophagia, headache, and abdominal pain. The pharyngeal and tonsillar mucosa are typically erythematous and occasionally edematous, with exudate present in 50–90% of cases. Cervical adenopathy is also common, seen in 30–60% of cases. Most patients improve spontaneously in 3–5 days, unless otitis media, sinusitis, or peritonsillar abscess occur secondarily.

The risk of rheumatic fever following GABHS infection of the pharynx is approximately 0.3% in endemic situations, and 3% under epidemic circumstances *(4)*. A single episode of rheumatic fever places an individual at high risk for recurrence following additional episodes of GABHS pharyngitis *(4)*. Acute glomerulonephritis occurs as a sequela in 10–15% of those infected with nephritogenic strains *(4)*. In patients who develop these sequelae, there is usually a latent period of 1–3 weeks.

Recently, PANDAS (pediatric autoimmune neuropsychiatric disorder associated with Group A streptococcal infection) has been described as an immune-mediated illness associated with GABHS infection, similar to Sydenham's chorea. In a recent prospective study identifying children with PANDAS, the most common presentation was the abrupt onset of severe obsessive-compulsive disorder behaviors including hand washing, preoccupation with germs, and daytime urinary urgency or frequency in the absence of infection *(5)*. These behaviors resolved with treatment of the accompanying sentinel GABHS pharyngitis. Recurrences of obsessive-compulsive behaviors were seen in 50% of patients reinfected with GABHS and resolved with antibiotic treatment. However, the association of PANDAS with GABHS infection remains unproven.

Carriage of GABHS may be defined as a positive culture for the organism in the absence of a rise in ASO convalescent titer, or in the absence of symptoms. The prevalence of GABHS carriers has been estimated at 10–50%. Carriers appear to be at little risk to transmit GABHS, or to develop sequelae of the disease. It is unlikely that these individuals are at increased risk for recurrent pharyngitis. The importance of this condition is in the diagnosis of true acute streptococcal pharyngitis; when this disorder must be distinguished from nonstreptococcal disease in a carrier.

Early diagnosis of streptococcal pharyngitis has been a priority in management of the disease, primarily due to the risk of renal and cardiac sequelae. Adenopathy, fever, and pharyngeal exudate have the highest predictive value for a positive culture and rise in ASO titer, and absence of these findings in the presence of cough, rhinorrhea, hoarseness, or conjunctivitis most reliably predicts a negative culture, or positive culture without rise in ASO *(6)*.

Most clinicians advocate throat culture as the gold standard to determine appropriate treatment for GABHS. However, the tonsils, tonsillar crypts, or posterior pharyngeal wall must be swabbed for greatest accuracy. The decision whether to treat pending culture results or to delay treatment until the results are available remains controversial, although some studies suggest that early treatment hastens the clinical response to antibiotics *(7,8)*.

In the mid-1980s, tests for rapid detection of the group-specific carbohydrate became available. Such assays have simplified the decision to treat at the time of the office visit and have eliminated the need for additional postvisit communication. However, while these tests have demonstrated a specificity of greater than 95%, their sensitivity is 70–90% *(9)*. As a result, many clinicians advocate throat culture for children with suspected streptococcal disease and negative rapid strep tests. Rapid antigen detection is usually more expensive than throat culture, and this technique must still be interpreted with care given the high incidence of post-treatment carriers. Studies also suggest a "learning curve effect" associated with this diagnostic modality. Serologic tests for ASO are the definitive means for diagnosing acute streptococcal infection.

Although most upper respiratory infections by GABHS resolve without treatment, antimicrobial therapy prevents suppurative and nonsuppurative sequelae including rheumatic fever and may also hasten clinical improvement *(7,8,10)*. Treatment is therefore indicated for positive rapid tests for the Group A antigen. When the test is negative or not available, one may treat empirically for a full course, assuming the test was falsely negative or for a few days pending throat culture results.

GABHS is sensitive to a number of antibiotics, including penicillins, cephalosporins, macrolides, and clindamycin. Expert panels have designated penicillin the drug of choice in managing GABHS owing to its track record of safety, efficacy, and for having a narrow spectrum *(11–14)*. To date, no strains of GABHS acquired in vivo have demonstrated penicillin resistance or increased minimum inhibitory concentrations in vitro *(15)*. Amoxicillin appears to have efficacy equal to that of penicillin *(13)*. When poor compliance is anticipated, azithromycin dosed once daily for 5 days may be a reasonable alternative. Erythromycin remains the drug of choice for patients with penicillin allergy.

Most patients with positive cultures following treatment are GABHS carriers; these individuals need not be retreated if their symptoms have resolved. For patients in whom complete bacteriologic clearance is desirable, such as those with a family member with a history of rheumatic fever, a course of clindamycin or a second course of penicillin combined with rifampin may yield increased success. In patients with recurrent symptoms, serotyping may aid in distinguishing bacterial persistence from recurrence. There are no data available regarding the use of antibiotic prophylaxis in these patients, and in such cases tonsillectomy may be most advantageous.

During antimicrobial therapy, patients must be monitored carefully for fluid intake, pain control, and impending suppurative complications such as peritonsillar abscess. Small children may become dehydrated rapidly, and may require hospitalization for administration of fluids intravenously.

Removal of the tonsils as prevention against infection has been a popular concept for decades. During the 1960s and 1970s, the procedure finally came under attack for its lack of scientific basis. A recent resurgence of interest in the procedure has resulted from a series of trials by Paradise and colleagues at the University of Pittsburgh supporting the use of tonsillectomy in cases of recurrent pharyngitis ***(16,17)***. However, the results of these studies must be interpreted with caution, and the procedure offered only to those children who meet the agreed criteria of seven episodes of GABHS in 1 year, five episodes a year for 2 years, or three episodes a year for 3 years ***(16)***.

Infectious Mononucleosis

Pharyngitis is one of the hallmarks of infectious mononucleosis, a disorder associated with primary infection by the Epstein–Barr virus (EBV), a member of the herpes virus family. Serologic reactivity to EBV antigens has been demonstrated in 80–95% of adults ***(18)***. However, while primary infection by EBV occurs during the second and third decade in developed nations and regions of high socioeconomic status, young children are more commonly affected in developing countries and regions of low socioeconomic status. When the virus is acquired at a younger age, symptoms are generally less severe. The incidence of infectious mononucleosis in the United States is approximately one per 50–100,000 per year, but increases to about 100 per 100,000 among adolescents and young adults ***(19)***. Infected individuals transmit EBV by way of saliva exchanged during kissing or other close contact.

EBV preferentially infects and transforms human B lymphocytes. The virus enters the cell by attaching to a receptor designed for proteins of the complement chain, and its genetic material is transported by vesicles to the nucleus, where it dwells as a plasmid and maintains a "latent" state of replication. An incubation period of 2–7 weeks follows initial exposure, during which EBV induces a proliferation of infected B-cells. Infectious mononucleosis is characterized by a prodrome of malaise and fatigue, followed by the acute onset of fever and sore throat. Physical examination typically reveals enlarged, erythematous palatine tonsils, in most cases with yellow-white exudate on the surface and within the crypts. Cervical adenopathy is present in nearly all patients, and involvement of the posterior cervical nodes often helps distinguish EBV infection from that by streptococcus or other organisms. Between the second and fourth weeks of illness, approximately 50% of patients develop splenomegaly, and 30–50% develop hepatomegaly ***(20)***. Rash, palatal petechiae, and abdominal pain may also be present in some cases. The fever and pharyngitis generally subside within about 2 weeks, while adenopathy, organomegaly, and malaise may last as long as 6 weeks.

Diagnosis of infectious mononucleosis can usually be made on the basis of clinical presentation, absolute lymphocytosis, the presence of atypical lymphocytes in the peripheral smear, and detection of Paul-Bunnell heterophil antibodies. The latter is the basis of the Mono-Spot, Mono-Diff, and Mono-Test assays, which test for agglutination of horse erythrocytes. Children under 5 years of age may not develop a detectable heterophil antibody titer; in these patients, it is possible to determine titers of IgG antibodies to the viral capsid antigen, as well as antibodies to the "early antigen" complex. Antibodies to EBV nuclear antigen appear late in the course of the disease. In most cases, rest, fluids, and analgesics are adequate to manage the symptoms of infectious mononucleosis. In more symptomatic patients, particularly those with respiratory compromise due to severe tonsillar enlargement and those with hematologic or neurologic complications, a course of systemic steroids may hasten resolution of the acute symptoms. Placement of a nasopharyngeal trumpet or endotracheal intubation may be necessary on rare occasions when complete airway obstruction is imminent. Antibiotics may be useful in cases of concomitant Group A beta-hemolytic pharyngotonsillitis; however, ampicillin use is known to induce a rash in this setting. The use of antiviral agents in infectious mononucleosis has yielded disappointing results.

Exposure to EBV has been implicated in the development of post-transplantation lymphoproliferative disorder (PTLD). Immune-suppressed children who have received bone marrow and solid organ transplants, may develop abnormal proliferation of lymphoid cells. Approximately 80% of affected individuals have a history of EBV infection ***(23)***. The clinical presentation is variable and can mimic graft-versus-host disease, graft rejection, or more conventional infections. Signs and symptoms may resemble an infectious mononucleosis-like illness or an extranodal tumor, commonly involving the gut, brain, or the transplanted organ. Mononucleosis-like presentations typically occur in children, within the first year of transplant, and are often associated with primary EBV infection after transfer of donor virus from the grafted organ. Extranodal tumors are more common among EBV seropositive recipients several years after the transplant ***(24)***. Even after conventional lymphoma chemotherapies, mortality is over 50% ***(24)***. Novel forms of immunotherapy have been tested in PTLD, including both antibody and cell-mediated approaches.

Gonorrhea

Infection by *Neisseria gonorrhea* is a rare source of pharyngitis in children, occurring almost exclusively among those who are sexually abused. In one series, oropharyngeal gonorrhea was reported in 4–6% of sexually abused children ***(25)***.

Gonococcal pharyngitis most commonly presents as an exudative pharyngitis accompanied by fever and adenopathy, not unlike that associated with a number of other organisms. The physician must therefore remain cognizant of other possible manifestations of gonococcal infection, and of signs and symptoms of other sexually transmitted diseases. Cultures should be obtained to confirm the diagnosis in suspicious cases, and to direct antibiotic therapy that is most commonly a single parenteral administration of ceftriaxone. Treatment should also be offered to the offending individual, and the infections must be reported to the appropriate local and national authorities.

Diphtheria

With the development of diphtheria toxoid and aggressive immunization programs, diphtheria laryngotracheitis has become all but extinct in the developed world. Since 1980, new cases have been reported to the Centers for Disease Control at a rate of 0.001 per 100,000, or approximately three new cases per year ***(26)***. Nevertheless, the disease remains endemic in many nations throughout the world.

Diphtheria laryngotracheitis is caused by *Corynebacterium diphtheriae*, a club-shaped, Gram-positive bacillus. The bacterium is usually acquired via the respiratory passages or, rarely, the mucous membranes. Nasal congestion, pharyngitis, anorexia, and low-grade fever may be present. Cervical lymphadenitis and edema of the soft tissues of the neck are also common.

Following an incubation period of 2–4 days, diphtheria exotoxin is released by the organism, initiating local tissue necrosis and exudate. As the affected area expands, the exudate turns fibrinous and develops into an adherent gray membrane also containing inflammatory cells, epithelial cells, and red blood cells. Enlargement of the membrane and progressive edema cause airway compromise and stridor, and dislodgement of the membrane may cause frank obstruction. Systemic effects of the toxin include myocarditis, peripheral neuritis, and acute tubular necrosis of the kidneys.

Definitive diagnosis is made by culture of the membrane, but management should not be delayed for culture results. Severely compromised patients will require an artificial airway, usually tracheotomy, since the membranes are generally more tenacious than those in bacterial tracheitis. Once the airway is secure and a presumptive diagnosis is made, the patient is tested for sensitivity to horse serum and antitoxin is administered. Antibiotic therapy with penicillin or erythromycin is subsequently started, and nonimmune personal contacts are also treated. Prognosis depends on the immunization status of the host, the promptness of medical therapy, and the virulence of the infecting organism. Prevention of diphtheria is achieved through immunization during infancy.

Kawasaki Disease (Mucocutaneous Lymph Node Syndrome)

Kawasaki disease (KD) is a disorder of unknown etiology characterized by fever, rash, pharyngitis, conjunctival inflammation, edema of the extremities, and cervical adenopathy. KD has been linked over the last three decades to serious cardiac complications, arthritis, and a number of other manifestations.

KD is a disease of young children, with 80% of cases occurring in children under 5 years of age *(27)*. Fatalities are most common during infancy. The disease is slightly more common in males and among individuals of Asian extraction. Between 3,000 and 5,000 cases occur annually in the United States *(28)*.

Most investigators believe KD to be the result of an infectious agent or an immune response to an infectious agent. KD occurs in three distinct clinical phases. The acute phase lasts 1–2 weeks and is characterized by prolonged high spiking fever, oral and oropharyngeal changes, rash, erythema of the bulbar conjunctiva, swelling and erythema of the extremities, and adenopathy. In the subacute phase, days 10–25, most of these signs and symptoms resolve; however, conjunctival changes usually persist and the child remains irritable. The toes and fingers begin to desquamate and joint pain is present in about 30% of patients. Cardiac dysfunction typically becomes evident during this period. The third or convalescent stage begins when clinical signs of KD have completely resolved and ends when the sedimentation rate returns to normal.

Diagnosis of KD is based on the clinical presentation. Patients must have a history of persistent fever, elevation of the sedimentation rate, as well as four of the five other acute signs listed above. Therapy for KD in the acute phase is directed at prevention of cardiac complications. High-dose aspirin is usually administered, with a watchful eye for signs of Reye's syndrome, to decrease myocardial inflammation and prevent thrombosis. Addition of intravenous immune globulin (IVIG) to the protocol results in a more rapid anti-inflammatory effect than that seen with aspirin alone. IVIG also appears to lessen the risk of long-term coronary artery abnormalities. Other manifestations of KD are treated symptomatically. Once the convalescent phase is reached, patients are generally monitored at regular intervals for evidence of cardiac complications.

Peritonsillar Infection

Peritonsillar infection may present as either cellulitis or abscess (PTA). Peritonsillar infection occurs more commonly in adolescents and young adults than in young children. Affected patients present with symptoms of sore throat, odynophagia, fever, voice change, and otalgia. Common physical findings include fever, drooling, trismus, muffled "hot potato" voice, and pharyngeal asymmetry with inferior and medial displacement of the tonsil. Radiographic evaluation is usually not necessary, but may be useful in young or uncooperative children or in equivocal cases. Computerized tomography with contrast remains the imaging modality of choice in children *(29)*.

While patients with peritonsillar cellulitis may be treated with antibiotics alone, most abscesses require either aspiration or incision and drainage as definitive therapy. Evacuation of a PTA can be managed by needle aspiration, incision and drainage, or immediate ("quinsy") tonsillectomy with nearly equivalent efficacy *(30,31)*. In very young or poorly cooperative patients, or in those in whom an abscess has been inadequately drained, tonsillectomy is curative and essentially eliminates any chance of recurrence.

"Chronic" Tonsillitis

Chronic tonsillitis is a poorly defined condition that is usually a reference to a sore throat of at least 3 months' duration accompanied by physical findings of tonsillar inflammation. Affected individuals may report symptoms of chronic sore throat, halitosis, or debris or concretions in the tonsil crypts, and may have persistent cervical adenopathy. Throat culture in such cases is usually negative. Tonsillectomy may be useful for children who do not respond to improved oropharyngeal hygiene and aggressive antibiotic therapy.

Infectious and Inflammatory Disease of the Adenoid

Recurrent or Chronic Adenoiditis

Because the affected tissue resides on the posterior wall of the nasopharynx where visualization and culture are difficult, adenoiditis is usually diagnosed based on symptoms rather than physical findings. Most individuals in whom the diagnosis is made present with nasal stuffiness, mucopurulent rhinorrhea, halitosis, chronic cough, and "snorting" or "gagging" on the mucus throughout the day. There are no established criteria for making this diagnosis, or for differentiating it from viral upper respiratory illness or acute sinusitis.

Often the symptoms attributed to chronic adenoiditis may be the result of adenoid hyperplasia encroaching on the choanae and causing stasis of secretions within the nose. In such cases, it may be difficult to tell whether the adenoid size is causing the symptoms or whether the hyperplasia was induced by chronic inflammation within the adenoid pad *(32)*, but adenoidectomy is often curative. Organisms commonly isolated include *Haemophilus influenzae*, *Moraxella catarrhalis*, a variety of streptococci including Group A, *Staphylococcus aureus*, and *Streptococcus pneumoniae*.

Antibiotic therapy directed at common upper respiratory organisms is reasonable for patients with symptoms of chronic adenoiditis. However, recent data suggest that many organisms, particularly *H. influenzae*, are capable of forming bacterial biofilms within the adenoid that make them resistant to such therapy *(32,33)*. The adenoid may also become inflamed secondary to gastroesophageal reflux disease (GERD).

The relationship between chronic rhinorrhea, chronic adenoiditis, and recurrent rhinosinusitis is poorly understood. Recent data suggest that adenoidectomy may be efficacious in the management of children with persistent and recurrent sinonasal complaints, and most clinicians favor adenoidectomy prior to consideration of endoscopic sinus surgery *(34)*.

The proximity of the adenoid pad to the eustachian tube has prompted a number of clinicians to study the potential benefits of adenoidectomy and adenotonsillectomy in the management of otitis media. The effect of the adenoid on the eustachian tube is likely one of regional inflammation or infection rather than one of direct compression *(34)*. There is increasing evidence that adenoidectomy *(35–40)* has a role in the management of both recurrent acute and chronic otitis media. Based on the data, adenoidectomy should be considered along with the first set of tubes if the child has symptoms of nasal obstruction or recurrent rhinorrhea, or whenever a second set of tubes is necessary *(34)*. In children with a history of cleft palate, the procedure should be performed only when the otitis is relentless; in such cases, an inferior strip of adenoid should be preserved to avoid velopharyngeal insufficiency. Tonsillectomy is a reasonable additional procedure when indications such as airway obstruction or recurrent pharyngitis are also present.

Malignancy

The most common malignant neoplasm in the oropharyngeal cavity in children is lymphoma, usually non-Hodgkin B-cell *(41)*. Unilateral tonsillar enlargement or asymmetry of the tonsils in the absence of acute infection is a common finding in children. Although malignancy should always be considered as part of the differential diagnosis, other nonmalignant causes include: chronic infection, glycogen or lipid storage disorders, benign tumors, and pathologies of adjacent tissue *(27)*.

Unilateral tonsillar enlargement is generally a result of the asymmetry of the anterior tonsillar pillars or difference in depth of the tonsillar fossa rather than a true tonsillar enlargement *(41)*. Rapid unilateral enlargement of the tonsil is very suggestive of tonsillar lymphoma, especially when associated with local and systemic symptoms such as dysphagia, fever, weight loss, cervical lymphadenopathy, or hepatosplenomegaly *(41)*. Tonsillar lymphoma should also be considered when acute tonsillitis is asymmetric and asymmetry persists despite appropriate medical treatment *(41)*. The lesions are often bulky and large, gray-tan in color, and may extend into adjacent soft tissue or have ulceration *(27)*. Biopsy is necessary for histological diagnosis and involves tonsillectomy. Treatment options for non-Hodgkin lymphoma include radiotherapy and chemotherapy *(27)*.

Conclusions

The tonsils and adenoid are lymphoid tissues that participate in the development of regional immunity in the pharynx. As such, they are readily susceptible to disorders such as infection, neoplasia, or hyperplasia. Common infections include Group A streptococcal pharyngitis, infectious mononucleosis, peritonsillar abscess, and chronic adenoiditis. Neoplastic disease is far less common and is usually lymphoma arising primarily or as a result of a posttransplantation lymphoproliferative disorder. Resulting alterations in the tonsils and adenoid may affect their function and the function of neighboring structures and tissues.

References

1. Paulussen C, Claes J, Claes G, Jorissen M. Adenoids and tonsils, indications for surgery and immunological consequences of surgery. Acta Otorhinolaryngol Belg 2000;54:403–8.
2. Cherry JD. Pharyngitis. In: Feigin RD, Cherry JD, eds. Textbook of Pediatric Infectious Diseases, 4th edition. Philadelphia: W.B. Saunders Co. 1998:148–56.
3. Markowitz M. Changing epidemiology of Group A streptococcal infections. Pediatr Infect Dis J 1994;13:557–60.
4. Kaplan EL, Gerber MA. Group A streptococcal infections. In: Feigin RD, Cherry JD, eds. Textbook of Pediatric Infectious Diseases, 4th edition. Philadelphia: W.B. Saunders Co. 1998:1076–88.
5. Murphy ML, Pichichero ME: Prospective identification and treatment of children with pediatric autoimmune neuropsychiatric disorder associated with Group A streptococcal infection (PANDAS). Arch Pediatr Adolesc Med 2002;156:356–61.
6. Kline JA, Runge JW. Streptococcal pharyngitis: a review of pathophysiology, diagnosis, and management. J Emerg Med 1994;12:665–80.
7. Randolph MF, Gerber MA, DeMeo KK, Wright L. Effect of antibiotic therapy on the clinical course of streptococcal pharyngitis. J Pediatr 1985;106:870–5.
8. Krober MS, Bass JW, Michels GN. Streptococcal pharyngitis: placebo-controlled double-blind evaluation of clinical response to penicillin therapy. JAMA 1985;253:1271–4.
9. Gerber MA, Shulman ST. Rapid diagnosis of pharyngitis caused by Group A streptococci. Clin Microbiol Rev 2004;17:571–80.
10. Del Mar CB, Glasziou PP, Spinks AB. Antibiotics for sore throat. Cochrane Database Syst Rev 2006;4:CD000023.
11. Bisno AL, Gerber MA, Gwaltney JM, Kaplan EL, Schwartz RH. Practice guidelines for the diagnosis and management of Group A streptococcal pharyngitis. Clin Infect Dis 2002;35:113–25.
12. American Academy of Pediatrics Committee on Infectious Diseases. Red Book: Report of the Committee on Infectious Diseases, 27th edition. Elk Grove Village, IL: American Academy of Pediatrics. 2006:610–20.
13. Dajani A, Taubert K, Ferrieri P, Peter G, Shulman S. Treatment of acute streptococcal pharyngitis and prevention of rheumatic fever: a statement for health professionals. American Heart Association Committee on Rheumatic Fever, Endocarditis, and Kawasaki Disease of the Council on Cardiovascular Disease in the Young. Pediatrics 1995;96:758–64.
14. World Health Organization. Rheumatic Fever and Rheumatic Heart Disease. Geneva, Switzerland: World Health Organization. 1988. Technical Report Series No. 764.
15. Gerber MA. Diagnosis and treatment of pharyngitis in children. Pediatr Clin North Am 2005;52:729–47.
16. Paradise JL, Bluestone CD, Bachman RZ, et al. Efficacy of tonsillectomy for recurrent throat infection in severely affected children. N Engl J Med 1984;310:674–83.
17. Paradise JL, Bluestone CD, Colborn DK, Bernard BS, Rockette HE, Kurs-Lasky M. Tonsillectomy and adenotonsillectomy for recurrent throat infection in moderately affected children. Pediatrics 2002;110:7–15.
18. Henle W, Henle G. Epidemiologic aspects of Epstein–Barr virus (EBV)-associated diseases. Ann NY Acad Sci 1980;354:326–31.
19. Plotkin SA. Infectious mononucleosis. In: Behrman RE, Kliegman RM, Nelson WE, eds. Nelson' Textbook of Pediatrics, 14th edition. Philadelphia: W.B. Saunders Co. 1992:805–8.
20. Sumaya CV. Epstein–Barr virus. In: Feigin RD, Cherry JD, eds. Textbook of Pediatric Infectious Diseases, 4th edition. Philadelphia: W.B. Saunders Co. 1998:1751–64.
21. Andersson J, Britton S, Ernberg I, Andersson U, Henle W, Skoldenberg B, Tisell A. Effect of acyclovir on infectious mononucleosis: a double-blind, placebo-controlled study. J Infect Dis 1986;153:283–90.
22. van der Horst C, Joncas J, Ahronheim G, et al. Lack of effect of peroral acyclovir for the treatment of acute infectious mononucleosis. J Infect Dis 1991;164:788–92.
23. Shapiro NL, Strocker AM, Bhattacharyya N. Risk factors for adenotonsillar hypertrophy in children following solid organ transplantation. Int J Pediatr Otorhinolaryngol 2003;67:151–5.
24. Macsween KF, Crawford DH. Epstein–Barr virus-recent advances. Lancet Infect Dis 2003;3:131–40.
25. White ST, Loda FA, Ingram DL, Pearson A. Sexually transmitted diseases in sexually abused children. Pediatrics 1983;72:16–21.
26. http://www.cdc.gov/ncidod/dbmd/diseaseinfo/diptheria_t.htm
27. Cinar F. Significance of asymptomatic tonsil asymmetry. Otolaryngol Head Neck Surg 2004;131:101–3.
28. American Academy of Pediatrics Committee on Infectious Diseases. Red Book: Report of the Committee on Infectious Diseases, 27th edition. Elk Grove Village, IL: American Academy of Pediatrics. 2006:412–15.
29. Friedman NR, Mitchell RB, Pereira KD, Younis RT, Lazar RH. Peritonsillar abscess in early childhood. Presentation and management. Arch Otolaryngol Head Neck Surg 1997;123:630–2.

30. Johnson RF, Stewart MG, Wright CC. An evidence-based review of the treatment of peritonsillar abscess. Otolaryngol Head Neck Surg 2003;128:332–43.
31. Herzon FS. Peritonsillar abscess: incidence, current management practices, and a proposal for treatment guidelines. Laryngoscope 1995;105:1–17.
32. Lee D, Rosenfeld RM. Adenoid bacteriology and sinonasal symptoms in children. Otolaryngol Head Neck Surg 1997;116:301–7.
33. Galli J, Calo L, Ardito F, Imperiali M, Bassotti E, Fadda G, Paludetti G. Biofilm formation by Haemophilus influenzae isolated from adeno-tonsil tissue samples, and its role in recurrent adenotonsillitis. Acta Otolaryngol Ital 2007;27:134–8.
34. Zuliani G, Carron M, Gurrola J. Identification of adenoid biofilms in chronic rhinosinusitis. Int J Pediatr Otorhinolaryngol 2006;70:1613–17. Epub 2006 Jun 16.
35. Vandenberg SJ, Heatley DG. Efficacy of adenoidectomy in relieving symptoms of chronic sinusitis in children. Arch Otolaryngol Head Neck Surg 1997;123:675–8.
36. Maw AR. Chronic otitis media with effusion (glue ear) and adenotonsillectomy: prospective randomised controlled study. BMJ 1983;287:1585–8.
37. Gates GA, Avery CA, Prihoda TJ, Cooper JC. Effectiveness of adenoidectomy and tympanostomy tubes in the treatment of chronic otitis media with effusion. N Engl J Med 1987;317:1444–51.
38. Paradise JL, Bluestone CD, Rogers KD, et al. Efficacy of adenoidectomy for recurrent otitis media in children previously treated with tympanostomy-tube placement: Results of parallel randomized and nonrandomized trials. JAMA 1990;263:2066–73.
39. Coyte PC, Croxford R, McIsaac W, Feldman W, Friedberg J. The role of adjuvant adenoidectomy and tonsillectomy in the outcome of the insertion of tympanostomy tubes. N Engl J Med 2001;344:1188–95.
40. Paradise JL, Bluestone CD, Colborn DK, Bernard BS, Smith CG, Rockette HE, Kurs-Lasy M. Adenoidectomy and adenotonsillectomy for recurrent acute otitis media: parallel randomized clinical trials in children not previously treated with tympanostomy tubes. JAMA 1999;282:945–53.
41. Berkowitz RG, Mahadevan M. Unilateral tonsillar enlargement and tonsillar lymphoma in children. Ann Otol Rhinol Laryngol 1999;108:876–9.

Sleep-Disordered Breathing (SDB) in Children

Ron B. Mitchell

Key Points

- SDB is diagnosed with increasing frequency in children and is known to affect behavior, quality of life, and school performance.
- In the majority of children with SDB, the diagnosis is based on the presence of daytime and night-time symptoms along with adenotonsillar hypertrophy.
- Polysomnography (PSG) is the "gold standard" for the diagnosis and quantification of SDB and used when there is doubt about the diagnosis, in high-risk groups, or when there are persistent symptoms of SDB after surgical therapy.
- Children with obesity, craniofacial, neuromuscular, and genetic disorders are more likely to have SDB and persistent symptoms after surgery.
- Adenotonsillectomy (T&A) leads to resolution of SDB in majority of children including improvements in behavior, quality of life, and school performance.

Keywords: Sleep • Apnea • Children • Tonsils • Polysomnography

Sleep-disordered breathing (SDB) in children represents a spectrum of sleep problems ranging in severity from primary snoring to upper airway resistance to obstructive sleep apnea (OSA) *(1)*. SDB has been diagnosed in children with an increasing frequency over the past 20 years *(2)*. There is compelling evidence that SDB affects behavior, neurocognition, and quality of life in children. Adenotonsillar hypertrophy is the most common cause of SDB, and adenotonsillectomy has become the surgical therapy of choice for these sleep disorders *(3)*.

R.B. Mitchell
Division of Pediatric Otolaryngology, Department of Otolaryngology – Head and Neck Surgery, Cardinal Glennon Children's Medical Center, Saint Louis University School of Medicine, St. Louis, MO, USA
e-mail: rmitch11@slu.edu

Definition

Snoring – noisy breathing during sleep with normal oxygen saturation and no sleep disruption.

Upper airway resistance – snoring, labored breathing, paradoxical breathing, and disrupted sleep, without discrete obstructive apneas or hypopneas.

Obstructive sleep apnea – reduction (hypopnea) or cessation (apnea) of airflow through the nostrils and mouth that can be associated with oxygen desaturation and disruption of sleep.

Prevalence

Between 10 and 25% of children snore. OSA is present in 1–4% of children. The prevalence of OSA is highest in 4–6 year olds.

Diagnosis

Clinical evaluation – Diagnosis is based on a history of daytime and night-time symptoms in a child with adenotonsillar hypertrophy. These symptoms include loud snoring, witnessed apneas, periods when the child is gasping for air or choking, and possible enuresis. During the day the child may have hypersomnolence

R.B. Mitchell and K.D. Pereira (eds.), *Pediatric Otolaryngology for the Clinician,*

DOI: 10.1007/978-1-60327-127-1_25,

or hyperactivity. Attention problems that lead to reduced school performance are common. Healthcare utilization is higher in children with SDB and decreases after surgical therapy *(4)*. Although a clinical history is accurate at confirming the presence of snoring it is poor at diagnosing or quantifying OSA *(5)*.

Polysomnography – Objective assessment of the presence and severity of SDB is accomplished with overnight polysomnography (sleep study) *(6)*. It is the "gold standard" for diagnosing and quantifying SDB. This evaluation involves recording respiratory effort (oronasal airflow, movement of chest and abdomen, pulse oximetry, end tidal CO_2) and nonrespiratory (heart rate, electroencephalography, electrooculography) parameters. The number of obstructive apneas (total cessation of oronasal airflow for two or more respiratory cycles with persistence of respiratory effort) and hypopneas (50% or greater reduction in oronasal airflow for two or more respiratory cycles) is commonly reported. Apneas can also be categorized as obstructive, central, or mixed. SDB severity can be graded based on a number of factors. Most sleep laboratories report the respiratory distress index (RDI) or the apnea hypopnea index (AHI) as a measure of severity. The other commonly used measure of severity is the minimum oxygen saturation. The RDI or AHI typically includes the number of obstructive apneas and hypopneas as well as central apneas per hour. Although an accurate indicator for the diagnosis of SDB, polysomnography is expensive, time consuming, and is not available in all institutions.

Other diagnostic methods:

Questionnaires – Many are available but mostly used as research tools. The most commonly used is the OSA-18 quality-of-life survey *(7)*.

Oximetry – It is of limited diagnostic value because children with SDB do not necessarily have periods of desaturation. If an oximetry study is normal, a formal PSG is necessary. Oximetry may be used as a triage tool either to reassure parents who have a heightened concern about their child's breathing pattern with limited or no access to a sleep study or to identify children who have significant hypoxemia and need more urgent attention *(1)*.

Nap studies – The same monitoring sensors as overnight polysomnography are used but the test occurs during the day and has a short sampling time of less than 4 h. Nap studies have significant limitations. Children over 4 years rarely nap and rapid eye movement sleep is unlikely to occur during this limited study thus underestimating the severity of SDB. A negative nap study would require overnight polysomnography to rule out SDB *(1)*.

Others – Audiotapes and videotapes recorded by caregivers are useful, inexpensive ways of documenting SDB *(1)*.

High-Risk Groups

The factors determining high-risk group include:

Young children – Children under the age of 3 are more likely to have perioperative complications particularly respiratory compromise. They are also more likely to have poor oral intake and dehydration after surgery. Children with craniofacial, neuromuscular, or genetic disorders often present with SDB before the age of 3 and can form a high proportion of children in this category, especially in tertiary referral centers. A high proportion of these young children are routinely monitored overnight after surgery *(8)*.

Obesity – The prevalence of childhood obesity in the USA has risen from 6 to 14% over the last quarter century and the prevalence of SDB in children with obesity is 25–40%. SDB is more severe in these children and surgical therapy improves but does not always resolve the sleep disorder *(9)*. Children with obesity are at high risk of postoperative respiratory compromise.

Down syndrome – Multiple anatomic and physiologic factors predispose these children to SDB. The prevalence of SDB in children with Down syndrome is reported to be between 50 and 100%. Even though surgery may be successful initially, recurrence of symptoms of SDB is high.

Craniofacial problems – These deformities result from abnormal development of the brain, cranium, and facial skeleton, and include Apert, Crouzon, and Pfeiffer syndromes. SDB in these children is caused by structural abnormalities of the maxilla, mandible, and palate that lead to crowding of the nasopharynx and oropharynx. *This results in a complex clinical picture that may vary over time.*

Neuromuscular disorders – Children with neuromuscular diseases form a heterogeneous group based on the etiology of individual disorders. The symptoms of SDB in children with neuromuscular disease are probably underestimated and often difficult to distinguish from the underlying disease.

Mucopolysaccharidoses – These are a group of genetic disorders characterized by accumulation of mucopolysaccharides in the soft tissues of the body. SDB is common in these children because of upper airway narrowing caused by hypertrophy of the tongue, tonsils, adenoids, and mucous membranes. SDB is a severe and progressive consequence of mucopolysaccharidoses and not infrequently the cause of death in these children.

Others – Children with cerebral palsy, sickle-cell anemia, Arnold-Chiari malformations, Prader-Willi syndrome, and achondroplasia.

The prevalence of SDB is usually underestimated and surgical management is more complex in these children ***(10)***. These children are more likely to have upper airway obstruction that is multifactorial in etiology, and they more commonly have perioperative complications. In these cases, T&A may only lead to partial resolution of SDB. Additional procedures such as uvulopalatopharyngoplasty (UPPP) and tracheotomy may be necessary in selected children. In addition, some of these high-risk children will be candidates for continuous positive airway pressure (CPAP).

Treatment

T&A is the first-line treatment in the majority of children with SDB. Most children undergo T&A as an outpatient procedure. It is effective in resolving SDB in over 85% of children ***(3)***. Children with mild SDB or persistent symptoms after surgery may benefit from nonsurgical anti-inflammatory treatments including a nasal steroid spray and/or a leukotriene modifier (montelukast) ***(11)***. In children with craniofacial, neuromuscular, and/or genetic disorders, T&A results in improvement but usually not resolution of SDB. Other more extensive procedures such as UPPP, facial advancement, and tracheotomy may be required in selected cases. CPAP may be used in addition to surgical therapy in cases where compliance can be achieved ***(12)*** (Fig. 1).

Outcome

Polysomnography – Adenotonsillectomy, in the majority of children (>85%), leads to significant improvements

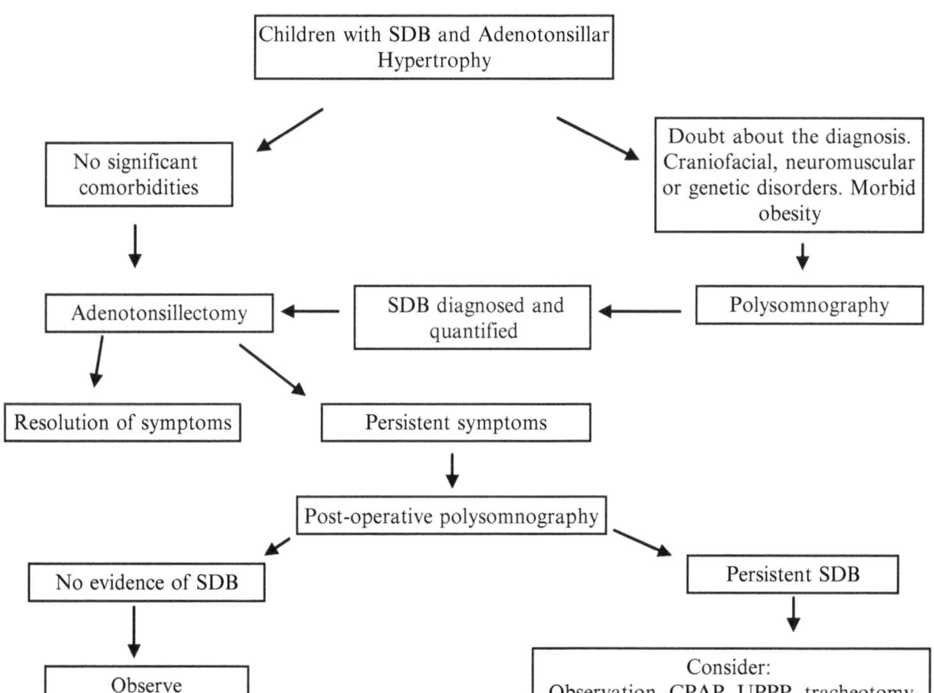

Fig. 1 SDB in children

in sleep parameters as measured by postoperative polysomnography *(3)*.

Quality of life – Caregivers report a dramatic improvement in sleep disturbance, physical symptoms, emotional symptoms, and daytime functioning in their children after T&A for SDB *(2)*.

Behavior – A high proportion of children with SDB have externalizing (hyperactivity and aggression) and internalizing (anxiety, depression, and somatization) behavioral problems. These problems improve significantly after T&A and are maintained for at least a year after surgery.

School performance and healthcare resources – There is evidence that the improvement in sleep after T&A leads to better school performance *(13)* and a decrease in healthcare utilization for children *(4)*.

References

1. Clinical practice guideline: diagnosis and management of childhood obstructive sleep apnea syndrome. *Pediatrics* 2002;109:704–12.
2. Mitchell RB, Kelly J. Behavior, neurocognition and quality-of-life in children with sleep-disordered breathing. *Int J Pediatr Otorhinolaryngol* 2006;70:395–406.
3. Mitchell RB. Adenotonsillectomy for obstructive sleep apnea in children: outcome evaluated by pre- and postoperative polysomnography. Laryngoscope 2007;117(10):1844–54.
4. Tarasiuk A, Simon T, Tal A, Reuveni H. Adenotonsillectomy in children with obstructive sleep apnea syndrome reduces health care utilization. Pediatrics 2004;113(2):351–6.
5. Brietzke SE, Katz ES, Roberson DW. Can history and physical examination reliably diagnose pediatric obstructive sleep apnea/hypopnea syndrome? A systematic review of the literature. Otolaryngol Head Neck Surg 2004;131(6):827–32.
6. American Thoracic Society. Cardiorespiratory sleep studies in children. Establishment of normative data and polysomnographic predictors of morbidity. Am J Respir Crit Care Med 1999;160(4):1381–7.
7. Franco RA Jr, Rosenfeld RM, Rao M. First place – resident clinical science award 1999. Quality of life for children with obstructive sleep apnea. Otolaryngol Head Neck Surg 2000;123(1 Pt 1):9–16.
8. Mitchell RB, Kelly J. Outcome of adenotonsillectomy for obstructive sleep apnea in children under 3 years. Otolaryngol Head Neck Surg 2005;132(5):681–4.
9. Mitchell RB, Kelly J. Outcome of adenotonsillectomy for obstructive sleep apnea in obese and normal-weight children. Otolaryngol Head Neck Surg 2007;137(1):43–8.
10. Mitchell RB, Kelly J. Pediatric SDB: high-risk populations and special circumstances. Richardson M, Friedman N, editors. In: Pediatric Sleep-Disordered Breathing. Marcel Dekker, Inc. 2006.
11. Goldbart AD, Goldman JL, Veling MC, Gozal D. Leukotriene modifier therapy for mild sleep-disordered breathing in children. Am J Respir Crit Care Med 2005;172(3):364–70.
12. Marcus CL, Rosen G, Ward SL, Halbower AC, Sterni L, Lutz J, Stading PJ, Bolduc D, Gordon N. Adherence to and effectiveness of positive airway pressure therapy in children with obstructive sleep apnea. Pediatrics 2006;117(3):e442–51.
13. Gozal D. Sleep-disordered breathing and school performance in children. Pediatrics 1998;102(3 Pt 1):616–20.

Pediatric Vascular Tumors

Scott C. Manning and Jonathan A. Perkins

Key Points

- Hemangiomas, lymphatic and venous malformations comprise the most common head and neck tumors of the pediatric age group.
- The majority of these lesions that require treatment are located in the head and neck region.
- Otolaryngologists occupy a central position in the team management of these challenging problems. Various other specialists from other fields including dermatology, plastic and general surgery, diagnostic and interventional radiology, orthopedics, psychiatry, pathology, and ophthalmology play a role in the management of these problems.
- Primary care providers should be encouraged to refer all suspected vascular anomalies as early as possible since timely diagnosis and treatment are often the keys to optimal management.

Keywords: Vascular anomaly • Hemangioma • Venous malformation • Lymphatic malformation • Arterio-venous malformation • Klippel–Trenaunay syndrome • syndrome • Kasabach–Merritt phenomenon

Introduction

The modern era of vascular anomaly understanding is based upon the clinical, histologic, and biochemical differences among these lesions. For example, Mulliken and Glowacki *(1)* described differences between hemangioma of infancy and other vascular anomalies. Subsequently, North et al. *(2)* described the hemangioma endothelial marker glucose 1 transporter (GLUT1) as a histologic way to differentiate these lesions from other vascular anomalies. Better understanding of the biochemical makeup and clinical differences between these lesions has led to better prognostication, more appropriate treatment, better timing of treatment, and ultimately better outcomes. New research exploring the fundamental aspects of angiogenesis and its inhibition treatments for cancer and chronic inflammatory processes promises to bring new treatment options to parents of children with vascular anomalies.

Since a large fraction of these lesions involve the head and neck region, otolaryngology plays a central role in the team management of these children along with dermatology, plastic and general surgery, diagnostic and interventional radiology, orthopedics, psychiatry, pathology, and ophthalmology. Primary care providers should be encouraged to refer all suspected vascular anomalies as early as possible (including direct communication to vascular anomaly centers to ensure that suspected hemangiomas are seen as soon as possible) since timely diagnosis and treatment are often the keys to optimal management.

Definitions

The definitions of pediatric vascular anomalies have changed over the past decade and continue to evolve as new research provides increasing understanding of these lesions. The main differentiation in current classification models is now between vascular tumors (new cell growth) and vascular malformations (disorganized

S.C. Manning (✉)
Department of Otolaryngology, University of Washington, Division of Pediatric Otolaryngology, Seattle Children's Hospital, Seattle, WA, USA
e-mail: scott.manning@seattlechildrens.org

J.A. Perkins
Department of Otolaryngology, University of Washington, Vascular Anomalies Service, Settle Children's Hospital, Seattle, WA, USA

R.B. Mitchell and K.D. Pereira (eds.), *Pediatric Otolaryngology for the Clinician,*
DOI: 10.1007/978-1-60327-127-1_26, © Humana Press, a part of Springer Science + Business Media, LLC 2009

Table 1 International society for the study of vascular anomalies (ISSVA) classification (http://www.issva.org/)

Vascular Tumors
• Hemangioma at infancy
• Congenital hemangioma
• RICH (rapidly involuting congenital hemangioma)
• NICH (noninvoluting congenital hemangioma
• Tufted angioma
• Kaposiform hemnagioendothelioma
Vascular malformations
Slow flow:
• Capillary
• Port-wine (venular)
• Venous malformation
• Lymphatic malformation
• Complex combined
• Klippel–Trenaunay syndrome
• Proteus syndrome
Fast flow:
• Arterial malformation
• Arteriovenous fistula
• Arteriovenous malformation

vasculature without new growth). But even this differentiation may not be clear-cut as evidenced by new research demonstrating possible neoplastic endothelial cell growth in lymphatic malformations *(2)*. A current classification from the International Society of the Study of Vascular Anomalies (ISSVA) is outlined in Table 1. Practitioners involved in the management of children with vascular anomalies must strive to use current terminology in order to achieve coherence and consistency among team members.

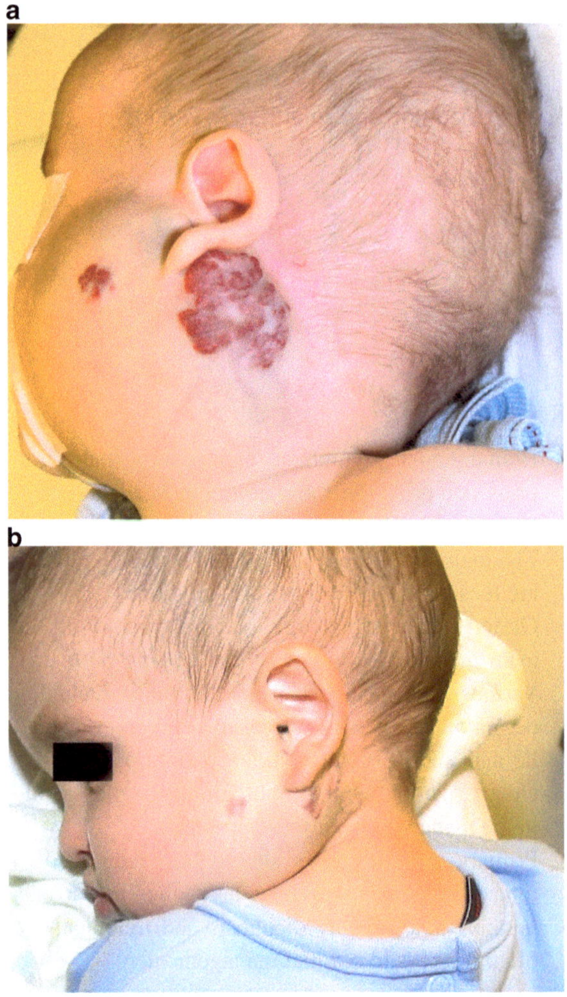

Fig. 1 (**a**) Four-month-old male with compound left parotid hemangioma. Note areas of gray involution mixed with areas of red proliferation. (**b**) Same patient at age 1 with significant involution. No treatment was undertaken

Vascular Tumors

Hemangioma of Infancy

History, Physical Appearance, and Pathology

Hemangiomas of infancy are, by definition, not present at birth but up to 30% may have a sentinel macule or telangiectasia. They proliferate mostly in the first 9 months of life and then undergo variable amounts of involution (Fig. 1a,b). They are the most common tumors of infancy. Hemangiomas are more common in Caucasians, infants of older mothers and those with placental abnormalities or pre-eclampsia, in premature babies, multiple births, and after chorionic villus sampling. The female to male ratio of hemangioma of infancy is approximately 1:6. Up to 10% of female Caucasians will have a hemangioma. Histologically, proliferating hemangiomas are characterized by plump, densely packed endothelial cells with increased mitotic figures and surrounding pericytes and fibroblasts. Involuting hemangiomas show increased mast cells, flattening of endothelial cells with apoptosis, and an increase in fibro-fatty tissue. Biochemical markers of proliferating hemangiomas are similar to that of placental endothelium with glucose transporter isoform 1 (GLUT 1) and Lewis antigen (LeY).

Superficial hemangiomas are generally cherry red macules and papules; deep hemangiomas are firm rubbery subcutaneous masses sometimes with a bluish skin hue. Compound hemangiomas obviously combine aspects of both types. Clinically, the overall footprint size of the hemangioma does not tend to change much during proliferation but the volume (as indicated by a hemi-circumferential measure) enlarges. Involution clinically occurs between ages 1 and 12. Approximately 60% of children are good involuters defined as near-total resolution of mass effect before age 4. However, even the so-called good involuters can have a poor cosmetic result due to fibro-fatty skin changes.

Recently, the multicenter Hemangioma Investigator Group (HIG) has prospectively categorized over 1,000 hemangioma children *(3,4)*. Of these, approximately 70% were solitary and 30% multiple. Three percent of children had six or more cutaneous hemangiomas, a marker for possible visceral or cerebral involvement and/or Kasabach–Merritt phenomena. Overall, 60% of hemangiomas were located in the facial, head and/or neck region, 23% in the trunk, 18% in the extremities, and 6% in the perineum. Thirteen percent of hemangiomas overall were segmental versus solitary but 22% of facial hemangiomas showed a segmental pattern. The most common segmental patterns on the face proved to be frontotemporal, maxillary, mandibular, and frontonasal (Fig. 2a,b). The patterns do not correspond directly to dermatomes but may represent embryologic prominences related to neuroectodermal development as neural crest cells directly influence vascular endothelial cell migration patterns.

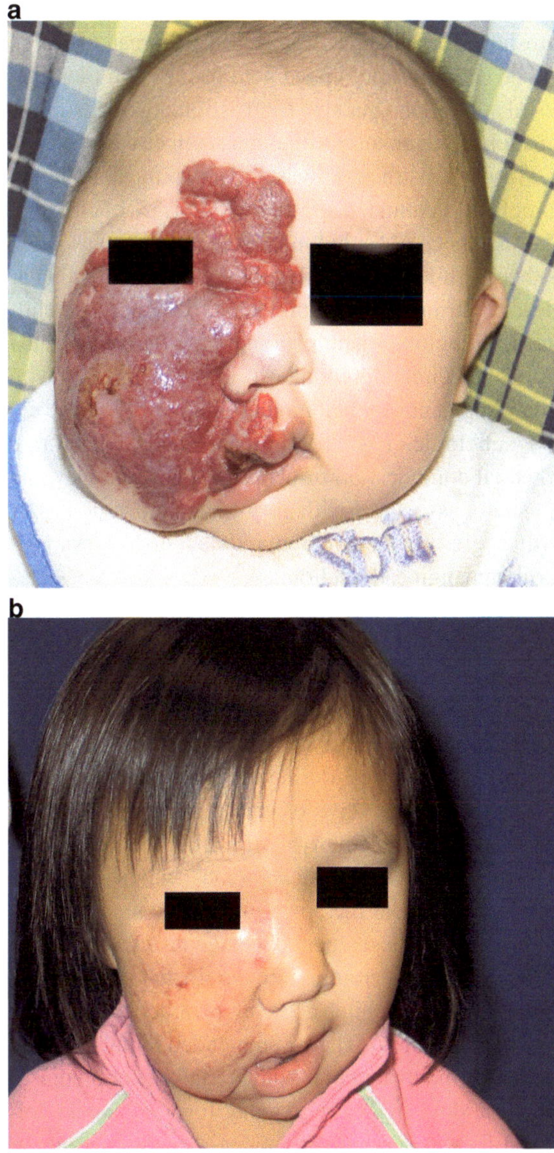

Fig. 2 (**a**) Four-month-old female with ulcerated right facial segmental hemangioma, treated with pulse dye laser, wound care, and systemic steroids. (**b**) Same patient at age 4 with extensive fibrofatty changes

Imaging

The typical computed tomographic appearance of an infantile hemangioma during proliferation is that of a fairly well circumscribed lobular mass with high flow, dilated feeding and draining vessels, and uniform enhancement. With magnetic resonance imaging, hemangiomas are isointense to muscle on T1-weighted images and hyperintense by T2 with flow voids. Ultrasound with Doppler will show a well-defined mass with numerous high flow vessels.

Complications

The HIG *(3,4)* found that approximately 25% of hemangioma children suffered some type of complication usually arising during the period of most rapid proliferation between 3 and 4 months of age. Of note, children with segmental hemangiomas were over ten times more likely to experience a complication compared to those with solitary lesions. Also, large hemangiomas, defined as greater than 37.3 cm^2, were found to generally have a much higher rate of complications.

The most common type of complication from hemangioma is ulceration (16% of children in the HIG series) and the incidence is greater with hemangiomas involving the perineum, oral commissure, nasal tip, external ear, and generally with segmental hemangiomas *(5)*. The second most common complication was threat to vision seen in approximately 6% of children. All children with periorbital hemangiomas should have an ophthalmologic examination and a low threshold for imaging the orbit. The threat to vision can be not only from visual field obstruction (deprivational amblyopia) but also from astigmatism or strabismus related to an intraorbital mass effect.

Airway obstruction was the next most common complication found in approximately 1.5% of children. The incidence of "subglottic" hemangioma was much higher in children with bilateral segmental mandibular (beard distribution) hemangiomas (65% of these children). "Subglottic" hemangiomas are often more transglottic and circumferential, especially in children with facial segmental hemangiomas, than truly localized and subglottic. High-output heart failure is a rare potential complication of hemangioma of infancy and is usually associated with very large hemangiomas or with aggressive hemangioma states such as kaposiform hemangioendotheliomas.

Treatment

A clinical characteristic of hemangioma of infancy is steroid responsiveness during the phase of proliferation and approximately 25% of children in the HIG *(3,4)* series were given some type of steroid therapy. About 90% of proliferating hemangiomas will show some response to steroid therapy although the response rate is lower for liver and other noncutaneous sites. Absolute indications for steroid treatment include ulceration, high-output heart failure, airway obstruction, threat to vision, and pain *(6)*. The recommended initial systemic corticosteroid treatment is with prednisone or prednisolone at a dose of 2–5 mg/kg/day for 4–12 weeks followed by a gradual dosing taper. Antacids or proton pump inhibitors are administered in order to reduce gastrointestinal symptoms. Compliance is hampered in some children because of its bad taste and in those instances, a compounding pharmacy capable of adding flavors (chocolate) is a significant asset.

Potential side effects and complications of steroid therapy include irritability, insomnia, gastric irritation, gastric ulcer, hyperglycemia, growth suppression, and adrenal suppression. Intralesional steroids offer the promise of higher lesional concentrations. A common dosing regimen for intralesional treatment is triamcinolone 3–4 mg/kg with a maximum of 20 mg per session *(7)*. Potential complications include dermal atrophy in addition to systemic side effects. Decisions for periorbital injections are probably best left up to experienced ophthalmologists because of the risk of retinal artery thrombosis.

An exciting new therapy for infantile hemangiomas has recently been described by Leaute-LaBreze et al *(8)*. The beta-blocker propranolol was noted by chance to be associated with significant improvements in involution in patients undergoing treatment for high blood pressure related to steroid therapy. Specifically, some patients were noted to show significant reductions in redness and mass effect. This observation has been supported by other case reports. The mechanism of action is unknown and the ideal dosing regimen is yet to be determined.

For rare life-threatening hemangiomas (heart failure, bleeding, infection) unresponsive to corticosteroids, chemotherapy can be considered. Vincristine at 1–1.5 mg/m^2/day and interferon alfa at 30,000,000 IU/m^2/day are two standard regimens. Interferon, especially in young infants, carries the risk of permanent neurologic sequelae including spastic diplegia.

Ulcerations should be treated early and aggressively in order to prevent development of infection with subsequent tissue loss and scarring. Ulcerations most commonly present at the peak of proliferation between 3 and 4 months of age, therefore newly diagnosed children with hemangioma patterns associated with increased risk for ulceration need early referral to vascular anomaly clinics. Treatment options for ulcerations include topical antibiotics and hydrating ointments, systemic antibiotics, systemic steroids, and occlusive dressings where feasible *(9)*. Pulse dye laser is sometimes advocated as a treatment for superficial ulcerations although there are reports of segmental lesions worsening after laser. Ulcerations should be treated aggressively as they will almost inevitably lead to significant scarring and a potential need for surgery later *(9)*.

During the proliferation phase of hemangioma of infancy, surgery is considered when medical therapy is not effective. Indications include airway obstruction, loss of vision with concern for amblyopia, ulceration, bleeding, and heart failure *(6)*. Biphasic stridor developing over the first 6–12 weeks of life should elicit concern for laryngeal hemangioma and should initiate endoscopy for diagnosis. In children with laryngeal hemangiomas that are not responsive to systemic steroid treatment, endoscopic steroid injection is often attempted, keeping the child intubated for at least 1 day post-procedure. When steroid injection fails, endoscopic ablative treatment with a carbon dioxide laser is usually recommended for isolated subglottic lesions and open excision is increasingly recommended for circumferential lesions such as those seen in association with beard distribution segmental facial hemangioma *(10,11)*.

Pediatric patients begin to show self awareness in terms of how people react to their appearance by age 2–3 and vascular anomaly teams often consider surgical intervention at this time for facial hemangiomas with poor involution or significant skin changes. Surgical options include elliptical excision oriented along relaxed skin tension lines (forehead, preauricular, eyelid, neck), circular excision with pulse string (cheek), wedge excision (lip), and open rhinoplasty (small nasal tip) *(12)*. Pulse dye laser can be used to treat residual superficial telangiectasias (Fig. 3a,b).

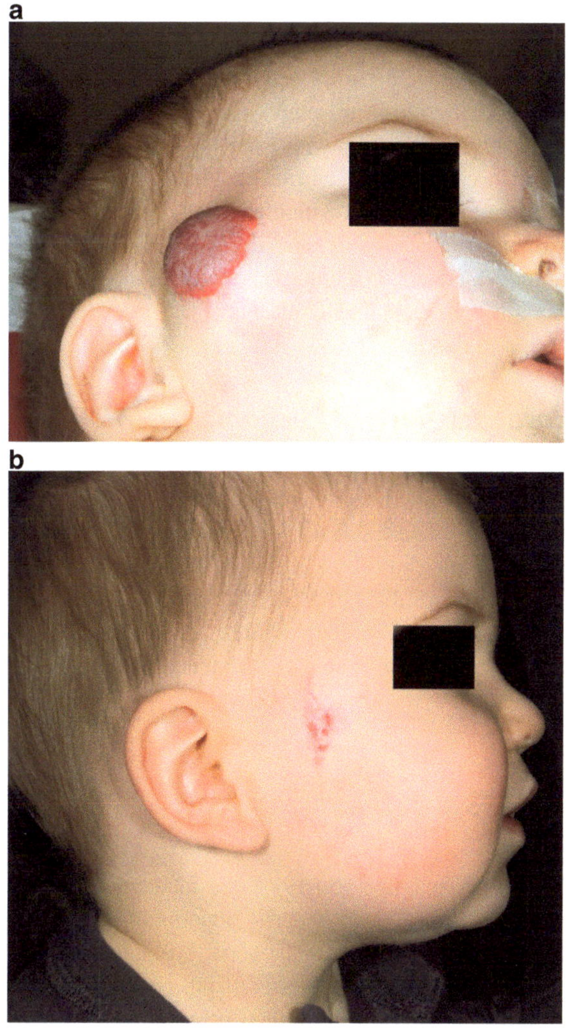

Fig. 3 (**a**) One-year-old male with proliferating right cheek hemangioma despite one course of systemic steroids. (**b**) Post-excision. Some areas of cutaneous involvement were purposefully left in order to close the wound without tension. Pulse dye laser will be performed in the future if the skin redness persists

Congenital Hemangiomas: NICH and RICH

In general, noninvoluting congenital hemangiomas (NICH) and rapidly involuting congenital hemangiomas (RICH) differ from hemangiomas of infancy by being present at birth and by the absence of gluc-1 staining histologically *(13)*. RICH generally presents as a large ulcerating solitary mass with histology similar to hemangioma of infancy but with a tendency toward more involuting zones at an earlier stage. Both RICH and NICH differ from infantile hemangiomas by demonstrating larger and more irregular feeding vessels, sometimes with direct arterial-venous shunts and arterial aneurysms. By imaging, RICH and NICH are difficult to distinguish from congenital arteriovenous anomalies or malignant vascular neoplasms. Not surprisingly, both RICH and NICH are associated with a significant incidence of high-output cardiac failure. Treatment often includes vincristine or surgery if high-dose steroid therapy is unsuccessful.

Diffuse Neonatal Hemangiomatosis

Diffuse neonatal hemangiomatosis is a rare condition that should be suspected in any infant with multiple cutaneous hemangiomas. This condition is associated with visceral involvement especially in the liver and with central nervous system involvement. All infants with multiple cutaneous hemangiomas (some authors recommend six or greater as the threshold) should have a liver ultrasound and head imaging. If visceral involvement is confirmed, the evaluation should include electrocardiogram, echo, chest X-ray, complete blood count, thyroid function, and liver function tests. The disease process has a high mortality rate and early diagnosis and systemic treatment with steroids, interferon, or vincristine is critical. Children with hepatic and cutaneous lesions can frequently have profound hypothyroidism.

Tufted Angioma and Kaposiform Hemangioendothelioma

Tufted angioma is a rare tumor usually appearing shortly after birth. The lesions may present as isolated masses or cutaneous plaques. The natural history is unpredictable with some cases regressing and some progressing. A minority of cases are associated with Kasabach–Merritt phenomenon (KMP – see below). Kaposiform hemangioendothelioma is an aggressive vascular neoplasm with a high association with KMP. A majority of cases occur in early infancy and histologically they demonstrate endothelial cells with high mitotic indices. KMP is often associated with kaposiform hemangioendothelioma. Vincristine is a common treatment modality but mortality rates remain significant.

Kasabach–Merritt Phenomenon (KMP)

KMP is characterized by a consumptive coagulopathy with low platelets and low fibrinogen, elevated D-dimers and prothrombin and partial thromboplastin times, and hemolytic anemia associated with a vascular tumor or malformation. Mortality rates are as high as 20% even with systemic treatments including vincristine and cytoxan.

PHACES Syndrome

PHACES stands for posterior fossa intracranial abnormalities, hemangiomas, arterial abnormalities, cardiac defects and coarctation of the aorta, eye abnormalities, and sternal clefting (sometimes with other ventral clefting abnormalities). Central nervous system symptoms can be progressive and include developmental delays, seizures, and stroke. Children with suspicion for PHACES need to undergo head imaging, ophthalmologic, and cardiac evaluation. Some clinicians recommend antiplatelet therapy for children with abnormal cerebral vasculature in order to try to prevent a congenital stroke.

Vascular Malformations

Lymphatic Malformations

Etiology and Clinical Course

The exact etiology of lymphatic malformations remains unknown. The principle theories involve failure of the lymphatic system to separate from or adequately connect to the venous system. As mentioned previously, new research supports the concept of possible dysregulation of lymphatic endothelial cell growth in these lesions and therefore they may not be simple malformations. Seventy-five percent of lymphatic malformations involve the head and neck (Fig. 4a,b) and 50–60% are diagnosed antenatally or at birth ***(14)***. Other common areas of involvement include the axilla and the abdominal wall. Lymphatic malformations not noted at birth can present later in life with enlargement due to infection or trauma ***(15)***.

MRI is arguably the best imaging modality with T1-weighted imaging showing nonenhancing muscle signal and T2 demonstrating nonenhanced high signal but without the feeding and draining vessels seen with hemangiomas. Computed tomography will show nonenhancing fluid density areas. Either modality is useful for classifying the lesion as macrocystic (2-cm or greater cystic spaces), microcystic, or mixed.

With increasing use of diagnostic ultrasound, a larger percentage of lymphatic malformations are being diagnosed prenatally. Antenatal lymphatic malformations can be associated with polyhydramnios and chromosomal abnormalities including Turner's syndrome and trisomy 21, 18, or 13 ***(16)***. Early diagnosis via ultrasound has led to improved survival in children with massive cervicofacial lesions and airway obstruction via a two-team planned Cesarean section and bronchoscopy (or tracheotomy) procedure involving delaying of placental separation ***(17,18)***.

Several staging systems have been proposed for head and neck lymphatic malformations and several common themes have emerged ***(19,20)***. Infrahyoid, unilateral lesions tend to be macrocystic with better response rates to surgery or sclerotherapy. In contrast, bilateral suprahyoid lesions tend to be microcystic or mixed, with much poorer response to treatment and with much higher complication and long-term sequelae rates. Mucosal involvement is a bad predictor for outcomes and the worst lesions are the large bilateral "beard distribution" malformations that involve the parotid glands, floor of mouth, and tongue. The best prognosis is found in the macrocystic, unilocular posterior inferior lesions. A small proportion of these lesions may even show complete or nearly complete spontaneous resolution with time.

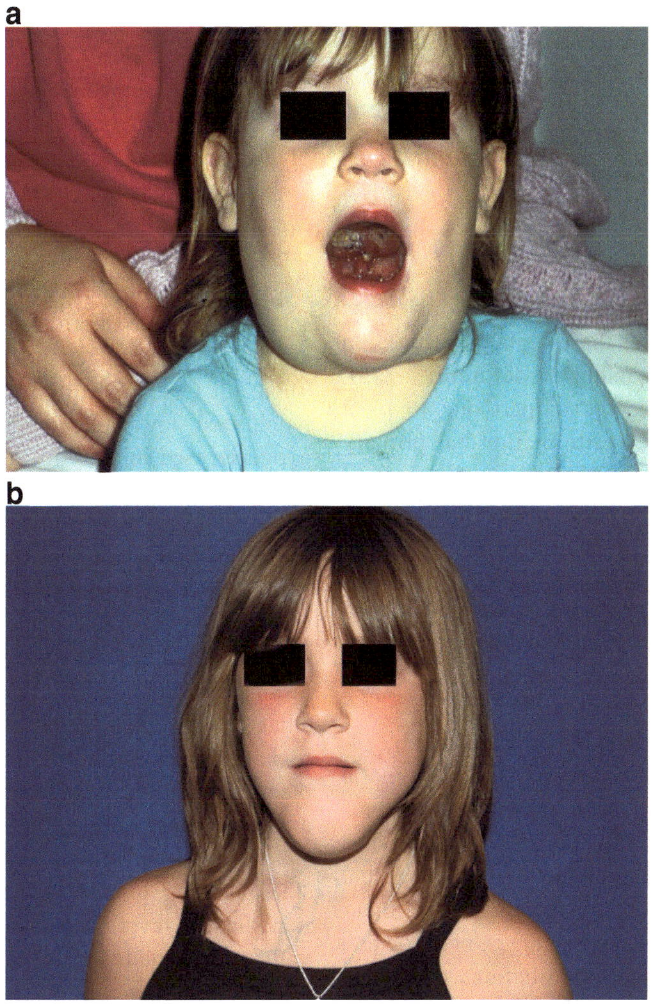

Fig. 4 (**a**) Three-year-old female with beard distribution lymphatic malformation with oral mucosal and tongue involvement. The patient's airway up to this point had been managed with intravenous antibiotics and steroids, and tonsillectomy and adenoidectomy. (**b**) Same patient at age 8 after staged right and left total partotidectomy and neck dissections at ages 4 and 6 years, respectively. The patient has excellent articulation and mandibular symmetry is improving with growth. The plan is for mandibular osteotomies in the near future

Infection and Immunodeficiency

Infection is a common problem with lymphatic malformations especially the suprahyoid microcystic or mixed variety with mucosal involvement. Infection can trigger marked swelling and thereby aggravate airway and feeding issues and recurrent infection is often an indication for surgical excision. Infection is treated acutely with appropriate broad spectrum antibiotics and the addition of systemic corticosteroids seems to offer a significant treatment benefit *(21)*.

Recent studies have shown that children with large bilateral or microcystic lymphatic malformations have significant lymphocytopenia involving T, B, and NK cell subsets. The lymphocytopenia does not appear to be related to lymphocyte sequestration within the malformations as histologic examination of surgical specimens does not demonstrate unusual lymphocyte density *(22)*. The lymphocytopenia may be part of the fundamental developmental process of lymphatic malformations. In a follow-up study, children with large bilateral or microcystic lesions with lymphocytopenia were found to have more hospitalizations, more central line placements for antibiotics, and more treatment complications versus lymphatic malformation children without lymphocytopenia *(23,24)*.

Skeletal and Ssoft Tissue Malformation and Hypertrophy

Primary bone involvement of the mandible is common with larger beard distribution suprahyoid lesions and a large percentage of these high-stage children will have significant mandibular deformities *(25)*. Skeletal overgrowth may be in part due to local effects of the lymphatic malformation but primary histologic lymphatic malformation involvement of the bone is also common. Early surgical excision of the soft tissue lymphatic malformation does not appear to change the rate or incidence of bony involvement. In some series of beard distribution lymphatic malformations, a large percentage of children undergo mandibular osteotomies as part of treatment *(25)*.

Tongue involvement with hypertrophy and bleeding is also common with large suprahyoid lymphatic malformations and can result in severe problems with airway compression, feeding, and speech. The pendulum appears to be swinging away from radical early surgery toward more conservative initial management followed by surgery in stages, one side at a time, if necessary. Acute exacerbations of tongue edema are treated initially with antibiotics and steroids and bleeding from mucosal blebs can be managed with cautery or laser. With time, flare ups of infection tend to diminish perhaps due to maturation of systemic immunity, and often mandibular growth starts to catch up with tongue size. Aggressive tongue reduction surgery is a last resort in refractory cases.

Treatment Options: Sclerotherapy Versus Surgery

Favorable stage lymphatic malformations, such as unilocular macrocystic posterior lateral malformation, can be observed over time if problems such as infection do not occur. A decision for intervention is usually triggered by concerns for airway, feeding, speech, infection, or appearance.

Sclerotherapy

Sclerotherapy for macrocystic (greater than 2-cm spaces) lymphangiomas is not new but the popularity of this intervention appears to be on the rise. The technique of sclerotherapy usually involves percutaneous needle aspiration of the macrocystic spaces under fluoroscopic guidance with subsequent injection of the sclerosing agent. Part of the increased interest in sclerotherapy derives from the promise of decreased toxicity and scarring risk with the use of OK-432 (picibanil, Chugai Pharmaceuticals). This product is a lyophilized low-virulence Group A streptococcus pyogenes used initially for treatment of pleural effusions and first recommended for lymphatic malformations by Ogita *(26)*. It is not commercially available at present in the US but published reports are promising with complete or near-complete response rates for macrocystic disease, usually achieved after multiple treatments *(27,28)*. Similar efficacy for macrocystic lesions has been reported for doxycycline, bleomycin, ethanol, and sodium tetradecyl sulfate *(29,30)*. Major toxicity issues including pulmonary fibrosis with bleomycin and permanent nerve injury with ethanol are rare. Other rare complications include sepsis, shock, stroke, and seizures. More minor issues such as skin blistering, fever, erythema, and pain at the injection site and fever are more common. Sclerotherapy with all reported agents is usually ineffective for microcystic lesions.

Surgery

Surgical excision has been the traditional treatment of choice for most types of lymphatic malformation. A recent inpatient pediatric hospital data base review demonstrated an estimated 1,600 admissions per year related to lymphatic malformation in the U.S. with surgical excision the most common procedure performed as recently as the year 2000 *(31)*. However, complication rates, especially for high-stage mixed suprahyoid lesions, are high and include cranial nerve injury, tongue edema requiring tracheotomy, bleeding, and infection *(25)*. Macrocystic lesions in the posterior inferior neck, and circumscribed parotid and submaxillary lesions have a high rate of complication-free surgical success *(21)*, but these are also the most favorable lesions to treat with sclerotherapy.

When surgery is contemplated, the goal should be total excision with preservation of vital structures. The approach for large lesions is similar to that with squamous cell carcinoma in the head and neck; begin with identification and preservation of vital nerves and vessels, then perform en bloc excision of the involved lymphatic envelope. Subtotal excision, not surprisingly, results in more post-operative persistent problems *(31)*. Lymphatic malformations present difficult surgical challenges because of their infiltrating nature. It is not uncommon in large facial malformations to have branches of the facial nerve weave back and forth on the linings of cystic spaces resulting in attenuation and much greater nerve length. Dissection is extremely difficult in these cases and intraoperative electromyographic nerve mapping can be beneficial. For suprahyoid beard distribution lesions with mucosal involvement, waiting as long as possible before surgery and doing staged excision, one side at a time, can possibly reduce the potential for permanent tongue enlargement.

Lymphangioma involvement of the face poses significant cosmetic and functional challenges. Lymphatic malformations lateral to the lateral canthal line tend to be more macrocystic and can be approached via a total parotidectomy (or sceroltherapy) while lesions in the middle third of the face tend to be more mixed macro- and microcystic. Extensive involvement of the medial one third of the face is rare and usually is completely microcystic. These melolabial malformations may represent a special type of lymphatic malformation pathophysiology and treatment requires facial incisions along aesthetic lines *(32, 33)*.

Treatment Option Conclusions

A few consensus views appear to be emerging. The wisdom of waiting for spontaneous resolution for unilocular or nearly unilocular lesions especially in the posterior inferior neck is increasingly debated. Also, most large vascular anomaly centers treat macrocystic disease initially with sclerotherapy. Most authors recommend using systemic steroids in addition to antibiotics to treat severe infection, at least in children beyond the age of infancy, although controlled studies are lacking. There is less agreement regarding the benefit of waiting as long as possible before considering surgery for large lesions. Many clinicians believe that delaying surgery and performing surgery in stages can reduce the rate of complications such as tongue edema especially in large suprahyoid lesions. Debate continues about early versus late surgery for large suprahyoid lymphangiomas and the ultimate impact of the timing of intervention on mandibular and other facial growth and asymmetry potential.

Venous Malformations

The second most common type of slow flow vascular malformation after lymphatic malformation is venous malformation. In the head and neck, these lesions usually have a bluish overlying skin or mucosal hue and they compress easily and enlarge with a valsalva maneuver. They are present at birth but may not be recognized until growth is triggered by trauma, infection, or hormonal influences during puberty or pregnancy. Lesions often slowly enlarge with time and they do not produce a bruit on auscultation. Doppler ultrasound shows slow flow and MRI scans show a bright signal on T2 imaging and are the most useful imaging modalities. Large venous malformations, especially involving the extremities, can present with chronic pain related to intralesional coagulopathy with development of inflammation and phlebolith formation. Elevated D-dimers and low fibrinogen are often associated laboratory findings.

Venous malformations do not undergo spontaneous resolution. Surgical excision when feasible can be effective but recurrences are common. Intravascular laser with YAG via ultrasound-guided venapuncture is sometimes effective. Also, percuntaneous sclerotherapy is gaining popularity as interventional radiologists gain experience and expertise.

Arteriovenous Malformations

Arteriovenous malformations (AVMs) are fast flow lesions with direct arteriovenous shunting. Like other vascular malformations, they can be triggered by infection, trauma, or hormonal changes. AVMs can be devastatingly destructive and present extreme management problems (Fig. 5). Imaging with Doppler ultrasound

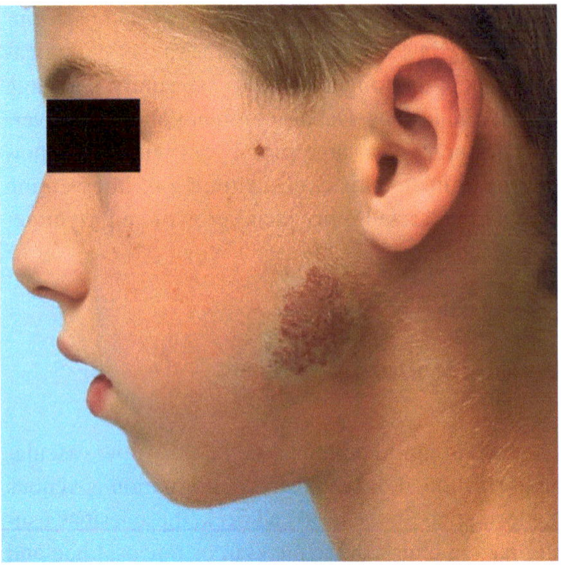

Fig. 5 Twelve-year-old male with a left cheek arteriovenous high flow malformation. The lesion was enlarging and causing pain. It was treated with wide excision including the overlying skin

and MR angiography is usually sufficient for diagnosis but conventional angiography is usually necessary to delineate the full extent of the lesions. AVMs can be classified into four potential stages: dormancy, expansion, destruction, and heart failure. During dormancy, they can be easily mistaken for other vascular anomalies.

Once an AVM is diagnosed, embolization and aggressive surgery is the only known potentially effective therapy although prognosis, especially for facial and extremity lesions, is guarded and recurrences are common. Excision must be radical and involve the overlying skin.

Summary

Vascular tumors and malformations are among the most common head and neck masses of infancy and childhood. The management of these lesions is increasingly delivered through a multidisciplinary team approach. The majority of these lesions in the head and neck area will benefit from some type of intervention and the care of this population can be extremely fulfilling.

References

1. Mulliken JB, Glowacki J. Hemangiomas and vascular malformations in infants and children: a classification based on endothelial characteristics. Plast Reconstr Surg 1982;69:412–427.
2. North PE, Waner M, Mizeracki A, Mihm MC Jr. GLUT1: a newly discovered immunohistochemical marker for juvenile hemangiomas. Hum Pathol 2000;31:11–22.
3. Sidle DM, Maddulozzo J, Crawford SE, et al. Altered pigment epithelium-derived factor and vascular endothelial growth factor levels in lymphangioma pathogenesis and clinical recurrence. Arch Otolaryngol Head Neck Surg 2005;131:990–995.
4. Haggstrom AN, Crolet BA, Baselga E, Chamlinn SL, Garzou MC, et al. Prospective study of infantile hemangiomas: clinical characteristics predicting complications and treatment. Pediatrics 2006;118:882–887.
5. Haggstrom AN, Lammer EJ, Schneider RA, Marcucio R, Frieden IJ. Patterns of infantile hemangiomas: new clues to hemangioma pathogenesis and embryonic facial development. Pediatrics 2006;117:697–703.
6. Friedan IJ, Haggstrom AN, Drolet BA, Mancini AJ, Friedlander SF, et al. Infantile hemangiomas: current knowledge, future directions. Proceedings of a research workshop on infantile hemangiomas. Pediatr Dermatol 2005;22:383–406.
7. Mulliken JB. Update on hemangioma. Int Pediatr 1999;14:132–134.
8. Leaute-Labreze C, Dumas de la Roque E, Hubiche T, Boralevi F, Thambo JB, Taieb A. Propranolol for severe hemangiomas of infancy. N Engl J Med 2008;358:2649–2651.
9. Frieden I, Enjolras O, Esterly N. Vascular birthmarks and other abnormalities of blood vessels and lymphatics. In: Schachner LA, Hansen RC, eds. Pediatric Dermatology, 3rd ed. Mosby 2003; Chapter 20: pp 833–862.
10. Thomas RE, Hornig RL, Manning SC, Perkins JA. Hemangioma of infancy: treatment of ulceration in the head and neck. Arch Facial Plast Surg 2005;7:312–315.
11. O-Lee TJ, Messner A. Open excision of subglottic hemangioma with microscope dissection. Int J Pediatr Otorrhinolaryngol 2007;71:1371–1376.
12. Vijayasekaran S, White DR, Hartley BEJ, et al. Open excision of subglottic hemangiomas to avoid tracheostomy. Arch Otolaryngol Head Neck Surg 2006;132:159–163.
13. Vlahovic A, Simic R, Kravljanac D. Circular excision and purse-string suture technique in the management of facial hemangiomas. Int J Pediatr Otorrhinolaryngol 2007;71:1311–1315.
14. Berenguer B, Mulliken JB, Enjoiras O, Boon LM, Wassef M, et al. Rapidly involuting congenital hemangioma: clinical and histopathologic findings. Pediatr Dev Pathol 2003;6:495–510.
15. Ozen IO, Moralioglu S, Karabulut R, Demirogullari B, Sonmez K, Tarkyilmaz Z, Kale N. Surgical treatment of cervicofacial cystic hygromas in children. ORL 2005;67:331–334.
16. Rahbar R, Rowley H, Perez-Atayde AR, McGill TJ, Healy GB. Delayed presentation of lymphatic malformation of the cervicofacial region: role of trauma. Ann Otol Rhinol Laryngol 2002;111:828–831.

17. Bloom DC, Perkins JA, Manning SC. Management of lymphatic malformations. Curr Opin Otolaryngol Head Neck Surg 2004;12:500–504.
18. Farrell PT. Prenatal diagnosis and intrapartum management of neck masses causing airway obstruction. Paediatr Anaesth 2004;14:48–52.
19. Bouchard S, Johnson MP, Flake AW, et al. The EXIT procedure: experience and outcome in 31 cases. J Pediatr Surg 2002;37:418–426.
20. de Serres LM, Sie KC, Richardson MA. Lymphatic malformations of the head and neck. A proposal for staging. Arch Otolaryngol Head Neck Surg 1995;121:577–582.
21. Kennedy TL, Whitaker M, Pellitteri P, Wood WE. Cystic hygroma/lymphangioma: a rational approach to management. Laryngoscope 2001;111:1929–1937.
22. Sires BS, Goins CR, Anderson RL, et al. Systemic corticosteroid use in orbital lymphangioma. Ophthal Plast Reconstructr Surg 2001;17:85–90.
23. Tempero RM, Hannibal M, Finn LS, Manning SC, Cunningham ML, Perkins JA. Lymphocytopenia in children with lymphatic malformation. Arch Otolaryngol Head Neck Surg 2006;132:93–97.
24. Perkins JA Tempero RM Hannibal MC Manning SC Clinical outcomes in lymphocytopenic lymphatic malformation children. Lymphat Res Biol 2007; 5: 169–174.
25. Padwa BL, Hayward PG, Ferraro NF, Mulliken JB. Cervicofacial lymphatic malformation: clinical course, surgical intervention, and pathogenesis of skeletal hypertrophy. Plast Reconstr Surg 1994;95:951–960.
26. Ogita S, Tsuto T, Tokiwa K, Takahashi T. Intracystic injection of OK-432: a new sclerosing therapy for cystic hygroma in children. Br J Surg 1987;74:690–691.
27. Banieghbal B, Davies MRQ. Guidelines for successful treatment of lymphangioma with OK-432. Eur J Pediatr Surg 2003;13:103–107.
28. Peters DA, Courtemanche DJ, Heran MK, Ludemann JP, Prendiville JS. Treatment of cystic lymphatic vascular malformations with OK-432 sclerotherapy. Plast Reconstr Surg 2006;118:1441–1446.
29. Alomari AI, Karian VE, Lord DJ, Padua HM, Burrows PE. Percutaneous sclerotherapy for lymphatic malformations: a retrospective analysis of patient-evaluated improvement. J Vasc Interv Radiol 2006;17:1639–1648.
30. Cordes BM, Seidel FG, Sulek M, Giannoni CM, Friedman EM. Doxycycline sclerotherapy as the primary treatment for head and neck lymphatic malformations. Otolaryngol Head Neck Surg 2007;137:962–964.
31. Harsha WJ, Perkins JA, Lewis CW, Manning SC. Pediatric admissions and procedures for lymphatic malformations in the United States: 1997 and 2000. Lymphat Res Biol 2005;2:58–65.
32. Reichelmann H, Muehifay G, Keck T, et al. Total, subtotal, and partial surgical removal of cervicofacial lymphangiomas. Arch Otolaryngol Head Neck Surg 1999;125: 643–648.
33. Witt PD Martin DS Marsh JL Aesthetic considerations in extirpation of melolabial lymphatic malformations in children. Plast Reconstr Surg 1995; 96: 48–57. .

Emergencies in Pediatric Otolaryngology

Foreign Body Management

Harlan Muntz

Key Points

- Children have a tendency to put things in their mouth, nose, and ear. If retained, the otolaryngologist is often called for retrieval.
- Vegetable matter and coins remain the most common foreign bodies (FBs). Death from airway or esophageal obstruction is very rare.
- A disk battery FB, regardless of location, should be considered an emergency. Every effort should be made to remove the FB before severe injury ensues.
- A variety of forceps are available. The use of the Hopkins rod technology has allowed for the development of optical FB forceps. This has significantly improved the successful and safe removal of FBs of the tracheobronchial tree and esophagus.
- Good communication between the surgeon and anesthesiologist is essential for airway FB retrieval. Careful planning before the child is in the operating room and continuous open discussion is imperative.

Keywords: Foreign body • Pediatric • Ear • Nose • Nasopharynx • Oropharynx • Hypopharynx • Esophagus • Larynx • Trachea • Bronchi

Principles of effective and safe foreign body (FB) management are applicable regardless of whether the location is the tracheobronchial tree, esophagus, nose, or ear. Children have the tendency to put things in their mouth, nose, and ear. If retained, the otolaryngologist is often called for retrieval. Unfortunately such events may not be isolated and multiple FBs or recurrent events are not unusual. Though there have been great strides made in the United States aimed at protecting the small child from toys and toy pieces that would be a potential choking hazard ***(1,2)***, a variety of other FBs are a problem. Vegetable matter and coins remain the most common FBs but anything that can be placed in the nose, ears, or mouth is a potential hazard. With significant improvement over the past century in the care of the child with a FB, death from airway or esophageal obstruction is very rare.

Education is of utmost importance. Arjamand et al. ***(3)*** suggested that parental education from a primary care provider resulted in a reduced risk of FB ingestion or aspiration. This highlights the importance of alerting the family to the risks of common FBs during well-child visits. In spite of excellent education, the incidence of FBs in children can never be eliminated ***(4)***.

Foreign Body Removal

Principles

When an object enters an orifice but is unable to exit, foreign body retention is a problem. Anatomical narrowings such as the isthmus in the ear canal, the nasal vestibule, or even the larynx (the narrowest part of the pediatric airway) prevent FBs from being expelled. There are also narrowed areas in the esophagus such as the cricopharyngeus, thoracic inlet, and the gastroesophageal junction that retain FBs; these can worsen by esophageal spasm. Larger objects may be pushed by the child's fingers, enter the esophagus with a swallow, or inhaled with a sudden inspiration. The shape and size of the FB determines how likely it is to become

H. Muntz
Division of Otolaryngology, The University of Utah School of Medicine, Salt Lake City, UT, USA
e-mail: Harlan.Muntz@intermountainmail.org

R.B. Mitchell and K.D. Pereira (eds.), *Pediatric Otolaryngology for the Clinician*,
DOI: 10.1007/978-1-60327-127-1_27, © Humana Press, a part of Springer Science + Business Media, LLC 2009

lodged. The sharp edge or point of a FB will usually trail during entry but will become impacted during attempts at exit. Disimpaction and sheathing of the sharp end allows safe removal. A small FB may traverse the esophagus when the spasm passes or be coughed from the airway. The larger the FB the less likely this is to happen. The FB that has entered the stomach is likely to traverse the gastrointestinal tract and be eliminated with the stool.

Careful attention to detail is required for removal of any FB. Good visualization, use of the proper forceps, and delicate retrieval should assist in the removal with minimization of injury to the surrounding tissues. As is important in most surgical techniques, experience is important to achieve patient safety. The use of a manikin simulator *(1)* or animal laboratory can be effective ways to learn and increase experience.

Forceps

Hundreds of forceps have been developed for removal of FBs. Many were developed for a specific FB, and were then rarely used. Most FB forceps can be classified into four major categories:

1. The forward-grasping or "alligator" forceps have jaws that open to grasp the FB (Fig. 1). There are often serrations on the blades to increase the friction between the jaws and the FB to allow improved retention. The "alligator" can be used in small spaces as the joint is close to the end of the forceps. These are ideal for vegetable matter and irregular or disk-shaped hard objects. They can also be used for disimpaction and sheathing of the sharp point on a FB such as a pin. The very smooth round FB may be difficult to remove with these forceps because of slippage. The "Hartman" foreps is also a forward-grasping forceps with a joint near the handle (Fig. 2). This allows the forceps to be opened more widely and therefore used with larger FBs and in larger spaces such as the nose. In a similar way, the Magill forceps (Fig. 3) can be used in retrieving a hypopharyngeal and upper esophageal FB.
2. The globular grasping forceps can be used for round or soft objects (Fig. 4). The standard in this category is the peanut forceps. The forceps blades surround

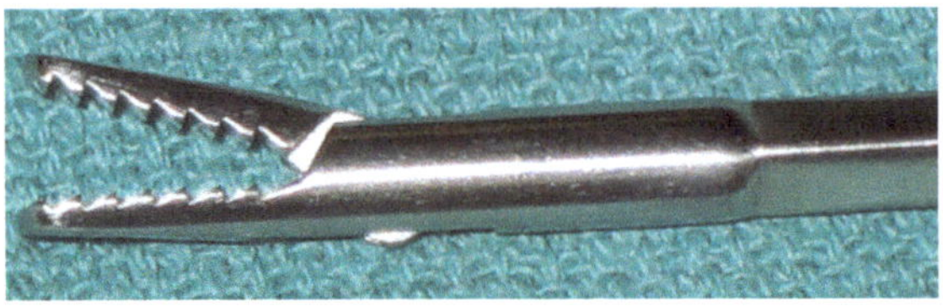

Fig. 1 The forward-grasping forceps has a distal joint. The serrations increase the friction to assist in the removal of many irregularly shaped FB

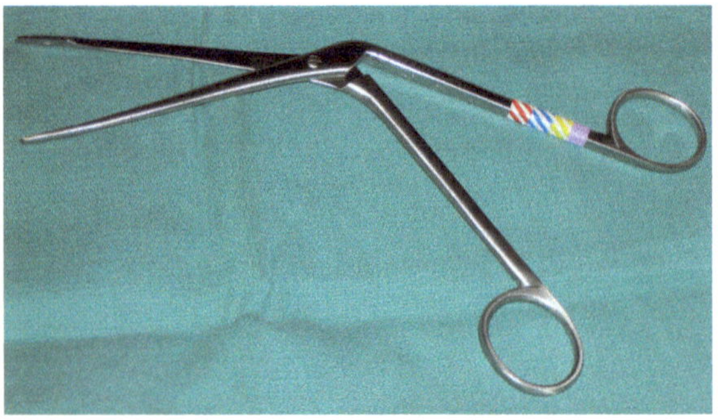

Fig. 2 The Hartman forceps has a proximal joint. This allows the removal of larger FB and is especially useful in the nose and ear

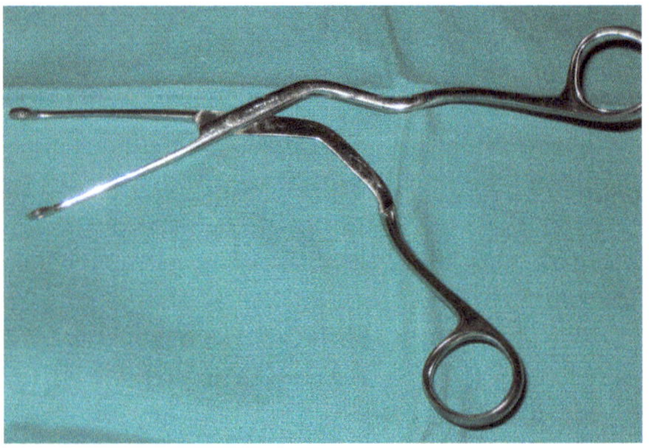

Fig. 3 The Magill forceps is often used to assist intubation. As such it has a proximal joint. It is useful for the removal of hypopharyngeal and proximal esophageal FB. It may also be used for appropriately shaped laryngeal FB

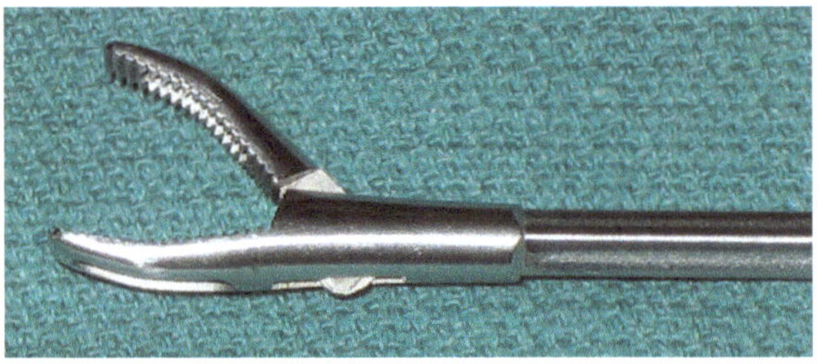

Fig. 4 The globular grasping forceps can be used for round FB. The classic case is the peanut. It has a distal joint allowing retrieval in small airways and the esophagus. The rounded jaws help prevent crushing of the nut

the FB. The jaws are curved to accomplish this. In removing a nut, the curved jaws decrease the chance of the nut or seed being broken into multiple pieces.

3. The rotational forceps were designed for retrieval of an impacted sharp FB. The distal portion of the jaws has a sharp point. The FB is grasped and as the FB is pulled out, the impacted sharp end fixes the FB so that the distal blunt end tumbles. This allows the blunt end to rotate into a proximal orientation and the sharp end will disimpact as the FB is safely removed.
4. Hollow tube forceps are exceptionally handy for the removal of cylindrical hollow FB such as pen caps. The serrations are on the outside and the forceps open in such a way that the jaws are parallel not angular. This allows introduction of the forceps into the lumen, engaging the internal walls of the object and facilitating retrieval.

The use of the Hopkins rod technology has allowed for the development of optical FB forceps (Fig. 5). This has significantly improved the ability of both the experienced and inexperienced surgeon to successfully and safely remove FBs. Distal illumination, magnification, and FB control are the key. Though not all of the above forceps are available as optical forceps, it is wise to use them if possible. The nonoptical forceps have been the standard for most of the past century and are still very useful today but because there are difficulties visualizing the FB as the forceps are introduced, it can become technically more challenging especially for the inexperienced.

In all cases, one should be prepared for difficulties in retrieving the FB. Knowing the shape and size of the FB and having a sample to practice with before the case is in progress, can reduce the risk and stress in the operating room. Additionally, even if one feels the FB could likely be removed with one type of forceps, one should have other options immediately available in the event of an unforeseen problem such as an additional FB.

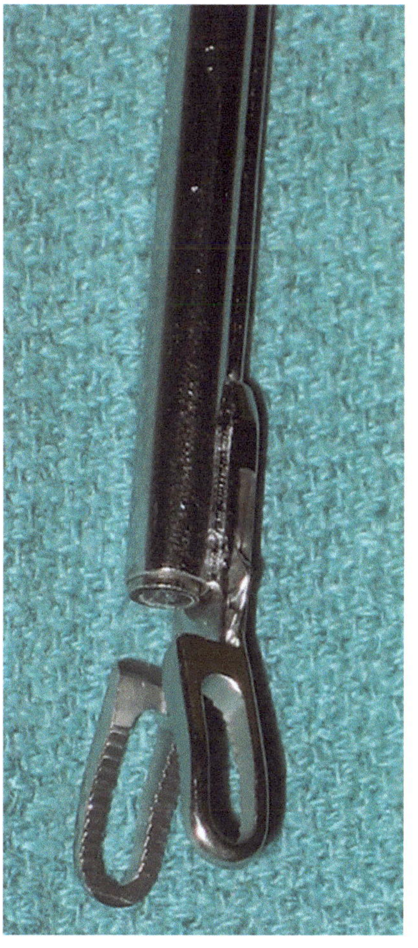

Fig. 5 The addition of the magnifying telescope to the FB forceps has allowed distal lighting with direct observation of the FB as it is being grasped. This has improved the success and ease of FB removal

Other Approaches

Many other approaches have been introduced for removal of FBs in an attempt to allow those without endoscopy experience or those with only flexible endoscopy experience to remove FBs.

Balloon retrieval has been widely used. In the esophagus this is often accompanied by radiographic documentation of the FB and balloon location. The concept is to pass the catheter beyond the FB and then inflate the balloon. The balloon can then be inflated against the lumen, pulled, and the FB gently removed. This has been done with Foley catheters in the esophagus and Fogarty catheters in the bronchus, esophagus, nose, and ear *(5)*. In any balloon retrieval one must be prepared that the FB could be lost upon exit from the lumen. This is critical with an esophageal FB. If the FB is lost at the level of the larynx, the airway may become occluded. Additionally, the FB could become impacted in the nasopharynx. In the ear, there is the need for adequate space distal to the FB for the balloon inflation. The presence of multiple nonradio opaque

FBs can lead to problems. What appears to be a simple FB may be complicated by other FBs that are not visualized but are in the path. This is especially a problem with a nonvisualized sharp FB. Additionally, there is a heightened risk, that is, if the FB has been present for a long time as edema, tissue erosion or granulation tissue can hinder extraction.

In a simple uncomplicated case, balloon retrieval can be an effective approach. It should be avoided if there is evidence of edema, if the duration of impaction is uncertain or prolonged, or if there is any chance of additional FBs.

Bouginage has been suggested for food impactions and coins in the esophagus *(6)*. In this technique, the food bolus is pushed into the stomach where it can be digested, passed safely through the intestinal system, and eliminated. This has also been suggested for coins. Though it has been used and many promote its safety, a retained food bolus can be the result of an esophageal stricture. This increases the risk of injury as the bolus is pushed into the stomach. As in balloon removal, unexpected, multiple, or nonvisualized FBs could lead to mucosal damage. Even with rigid esophagoscopy one could consider, with care, pushing the FB into the stomach with either the endoscope or forceps.

Right-angle instruments can be used to remove FBs. These are most commonly used in the ear canal and nose though they can be used to retrieve FBs of the esophagus. It is important to move beyond the "equator" of the FB so that it does not roll in place. If there is a lumen in the FB as in a bead, the right angle can be placed in the lumen to facilitate removal. A sharp right angle can also penetrate the FB to assist in the removal. Care must be taken to avoid injury to the epithelial lining of the lumen.

The stone basket, used to remove urethral stones, has also been used to remove FBs of the airway and esophagus and has been popularized by those using flexible endoscopy. It may also be used through a rigid endoscope.

There have been specialty instruments developed over the years for unusual FBs. One such is the safety-pin-closing forceps (Fig. 6). The idea is to reduce the chance of mucosal injury by closing the safety pin before extraction. However, if specialty instruments are not used frequently the chance of successful manipulation of the FB can be lower than use of standard techniques. This was best illustrated by a child who presented for the removal of a FB and the entangled FB forceps used to retrieve it (personal communication Lauren Holinger).

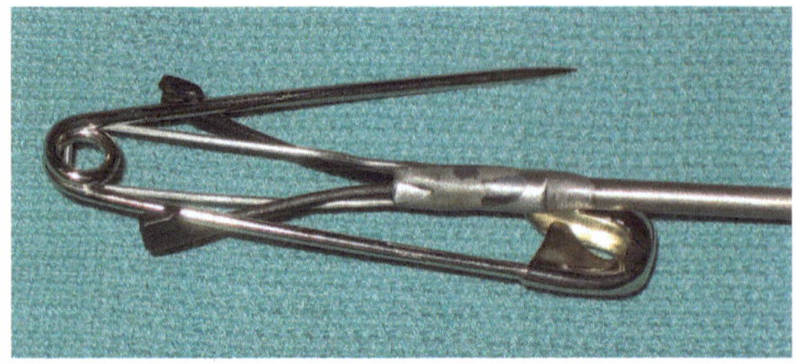

Fig. 6 In years before disposable diapers became a standard, safety pins were a common esophageal FB. As there is a sharp proximal point, many forceps and techniques were devised to remove the pin without an esophageal perforation. This illustrates one safety pin forceps that allows closure of the pin to facilitate extraction (**a**) and the safety pin within the forceps (**b**). As this is not an easy forceps to use, one should practice frequently before attempting to use this in a child

Special Considerations by Anatomical Site

Ear

FBs of the ear are commonly seen by primary care providers, emergency departments, and otolaryngologists. Except in the case of an expanding FB (e.g., a wet bean) or a live insect, these are rarely emergencies, though the associated family anxiety may make them seem as such. Studies suggest that nearly 80% of ear FBs can be successfully removed by emergency department staff *(7)*. The techniques used include forceps removal, balloon extraction, right-angled pick removal, and irrigation. Unfortunately irrigation does carry some risk if there is a tympanic membrane perforation as the irrigation flushes the middle ear as well as the ear canal. The use of sedation can be helpful in the very anxious child *(8)*. There is a greater chance of failure in removal by the emergency department if the FB is spherical and hard such as a ball or bead *(9)*. Additionally, if there have been multiple, failed attempts at removal, it is unlikely to be accomplished by continued attempts. In these situations it would be wise to refer for otolaryngologic consultation before a likely unsuccessful attempt. In some cases general anesthesia will be needed for removal. In all cases care must be taken to adequately visualize the FB. Delicate technique should be used to avoid laceration of the ear canal and more importantly the tympanic membrane or ossicular chain.

Nose

FBs in the nose are common. These can present early with an observed placement or delayed with the findings of foul, unilateral nasal drainage. Commonly seen are food or toy pieces, but occasionally there can be an extruded tooth or even a button battery (see below). As with any FB retrieval, adequate visualization is the key. Using a headlight and nasal speculum, the FB can usually be seen and grasped. A Hartman's forceps is an ideal instrument. Other possible techniques include the use of an operating microscope or sinus endoscopes for visualization in conjunction with any of the abovementioned forceps or techniques. It is important to realize that a nasal FB may easily become a lower airway FB if pushed to the nasopharynx and aspirated. A novel approach has been the "parental kiss." In this, the parent or physician opens the child's mouth and blows to attempt to dislodge the nasal FB. In a similar way, an ambu bag can be used *(10)*. An acute nasal FB is a potential airway emergency and should be addressed in a timely manner. If this is a chronic situation, it is unlikely to dislodge and become lodged in the lower airway. Occasionally, in the very anxious child, general anesthesia or conscious sedation may be required for FB removal. Epistaxis can be a complication of removal but will usually stop quickly.

Nasopharynx, Oropharynx, and Hypopharynx

FBs in the nasopharynx, oropharynx, and hypopharynx in children are usually best addressed under general anesthesia. The nasopharynx is best observed by retraction of the palate and a mirror or a 70–90° endoscope. Curved forceps can then be used for retrieval. It can also be dislodged through a nasal approach and retrieved from the oral cavity with the airway protected. Delayed removal may cause nasopharyngeal stenosis and severe airway obstruction.

In the oropharynx and hypopharynx, FBs are usually large or sharp. In older children, fish bones can lodge in this area leading to significant discomfort. They will most often be nonradio opaque and have a tendency to become deeply imbedded in the base of the tongue or pyriform fossa. Adolescents may tolerate retrieval with topical anesthesia and visualization with a mirror or an endoscope and curved forceps removal. Younger children will require general anesthesia.

Larger toys or toy pieces can be trapped in the oropharynx or hypopharynx. They are by nature airway FBs and should be emergently removed. Often the location is unknown. Care must be taken in the initial evaluation of the airway to make sure a nonobstructive FB does not become obstructive.

Larynx

Laryngeal FBs can be rapidly fatal. The child may have a croupy cough, hoarseness, and symptoms and signs of airway compromise. The laryngeal FB will commonly lodge in the sagittal plane. If the FB appears in the coronal plane on X-ray it is likely to be esophageal. This is an airway emergency and must be dealt with immediately in the OR. The ideal forceps as well as multiple FB forceps should be available based on an understanding of the shape of the FB and especially if the nature of the FB is unknown. The most deadly FB is the latex balloon *(11)*. The child pops the balloon and inhales a fragment. It drapes over the larynx and occludes the airway. In a similar way, but less deadly, one may see small pieces of plastic from containers or covers in the larynx.

Tracheobronchial Tree

An acute FB in the tracheobronchial tree is an emergency. Though the FB may have lodged in the bronchus, it could be dislodged and become tracheal or laryngeal and cause complete obstruction. If the diagnosis of a FB in the tracheobronchial tree is in doubt, the need for an emergency bronchoscopy is less critical. If there has been an observed aspiration event, even in the absence of signs or radiographic images suggestive of the FB, a bronchocopy is often indicated *(12,13)*. There is frequently a quiescent period after the FB has been aspirated where there is no cough or wheeze. Radiographic findings of air trapping, asymmetric chest movement, and atelectasis may be late findings or absent in the immediate presentation. The FB may also move and cause variation in location of the wheeze. Bilateral FBs can also lead to bilateral wheezing.

The following can assist in determining the need for a bronchoscopy: radiologic findings suggestive of FB; unilateral wheeze; an asymmetric chest rise; hemoptysis; chronic cough; deterioration of respiratory status. Certainly it is far better to have a negative bronchoscopy than suffer the complications of pneumonia, chronic mucosal changes, or even broncho-pleural fistula from a late diagnosis of a FB in the tracheobronchial tree. The greater the delay in diagnosis of a FB, the greater the chances of complications *(14,15)*.

Though some have used the flexible bronchoscope successfully in the management of airway FB, the use of a rigid bronchoscope under general anesthesia offers the advantages of controlled respiration, a more varied assortment of forceps, and control of the FB that is much more difficult with other techniques. It is important for the endoscopist to be familiar with a variety of techniques for tracheobronchial FB retrieval. Occasionally, especially in very distal airway FB retrieval, one may need to use a combination of techniques, using both flexible and rigid endoscopy as well as fluoroscopy.

Esophageal

There is debate over the ideal way to retrieve esophageal FBs. Fortunately there are many techniques available and the probability of a child dying by slow starvation because of esophageal obstruction or mediastinitis because of erosion through the esophageal wall is very small. Often FB ingestion is not witnessed. Dysphagia may be a prominent finding. Interestingly, cough and wheeze may be the primary symptom if there is a delay in diagnosis *(16,17)*. This is usually due to compression of the trachea leading to edema.

An esophageal FB is considered urgent but not an emergency unless there is airway obstruction or other significant symptoms. Attempts at bouginage or foley catheter extraction have been successfully described but these techniques should be approached with great caution especially if there is edema, a delayed presentation, or the possibility of multiple FBs. The procedure is considered less costly but the child is often strapped into position for a very uncomfortable procedure. Additionally, the airway is placed at risk as the FB is retrieved through the hypopharynx. The risk of losing the airway is also significantly higher if the procedure is done with conscious sedation.

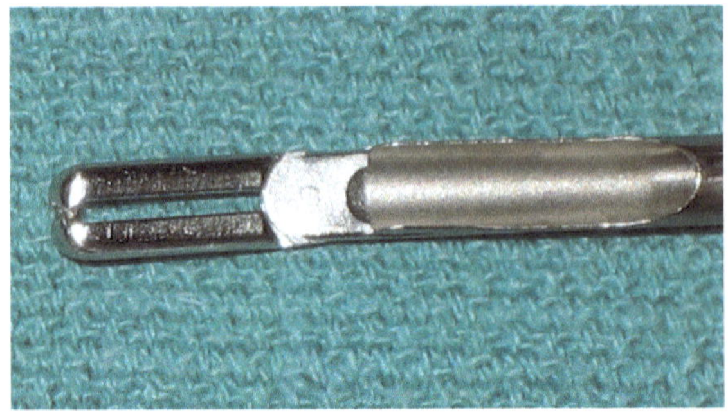

Fig. 7 The coin forceps was designed with Karl Stortz to focus on the most common esophageal FB. Here the distal end of the jaws will come together leaving a proximal gap. This allows the coin to be firmly grasped and reduces the risk of the coin slipping especially as it comes by the larynx

The most commonly seen esophageal FBs are coins. Over 20% of the time coins will pass spontaneously and to that end a 12–24-h observation period has been advocated before an attempt at retrieval *(18)*. Attempts to facilitate release of esophageal spasm by glucagon have been largely unsuccessful *(19)*. Special coin forceps are available that allow the forceps to engage the coin with a more parallel position of the jaws (Fig. 7).

Considerations for Anesthesia

Good communication between the surgeon and anesthesiologist is essential for airway FB retrieval. Careful planning before the child is in the operating room and continuous open discussion are imperative. Routine anesthetic procedures such as the need for the child to be without food or drink for several hours may be dangerous to a child with an airway FB. Rapid sequence is not recommended. Paralysis may make a partially obstructed airway completely obstructed. Before any paralysis is used it is imperative to know that the child will ventilate well with mask anesthesia. Spontaneous ventilation is always preferred. When the airway is obstructed, there is usually significant hypoventilation. Inhalation anesthesia is often the ideal way to proceed but this will take much longer with decreased minute

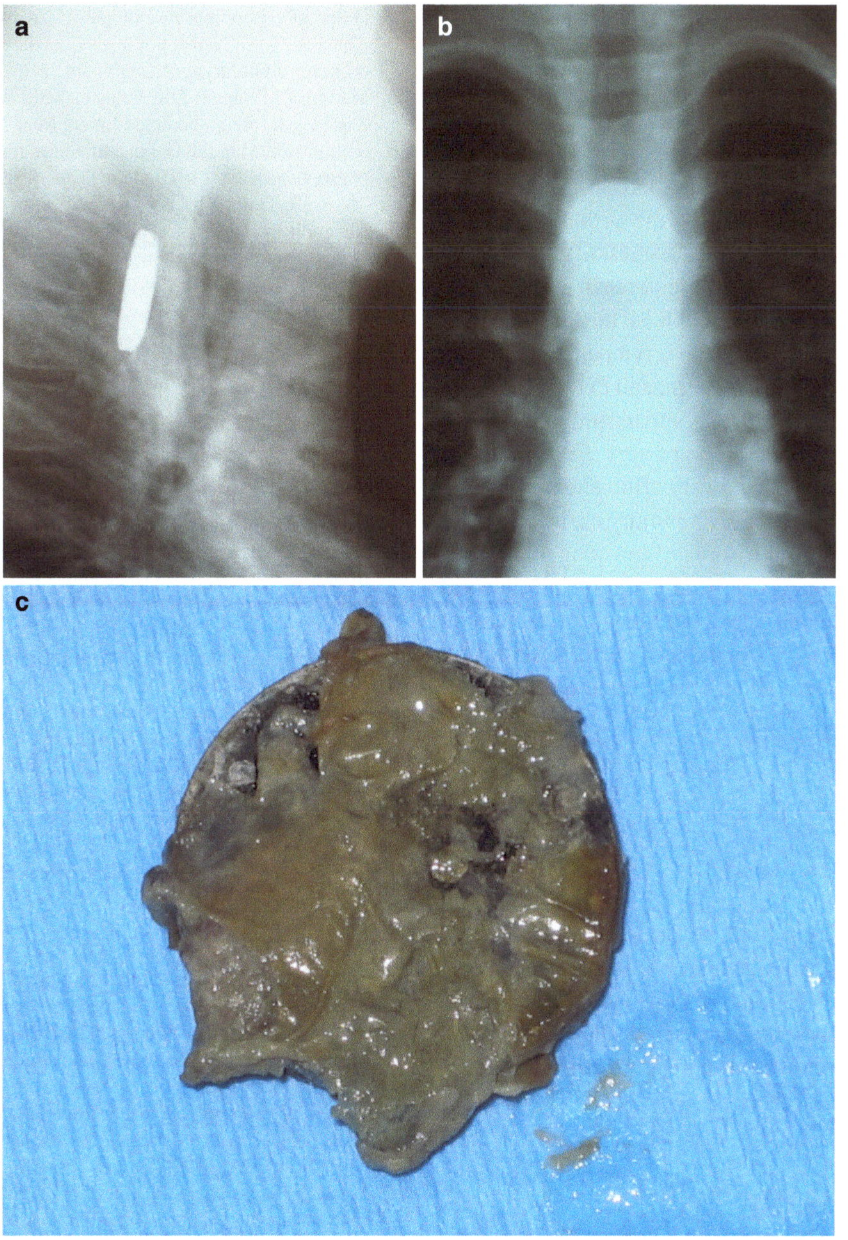

Fig. 8 The esophageal disk battery is an acute emergency because of the risk of esophageal injury. Here the radiograph shows the double density suggesting the battery. The extracted battery is seen caked with debris from the injured mucosa and muscle

ventilation. Rigid endoscopy allows for constant ventilation while the bronchoscope is in place. This is much more difficult when dealing with a laryngeal or hypopharyngeal FB. The optical telescopes can be attached to a video system so that the anesthesiologist can visualize the entire procedure.

The Disk Battery

Small batteries are widely used in a variety of devices. They are also a potentially damaging FB. The larger the battery, the greater the probability of retention ***(20)***.

The longer the retention the greater the risk of injury. Often the caregivers report the size and nature of the FB. Radiographic evaluation will show a double-density FB (Fig. 8). There has been a suggestion that a metal detector may also distinguish a coin from a battery. If the seal on the battery has been broken, the disk acts as a solid caustic source exposing the strong base to the epithelial surface. Early studies suggest that esophageal retention of a disk battery for greater than 2 h can cause a transmural injury *(21)*. In the nose this could lead to septal perforation, in the ear to a tympanic membrane perforation similar to a slag burn, and in the esophagus to a tracheoesophageal fistula, mediastinitis, or severe stricture. In general, a disk battery FB should be considered an emergency. Every effort should be made to remove the FB before severe injury ensues. Usually it can be removed with forward-grasping forceps or coin forceps. If there has been a significant mucosal injury, the FB may be "stuck" to the lumen, increasing the likelihood of injury with removal. In these situations, intraluminal stenting should be considered to prevent stenosis.

Conclusion

The otolaryngologist will be presented with a wide variety of FBs. The systematic approach to the removal is similar across locations. Understanding these issues and the methods used for removal will allow the clinician to approach each case with appropriate care and safety.

References

1. Deutsch ES, Dixit D, Curry J, Malloy K, Christensen T, Robinson B, Cognetti D. Management of aerodigestive tract foreign bodies: innovative teaching concepts. Ann Otol Rhinol Laryngol. 2007;116(5):319–23.
2. Milkovich SM, Rider G, Greaves D, Stool D, Chen X. Application of data for prevention of foreign body injury in children. Int J Pediatr Otorhinolaryngol. 2003;67 (Suppl 1):S179–82.
3. Arjmand EM, Muntz HR, Stratmann SL. Insurance status as a risk factor for foreign body ingestion or aspiration. Int J Pediatr Otorhinolaryngol. 1997;42(1):25–9.
4. Despres N, Lapointe A, Quintal MC, Arcand P, Giguere C, Abela A. 3-year impact of a provincial choking prevention program. J Otolaryngol. 2006;35(4):216–21.
5. Mariani PJ, Wagner DK. Foley catheter extraction of blunt esophageal foreign bodies. J Emerg Med. 1986;4(4):301–6.
6. Soprano JV, Mandl KD. Four strategies for the management of esophageal coins in children. Pediatrics. 2000;105(1):e5.
7. Marin JR, Trainor JL. Foreign body removal from the external auditory canal in a pediatric emergency department. Pediatr Emerg Care. 2006;22(9):630–4.
8. Brown L, Denmark TK, Wittlake WA, Vargas EJ, Watson T, Crabb JW. Procedural sedation use in the ED: management of pediatric ear and nose foreign bodies. Am J Emerg Med. 2004;22(4):310–14.
9. Thompson SK, Wein RO, Dutcher PO. External auditory canal foreign body removal: management practices and outcomes. Laryngoscope. 2003;113(11):1912–15.
10. Botma M, Bader R, Kubba H. 'A parent's kiss': evaluating an unusual method for removing nasal foreign bodies in children. J Laryngol Otol. 2000;114(8):598–600.
11. Ryan CA, Yacoub W, Paton T, Avard D. Childhood deaths from toy balloons. Am J Dis Child. 1990;144(11):1221–4.
12. Barrios Fontoba JE, Butierrez C, Lluna J, Vila JJ, Poquet J, Ruiz-Company S. Bronchial foreign body: should bronchoscopy be performed in all patients with a choking crisis? Pediatr Surg Int. 1997;12(2-3):118–20.
13. Reilly J, Thompson J, MacArthur C, Pransky S, Beste D, Smith M, Gray S, Manning S, Walter M, Derkay C, Muntz H, Friedman E, Myer CM, Seibert R, Riding K, Cuyler J, Todd W, Smith R. Pediatric aerodigestive foreign body injuries are complications related to timeliness of diagnosis. Laryngoscope. 1997;107(1):17–20.
14. Byard RW. Mechanisms of unexpected death in infants and young children following foreign body ingestion. J Forensic Sci. 1996;41(3):438–41.
15. Zerella JT, Dimler M, McGill LC, Pippus KJ. Foreign body aspiration in children: value of radiography and complications of bronchoscopy. J Pediatr Surg. 1998;33(11):1651–4.
16. Louis JP, Alpern ER, Windreich RM. Witnessed and unwitnessed esophageal foreign bodies in children. Pediatr Emerg Care. 2005;21(9):582–5.
17. Rimell FL, Thome A, Stool S, Reilly JS, Rider G, Stool D, Wilson CL. Characteristics of objects that cause choking in children. JAMA. 1995;274(22):1763–6.
18. Soprano JV, Fleisher GR, Mandl KD. The spontaneous passage of esophageal coins in children. Arch Pediatr Adolesc Med. 1999;153(10):1073–6.
19. Mehta D, Attia M, Quintana E, Cronan K. Glucagon use of esophageal coin dislodgment in children: a prospective, double-blind, placebo-controlled trial. Acad Emerg Med. 2001;8(2):200–3.
20. Yardeni D, Yardeni H, Coran AG, Golladay ES. Severe esophageal damage due to button battery ingestion: can it be prevented? Pediatr Surg Int. 2004;20(7):496–501.
21. Maves JD, Carithers JS, Birck HG. Esophageal burns secondary to disc battery ingestion. Ann Otol Rhinol Laryngol. 1984;93(4 Pt 1):364–9.

Deep Space Neck Infections in the Pediatric Population

Ryan Raju and G. Paul Digoy

Key Points

- Deep space neck infections are commonly seen in the pediatric population.
- Characteristic findings include fever, sore throat, and a warm, tender neck mass.
- A computed tomography (CT) scan is the gold standard for diagnosis and surgical planning, but the specificity of these studies is low. Ultrasonography is a less invasive alternative that may be equally effective in certain cases.
- Infections are typically polymicrobial, with Staphylococcus and Streptococcus being the most commonly isolated pathogens.
- A neck abscess is usually treated with surgical drainage and intravenous antibiotics.
- Intravenous antibiotics without surgical drainage in a clinically stable neck may be effective in selected cases.
- Diagnosis may be more challenging in younger children and in retropharyngeal infections.
- Retropharyngeal infections, peritonsillar abscesses, and atypical mycobacterium infections represent unique manifestation of deep neck infections that require special consideration.
- Complications of deep neck infections are uncommon, and carry severe sequelae.

Keywords: Deep space neck infection • Abscess • MRSA • Computed tomography • Retropharyngeal infection • Peritonsillar abscess • Mycobacterium

R. Raju and G.P. Digoy (✉)
Department of Otorhinolaryngology, University of Oklahoma College of Medicine, Oklahoma City, OK, USA
e-mail: gpaul-digoy@ouhsc.edu

Introduction

Deep neck infections are commonly encountered in both children and adults. However, the presentation, progression, and management differ greatly in these two groups. Diagnosis and treatment are dependent on the age of the child, the location of the infection, and the etiological agent involved. A review of the relevant anatomy, diagnosis, treatment options, and potential complications are discussed. The management of retropharyngeal infections, peritonsillar abscesses, and mycobacterial adenitis is discussed separately.

Anatomy of the Neck

An understanding of deep infections of the neck begins with knowledge of the anatomy of the superficial and deep cervical neck fascia. It is their relationship to each other that forms the potential neck spaces that can harbor infection and abscess formation. A detailed anatomical description is beyond the scope of this chapter, but can be found in many of the references listed ***(1–3)***.

The deep cervical fascia of the neck can be divided into a superficial, middle, and deep layer, which envelop various structures in the neck and dictate potential routes for spread of infections. Of primary importance for deep neck space infections are the submandibular, peritonsillar, parapharyngeal, and retropharyngeal spaces. Figure 1 demonstrates the fascia of the neck, as well as the relationship between the retropharyngeal space and the danger space. The danger space directly communicates with the mediastinum, creating a potential pathway for widespread infection.

R.B. Mitchell and K.D. Pereira (eds.), *Pediatric Otolaryngology for the Clinician*,
DOI: 10.1007/978-1-60327-127-1_28, © Humana Press, a part of Springer Science + Business Media, LLC 2009

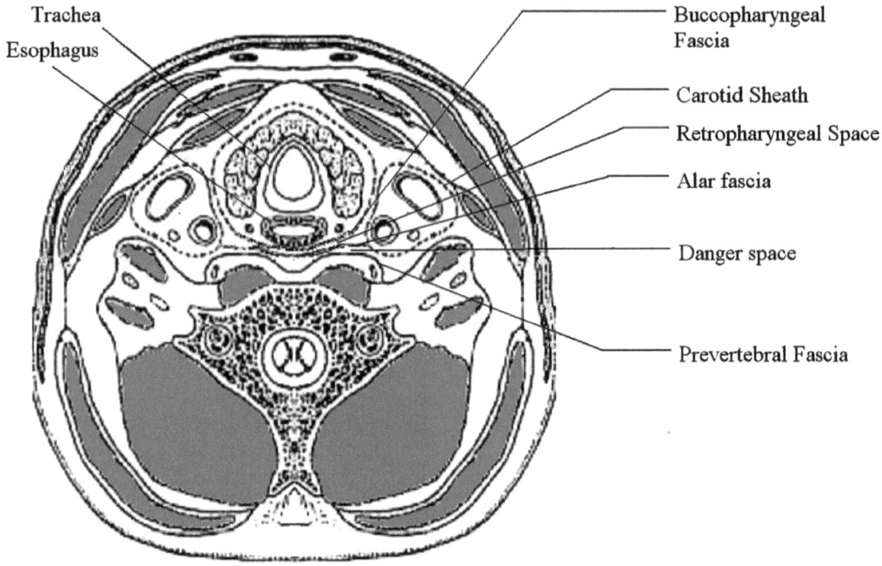

Fig. 1 Deep fascial spaces of the neck denoting the relationship of the retropharyngeal space to the esophagus and danger space ***(30)***

Diagnosis

History/Clinical Findings – Children with deep space neck infections more commonly present with fever, neck mass, odynophagia, dysphagia, sore throat, and decreased oral intake. These symptoms are usually present for approximately 3–5 days. Less common symptoms include agitation, cough, dehydration, drooling, snoring, stridor, torticollis, and neck stiffness ***(4,5)***. Important points in the history include the duration and progression of the symptoms, a recent upper respiratory tract infection, procedures performed to the neck (i.e., dental surgery, intubation), prior antibiotic therapy, risk factors for MRSA, recent travel, and a possible immunocompromised state. In children, a neck abscess can be present from shortly after birth to the late teenage years. The average age at presentation is 4–5 years, with peritonsillar abscesses typically presenting in older children and retropharyngeal abscesses seen in younger children ***(5–8)***.

Physical examination should assess for the presence of erythema, tenderness, and fluctuance of the neck mass, as well as lymphadenopthy, tracheal deviation, and neck stiffness. The examination of the oral cavity and pharynx should be performed with attention to the tonsillar size and symmetry, dentition, palatal edema, and uvular deviation. Though potentially life-threatening, airway compromise secondary to a deep neck infection is very rare. An important sign of airway compromise is "tripoding," which refers to a child in the seated position with their elbows or hands on their knees, leaning forward with the neck extended and head tilted slightly backward. This position gives the accessory muscles of respiration their most advantageous position, opens the upper airway, and makes breathing easier ***(4,9)***.

Though not mandatory, laboratory tests may be helpful in the work-up of a child with a potential deep neck infection. Leukocytosis, with or without a left shift, is typically seen on a complete blood count. Other helpful laboratory tests include a C-reactive protein (which can aid in determining progression of infection over time), a monospot test, and Epstein-Barr virus (EBV) titers. In cases of more chronic infection, a PPD (Tuberculosis) skin test should be considered. It is also important to consider other causes of inflammation such as congenital, neoplastic, or inflammatory conditions (Table 1) ***(10)***.

Deep neck infections in infants present more of a diagnostic challenge. In recent studies, neck swelling, lymphadenopathy, and an elevated white blood cell count (greater than 16,000/μL) were the only findings strongly associated with the presence of a neck abscess. Furthermore, symptoms of airway compromise are

Table 1 Causes of pediatric neck inflammation

• Bacterial	• Fungal/Parasites
◦ Lymphadenitis	◦ Histoplasmosis
◦ Abscess (deep or superficial)	◦ Apsergillosis
◦ Cat-scratch disease	◦ Toxoplasmosis
◦ Lemeirre's disease	◦ Lymphatic filariasis
◦ Actinomycosis	• Benign neoplasms
◦ Brucella	◦ Hemagioma
◦ Syphillis	◦ Lymphangioma
◦ Tularemia	• Malignant neoplasm
◦ Mycobacterium (atypical)	◦ Lymphoma
◦ Mycobacterium tuberculosis	◦ Rhabdomyosarcoma
• Viral	• Inflammatory
◦ Viral adenitis	◦ Kawasaki syndrome
◦ EBV	◦ Sarcoidosis
◦ HIV (chronic or acute)	◦ Marshall's syndrome
◦ CMV	

more common in children under the age of 1, though emergent intubation is rarely required *(4,5)*.

Imaging

Most commonly, computed tomography (CT) with IV contrast is used to differentiate between lymphadenitis and an abscess in a deep neck infection. The classic image finding of an abscess is an area of low attenuation with a rim of contrast enhancement, surrounded by soft tissue swelling. Lymphadenitis presents as a soft tissue swelling with the obliteration of fat planes. CT scans have been shown to be highly sensitive in the detection of an abscess, with sensitivities ranging from 87 to 100% ***(8,11,12)***. An abscess is rarely present if a rim-enhancing lesion is not found on a CT scan. However, the specificity of CT scans in identifying an abscess is poorer, ranging from 60 to 100% ***(6,9–14)***. The inability to find purulence in a child with a CT-defined abscess during surgery is not an uncommon event. Roberson et al. ***(8)*** suggest that a scalloped contour of the abscess wall is a better indicator of the presence of purulence. Using scalloping solely as a criteria for determining abscess formation greatly improves the specificity of a CT scan, but reduced the sensitivity to 64% ***(8)***. Examples of abscesses with both scalloped borders and smooth borders are shown in Fig. 2. Despite low specificity, a CT scan of the neck with contrast remains the best available diagnostic tool in the evaluation and management of a neck abscess.

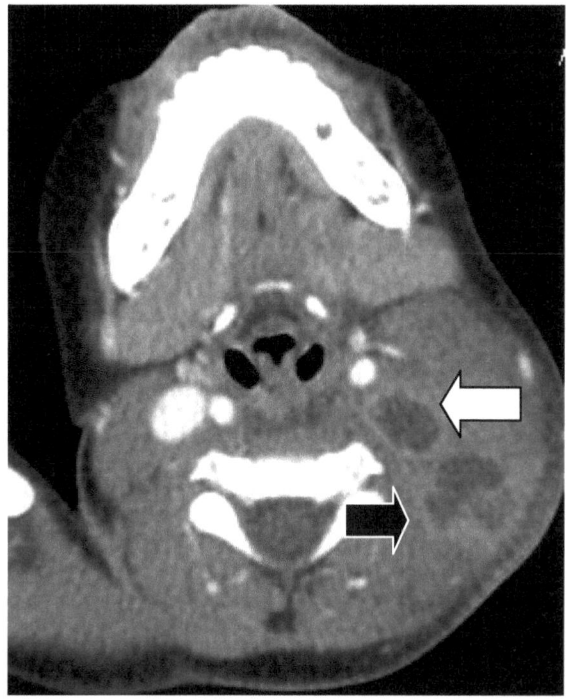

Fig. 2 CT scan of a 2-year-old female that shows two areas of hypodensity with rim enhancement. The *white arrow* shows a smooth bordered lesion. The *black arrow* shows an abscess with scalloped borders, which is more indicative of purulence

Though helpful in clinical diagnosis, the radiation exposure associated with a CT scan should always be considered. The decision to order CT scan should always be made with prudence and should never replace a thorough clinical exam.

Ultrasound scans may also aid in the diagnosis of an abscess. They can be performed at the bedside, do not require sedation, and can reliably predict the presence of a fluid-filled cavity. However, the quality of the scan is highly operator-dependent, and there is poorer visualization of structures in the upper oropharynx. Therefore, ultrasound scans are less commonly utilized compared to CT scans ***(8,9)***.

Microbiology

The types of bacteria found in neck infections vary regionally and continue to evolve over time. Group A beta-hemolytic streptococcus (GABHS), *Staphylococcus aureus*, and anaerobes are the most commonly isolated bacteria in neck abscess cultures *(5,7,10,14,15)*. GABHS has been reported to be rising in incidence and contributing to an overall increase in the number of neck abscesses *(14)*. Many infections are polymicrobial, containing Gram-positive, Gram-negative, and anaerobic organisms.

The location of the abscess has been correlated with specific bacteria. Peritonsillar, retropharyngeal, and parapharyngeal abscesses tend to be caused by GABHS, while submandibular and superficial neck abscesses are more commonly associated with *S. aureus*. Children under the age of 1 are commonly infected with *S. aureus(4,5,7)*.

The recent rise in the incidence of methicillin-resistant staphylococcus aureus (MRSA) has made the treatment of neck infections much more challenging. Community-acquired MRSA (CA-MRSA) rates have been rising rapidly in many areas, even in children without risk factors for MRSA infection *(16–18)*. In a 4-year period, Ossowski et al. *(19)* demonstrated an increase in the rate of CA-MRSA from 0% (1999–2001) to 34% (2002–2004).

Bartonella henslae is implicated as the cause of cat-scratch disease. As its name suggests, it is a pathogen that is common in cats and is typically transmitted to humans from a scratch. In an immunocompetent individual, inoculation results in a self-limiting but prominent lymphadenopathy that lasts over several weeks. The presence of small Gram-negative rods on a Warthin–Starry stain is pathognomonic for this disorder. Treatment is primarily supportive, though some improvement in the resolution of symptoms has been reported with a 5-day course of azithromycin *(10)*.

Other less common causes of neck infections and lymphadenopathy include atypical mycobacterium (discussed later), actinomycosis, fusobacterium necrophorum (Lemierre's syndrome), histoplasmosis, toxoplasmosis, aspergillosis, and lymphatic filariasis *(10)*.

Treatment

Medical Management

Medical management typically involves intravenous antibiotics followed by oral antibiotics once the child has been afebrile and clinically improving. Empiric therapy for deep neck infections varies greatly, but should include adequate coverage of Gram-positive, Gram-negative, and anaerobic organisms. Empiric coverage for MRSA may depend on the regional rates of resistance, though data show that MRSA is becoming more prevalent in deep neck infections *(19,20)*. Typical choices for empiric therapy include ampicillin-sulbactam, clindamycin with a third-generation cephalosporin, trimethoprimsulfamethoxazole, vancomycin with a third-generation cephalosporin, and linezolid. Table 2 lists some of the strengths and weaknesses of typical choices for empiric therapy. Clindamycin with a third-generation cephalosporin is a commonly used antibiotic choice, as it provides good Gram-positive and anaerobic coverage, and usually covers MRSA *(9,13,15,19)*.

The duration of time for continuing intravenous antibiotics varies based on clinical judgment, but fever, white blood cell count, and neck mobility are commonly used endpoints. Neck induration may take a few weeks to completely resolve.

Table 2 Empiric therapy for deep space neck infections

Antibiotic	Strengths	Weaknesses
Bactrim	• Covers MRSA • Cost effective	• Not available as IV • Side effect: Stephen-Johnson syndrome
Clindamycin	• Covers MRSA • Good Gram +/–, anaerobic coverage • IV/PO	• Increasing resistance • Erythromycin-inducible clindamycin resistance (need d-test) • Side effect: C dificile enterocolitis
Ampicillin-sulbactam	• Good Gram +/– coverage • Can switch to ampicillin/sulbactam for PO	• MRSA not covered
Vancomycin	• MRSA coverage	• Not available as PO • Nephrotoxicity • Must check levels • Side effect: red man syndrome
Linezolid	• IV/PO • Covers MRSA	• Expensive • Side effect: neutropenia, thrombocytopenia

Surgical Management

Children with clinical evidence of an abscess lateral to the great vessels typically undergo a transcervical incision and drainage under general anesthesia. The primary benefits of incision and drainage include obtaining cultures for culture-directed antibiotic therapy, removing free pus from the neck, and creating an external tract to prevent the re-accumulation of fluid. External incision and drainage has been reported to be 99% successful ***(9)***. The risks of the surgery depend on the location of the abscess, but primarily include injury to the marginal mandibular nerve, accessory nerve, vagus nerve, or great vessels ***(10)***.

Treatment Controversies

Treatment for deep neck abscesses depends on whether lymphadenitis or a suppurative abscess is suspected. As has been previously discussed, the uncertainty of making this distinction complicates decision making. In essence, lymphadenitis and cellulitis are treated with antibiotics, whereas a neck abscess in a clinically unstable child, is treated with immediate surgical drainage ***(7,8,11,13)***. Controversy exists over the best management of a clinically stable child with a neck abscess. Clinical stability typically implies the child is without signs of systemic toxicity, airway compromise, or evidence of spread to adjacent tissue spaces ***(11,13,21)***. Many studies have shown good treatment outcomes with medical management of a CT-defined neck abscess. McClay et al. found that 10 of 11 children (91%) with a CT-defined neck abscess improved with intravenous antibiotics alone ***(13)***. Sichel et al. ***(21)*** demonstrated 100% clinical improvement with IV antibiotics alone in a series of seven patients with parapharyngeal space infections.

Though the nonsurgical management of deep neck infections appears promising, a few caveats should be noted. These studies looked at only a small number of children that were closely monitored for worsening clinical symptoms and with a surgeon immediately available for drainage. Furthermore, given the aforementioned questions about the specificity of a CT scan in diagnosing an abscess, it is possible that some of the "abscesses" in these studies were actually lymphadentitis ***(9,13,21,22)***.

Complications

Complications of a neck abscess are uncommon but can carry severe morbidity and mortality. They are typically associated with a delay in diagnosis or treatment. Airway obstruction and death can occur. Rupture of a retropharyngeal or parapharyngeal abscess may result in severe pneumonitis. Septic venous thrombosis can occur, leading to septic emboli, septic shock, or neurovascular compromise. Carotid artery rupture may also result from an unresolved abscess. Spread of an infection along the danger space can rapidly lead to mediastinitis. It should be reinterated that though these catastrophic complications are very rare, they can occur if there is a delay in management ***(10,23)***.

Special Considerations

Retropharyngeal Infection – These infections are unique in their presentation, diagnosis, and treatment. Retropharyngeal infections tend to occur in a younger age group (26–42 months), possibly due to the regression of these nodes by the age of 5. These nodes receive drainage from the sinuses, nose, and nasopharynx, which may explain why these infections often follow an upper respiratory infection, and are more commonly caused by Streptococcus. Trauma to the pharynx and esophagus, either from foreign body ingestion or from an iatrogenic cause, such as intubation, may also result in the development of a retropharyngeal infection ***(6–8,10)***. A diagnosis may be difficult to make, given the children are typically younger and a neck mass is not always present on examination. Fever and malaise, the most common presenting symptoms, are nonspecific. However, symptoms such as torticollis, decreased range of movement of the neck, dysphagia, voice changes, or drooling should raise the clinical suspicion of a retropharyngeal infection. Though symptoms of airway obstruction while awake are rare, many children demonstrate an acute onset of snoring and obstructive apnea during sleep ***(9,10)***.

Lateral neck films and CT scans are both useful tests in the diagnosis of a retropharyngeal abscess. Lateral neck films are a good screening tool, with thickness of the posterior pharyngeal wall greater than 7 mm at C2 and 14 mm at C6 considered a positive finding in a child with a retropharyngeal abscess *(23)*. These films must be taken with the child in neck extension and at the end of inspiration, or a falsely positive thickening of the posterior pharyngeal wall may be diagnosed *(9)*. This may be difficult to achieve in a uncooperative child *(6,9,10)*. CT scanning is the imaging method of choice in the management of a retropharyngeal abscess *(9)*. However, the same concerns with the specificity of predicting purulence in other regions of the neck apply to the retropharynx.

Many studies demonstrate satisfactory outcomes with nonoperative management of retropharyngeal infections. However, prompt surgical drainage is necessary if no response to medical therapy is demonstrated, if there is evidence of airway compromise, if free pus is seen in the retropharyngeal space on imaging, or if the child appears toxic *(6,8,9,13)*.

Transoral drainage has been demonstrated to be safe for an abscess that is medial to the great vessels. External drainage is reserved for an abscess with spread lateral to the carotid artery. When intubating a child with a suspected retropharyngeal abscess, care must be taken to avoid possible rupture of the abscess and aspiration of its contents. Postoperative airway control with prolonged intubation or a tracheotomy are rarely required after drainage of a retropharyngeal abscess in children *(6,9)*.

Peritonsillar Abscess – A peritonsillar abscess is the most common complication of tonsillitis. It typically occurs in older children (10–13 years), although cases have been reported in children as young as 14 months *(7)*. Streptococcus is the most commonly isolated pathogen *(7)*. The classic history is that of a unilateral sore throat, odynophagia, dysphagia, fever, and a "hot potato" voice. Trismus, otalgia, and poor oral intake are common symptoms. A peritonsillar abscess is primarily diagnosed by physical examination. Findings include unilateral edema and erythema of the soft palate on the affected side, uvular deviation to the opposite side, and displacement of the tonsil medially and inferiorly. Rarely, a bilateral peritonsillar abscess may confound the diagnosis, as no uvular deviation is seen *(24)*. A CT scan may be helpful if the diagnosis is unclear or the child is too young for an adequate examination, though is not routinely necessary.

In older children and in adolescents, a peritonsillar abscess can often be drained under local anesthesia in an outpatient setting. Young children often require intraoperative drainage and hospital admission. The treatment recommendations for pediatric peritonsillar abscesses vary widely. A recent study showed that children 8 months to 6 years responded to intravenous antibiotics without drainage 68% of the time *(24)*. Needle drainage or incision and drainage under conscious sedation has been safely performed with minimal complications *(25,26)*.

Atypical Mycobacterium – Also known as scrofula, this is the most common cause of persistent cervicofacial masses in children and commonly affects children under the age of 5. These infections present as a slowly enlarging neck mass with a violaceous hue that persists for weeks after antibiotic therapy. Infected nodes often erupt and form draining fistulae. Chest X-ray and PPD are usually normal *(27)*. Scrofula is spread locally and is not life-threatening. Diagnosis is best made clinically, or by tissue biopsy and culture, that may take 3–6 weeks to obtain. Incision and drainage of these lesions results in a high rate of recurrence. Complete excision of the infected tissue is the treatment choice providing the best cosmetic result, and the lowest rate of reoperation *(10,27–29)*. A course of clarithromycin is usually given postoperatively for 3–6 months although its benefit is unclear. Successful treatment of these infections has been reported with antibiotics alone, and should be considered in cases where the location of the infection places critical structures at risk of surgical injury. Recurrence is common, especially when the infection has spread beyond a single node *(10,27)*.

Conclusion

Deep neck infections represent a commonly encountered problem in children. Though there is debate about various treatment methods, prompt diagnosis and intervention is the key to managing these infections. If treated appropriately, they tend to resolve with minimal sequelae. However, if diagnosis and intervention is delayed, life-threatening complications may occur. Changes in technology and antibiotic resistance may alter the principles of management in the future.

References

1. Byrne, M. and K.J. Lee, *Neck Spaces and Fascial Planes, in Essential Otolaryngology*. K.J. Lee, Editor. 2003, McGraw-Hill: New York. 422–439.
2. Moore, K. and A. Dalley, *Fascia of the Neck, in Clinically Oriented Anatomy*, K. Moore and A. Dalley, Editors. 1999, Lippincott Williams & Wilkins: Philadelphia. 998–999.
3. Standring, S. and B. Berkovitz, *Neck, in Gray's Anatomy: The Anatomical Basis of Clinical Practice*, S. Standring, Editor. 2005, Elsevier: Edinburgh. 531–566.
4. Cmejrek, R.C., J.M. Coticchia, and J.E. Arnold, *Presentation, Diagnosis, and Management of Deep-Neck Abscesses in Infants*. Arch Otolaryngol Head Neck Surg, 2002. **128**(12): 1361–1364.
5. Coticchia, J.M., et al., *Age-, Site-, and Time-Specific Differences in Pediatric Deep Neck Abscesses*. Arch Otolaryngol Head Neck Surg, 2004. **130**(2): 201–207.
6. Craig, F.W. and J.E. Schunk, *Retropharyngeal Abscess in Children: Clinical Presentation, Utility of Imaging, and Current Management*. Pediatrics, 2003. **111**(6): 1394–1398.
7. Dodds, B. and A.J. Maniglia, *Peritonsillar and Neck Abscesses in the Pediatric Age Group*. Laryngoscope, 1988. **98**(9): 956–959.
8. Roberson, D. and D. Kirse, *Surgical Management of Retropharyngeal Space Infections in Children*. Laryngoscope, 2001. **111**(8): 1413–1422.
9. Lalakea, M. and A. Messner, *Retropharyngeal abscess management in children: Current practices*. Otolaryngol Head Neck Surg, 1999. **121**(4): 398–405.
10. Roberson, D. and D. Kirse, *Infectious and Inflammatory Disorders of the Neck, in Pediatric Otolaryngology*, R.F. Wetmore, T.J. McGill, and H.R. Muntz, Editors. 2000, Thiene: New York. 969–991.
11. Lazor, J., et al., *Comparison of Computed Tomography Findings and Surgical Findings in Deep Neck Infections*. Otolaryngol Head Neck Surg, 1994. **111**(6): 746–750.
12. Ungkanont, K., et al., *Head and Neck Space Infections in Infants and Children*. Otolaryngol Head Neck Surg, 1995. **112**(3): 375–382.
13. McClay, J.E., A.D. Murray, and T. Booth, *Intravenous Antibiotic Therapy for Deep Neck Abscesses Defined by Computed Tomography*. Arch Otolaryngol Head Neck Surg, 2003. **129**(11): 1207–1212.
14. Nagy, M.M.D., et al., *Deep Neck Infections in Children: A New Approach to Diagnosis and Treatment. [Article]*. Laryngoscope, 1997. **107**(12): 1627–1634.
15. Cabrera, C.E., et al., *Increased Incidence of Head and Neck Abscesses in Children*. Otolaryngol Head Neck Surg, 2007. **136**(2): 176–181.
16. Purcell, K. and J. Fergie, *Epidemic of Community-Acquired Methicillin-Resistant Staphylococcus aureus Infections: A 14-Year Study at Driscoll Children's Hospital*. Arch Pediatr Adolesc Med, 2005. **159**(10): 980–985.
17. Fergie, J.E.M. and K.M.P.R. Purcell, *Community-Acquired Methicillin-Resistant Staphylococcus aureus Infections in South Texas Children. [Article]*. Pediatr Infect Dis J, 2001. **20**(9): 860–863.
18. Miller, L.G., et al., *Clinical and Epidemiologic Characteristics Cannot Distinguish Community-Associated Methicillin-Resistant Staphylococcus aureus Infection from Methicillin-Susceptible S. aureus Infection: A Prospective Investigation*. Clin Infect Dis, 2007. **44**(4): 471–482.
19. Ossowski, K., et al., *Increased Isolation of Methicillin-Resistant Staphylococcus aureus in Pediatric Head and Neck Abscesses*. Arch Otolaryngol Head Neck Surg, 2006. **132**(11): 1176–1181.
20. Marcinak, J.F. and A.L. Frank, *Treatment of Community-Acquired Methicillin-Resistant Staphylococcus aureus in Children. [Miscellaneous]*. Curr Opin Infect Dis, 2003. **16**(3): 265–269.
21. Sichel, J.-Y.M.D., et al., *Nonsurgical Management of Parapharyngeal Space Infections: A Prospective Study. [Article]*. Laryngoscope, 2002. **112**(5): 906–910.
22. Sichel, J., et al., *Redefining Parapharyngeal Space Infections*. Ann Otol Rhinol Laryngol, 2006. **115**(2): 117–123.
23. Gidley, P. and C. Stiernberg, *Deep Space Neck Infections, in Infectious Diseases and Antimicrobial Therapy of the Ears, Nose and Throat*, J. Gwaltney, J. Rubin Grandis, and A. Sugar, Editors. 1997, WB Saunders: Phialdelphia. 500–519.
24. Simons, J.P., B.F. Branstetter IV, and D.L. Mandell, *Bilateral Peritonsillar Abscesses: Case Report and Literature Review*. Am J Otolaryngol, 2006. **27**(6): 443–445.
25. Suskind, D.L., et al., *Conscious Sedation: A New Approach for Peritonsillar Abscess Drainage in the Pediatric Population. Arch Otolaryngol Head Neck Surg*, 1999. **125**(11): 1197–1200.
26. Bauer, P.W., et al., *The Safety of Conscious Sedation in Peritonsillar Abscess Drainage*. Arch Otolaryngol Head Neck Surg, 2001. **127**(12): 1477–1480.
27. Rahal, A.M.D., et al., *Nontuberculous Mycobacterial Adenitis of the Head and Neck in Children: Experience from a Tertiary Care Pediatric Center. [Article]*. Laryngoscope, 2001. **111**(10): 1791–1797.
28. Lindeboom, J.A., et al., *Surgical Excision versus Antibiotic Treatment for Nontuberculous Mycobacterial Cervicofacial Lymphadenitis in Children: A Multicenter, Randomized, Controlled Trial*. Clin Infect Dis, 2007. **44**(8): 1057–1064.
29. Tunkel, D.E., *Surgery for Cervicofacial Nontuberculous Mycobacterial Adenitis in Children: An Update*. Arch Otolaryngol Head Neck Surg, 1999. **125**(10): 1109–1113.
30. Espiritu, M.B. and J.E. Medina, *Complications of Heroin Injections in the Neck*. Laryngoscope, 1980. **90**(7): 1111–1119.

Complications of Acute Otitis Media

Kelley M. Dodson and Angela Peng

Key Points

- Complications of otitis media are much less frequent today than in the pre-antibiotic era, yet they remain a significant cause of pediatric morbidity from infectious disease.
- Complications of otitis media can be acute or chronic and further subdivided into intracranial and extracranial disease.
- Careful clinical evaluation and appropriate imaging studies are essential for the diagnosis of acute complications of otitis media. Oftentimes a high index of suspicion is required to recognize early complications.
- Management of complications typically involves culture of offending pathogens, appropriate intravenous antibiotic therapy, and surgical intervention.

Keywords: Otitis media • Complications • Mastoiditis • Meningitis • Brain abscess

Introduction

Otitis media is the most common bacterial infection in the pediatric population and can lead to both acute and chronic complications. Fortunately, acute emergent complications associated with otitis media are less frequent in the modern era due to effective antibiotic therapy, with rates declining from around 17 to 1% ***(1)***. In the past 10 years, several reports from the United States have suggested that complications of otitis media, especially acute mastoiditis, may be on the rise ***(2–4)***, while other reports abroad have disputed such a trend ***(5,6)***. Complications of acute otitis media may be further subdivided into intracranial and extracranial categories (Table 1). This chapter will review complications of acute otitis media and provide diagnostic and management principles for these potentially life-threatening disorders.

Complications of acute otitis media generally occur in otherwise healthy children and appropriate antibiotic treatment does not always prevent their occurrence ***(7–9)***. Offending organisms leading to complications of acute otitis media often include *Streptococcus pneumoniae*, *Hemophilus influenzae*, *Pseudomonas aeruginosa*, and *Staphylococcus aureus* ***(8,10)***. Although the microbiology of pediatric mastoiditis does not appear to have changed with the use of pneumococcal vaccine, the incidence of ceftriaxone resistance in pneumococci is on the rise in the postvaccine era ***(11)***.

Recent series indicate that intratemporal complications of otitis media far outnumber intracranial complications ***(5)***. Acute mastoiditis remains the most commonly encountered complication of acute otitis media ***(5,7)***. Meningitis is the most common intracranial complication of acute otitis media, while brain abscesses are more commonly associated with chronic otitis media and cholesteatoma. Multiple intracranial complications can be seen with the same episode of otitis media in a child ***(10)***.

Extracranial Complications

Acute Mastoiditis

Acute mastoiditis is the most frequent complication of acute otitis media. It is loosely defined as an

K.M. Dodson (✉) and A. Peng
Department of Otolaryngology – Head and Neck Surgery,
Virginia Commonwealth University Medical Center,
Richmond, VA, USA
e-mail: kdodson@vcu.edu

R.B. Mitchell and K.D. Pereira (eds.), *Pediatric Otolaryngology for the Clinician*,
DOI: 10.1007/978-1-60327-127-1_29,

Table 1 Acute complications of otitis media

Intracranial	Extracranial
Meningitis	Acute mastoiditis – Subperiosteal abscess – Bezold abscess
Intracranial abscess – Epidural – Subdural – Intraparenchymal	Petrous apicitis (Gradeningo syndrome)
Lateral sinus thrombosis	Facial nerve paralysis
Otitic hydrocephalus	Labyrinthitis
	Tympanic membrane perforation

infection of the mastoid spaces of the temporal bone, which are in continuity with the middle ear cavity through a channel known as the aditus ad antrum. It most often arises from direct extension of otitis media in a well-pneumatized temporal bone. The infectious process may then become localized within the mastoid air cell system, causing bony destruction and coalescence of air cells. The infectious process may spread beyond the confines of the temporal bone to postauricular soft tissues (subperiosteal or postauricular abscess) or may break through the mastoid tip to cause an abscess within the neck (Bezold abscess). Some recent case series have suggested an increasing incidence of acute mastoiditis *(2–4)*, while others suggest a decrease *(5,6)*. *Streptococcus pneumoniae* is the most common offending organism in acute mastoiditis and its role does not seem to be decreasing since the introduction of the polyvalent pneumococcal vaccine *(11)*.

In the pre-antibiotic era, acute mastoiditis was typically a disease of older children and adults *(12)*, but recent reports show an increased incidence in young children, particularly those less than 2 years of age *(6,8,12,13)*. Goldstein et al. *(7)* reported on 100 children with intratemporal complications of otitis media, of which 72% had acute mastoiditis. The most common symptoms were ear ache, postauricular pain, and fever for a mean of 3.5 days prior to presentation. Half of the children were 3 years of age or younger and 44% had received previous oral antibiotic therapy for otitis media, most commonly augmentin *(7)*. The higher incidence of acute mastoiditis in young children may be related to increasing antibiotic resistance, daycare, as well as nonspecific symptoms of acute otitis media in young children *(8,14)*. Indeed up to half of all young children presenting with acute mastoiditis have no previous diagnosis of acute otitis media *(15–17)*.

The diagnosis of acute mastoiditis involves a detailed history and physical examination, oftentimes revealing a bulging tympanic membrane. The most frequent sign is postauricular tenderness and erythema followed by protrusion of the auricle *(7)*. The diagnosis can be confirmed by a temporal bone CT scan, showing opacification and coalescence of the mastoid air cells, as well as possible extension or abscess formation elsewhere in the soft tissues or neck.

Treatment of acute mastoiditis may consist of appropriate intravenous antibiotics with conservative measures such as myringotomy with culture of offending pathogens *(6,7,16,18,19)*. More severe or unresolved cases may require a mastoidectomy *(13,15,2)*. Conservative treatment is often considered first for clinically stable children, with surgery reserved for those who fail medical management, or those who have underlying cholesteatoma or other suppurative complications. Predictors for the need for surgical therapy with mastoidectomy include symptom duration of 6 or more days prior to hospital admission, elevated white cell count above 20, or C-reactive protein above 150 *(18)*. The majority of children respond to conservative therapy of intravenous antibiotics and myringotomy with or without tube placement, with 22–36% requiring mastoidectomy *(3,6,7,18)*. Antibiotics are typically continued for a total of 6 weeks.

Facial Nerve Paralysis

Facial nerve paralysis (FNP) can account for 22% of intratemporal complications of acute otitis media in children *(7)*. In the pre-antibiotic era, FNP occurred in 0.6% of children with acute otitis media *(21)*. Up to 50% of facial nerves may have a dehiscence of the bony fallopian canal in the middle ear *(22)*, subjecting the nerve directly to inflammatory mediators during a suppurative infection. The majority of cases of facial nerve paralysis associated with acute otitis media are incomplete *(7)*. Half of children are aged 3 or younger with a mean duration of ear symptoms lasting 6 days prior to presentation *(7)*. Most patients with FNP secondary to acute otitis media respond with a complete recovery of function after treatment with intravenous antibiotics and myringotomy/tube placement *(21)*.

Labyrinthitis

Labyrinthitis is an inflammatory process, either serous or suppurative, within the inner ear. Labyrinthitis can occur in up to 5% of children with complications of acute OM *(7)*. Symptoms include otalgia, dizziness, hearing loss, and vomiting. A MRI scan may reveal enhancement of inner ear structures and imaging is important to investigate predisposing congenital malformations of the inner ear. Most children respond to intravenous antibiotics and myringotomy/tube placement. Exploratory tympanotomy to rule out a congenital fistula may be indicated *(7)*. Permanent sensorineural hearing loss may result despite successful treatment, particularly in cases of suppurative labyrinthitis.

Petrous Apicitis

Petrous apicitis, also known as Gradenigo's syndrome, is a suppurative infection of the petrous apex portion of the temporal bone with the classic triad of otorrhea, abducens nerve palsy (diplopia), and severe retro-orbital pain. In the pre-antibiotic era, petrous apicitis was a common sequelae of acute otitis media and mastoiditis, but is relatively rare today *(23,24)*. Although acute petrositis has been reported in 4–15% of intratemporal complications of acute otitis media in children *(7,8)*, the classic triad is rarely seen at presentation *(7,23)*. Half of the children have permanent hearing loss and palsy of the sixth cranial nerve that lasts around 3 weeks. Concomitant intracranial complications are common. Diagnosis is confirmed with CT or MRI demonstrating the inflammatory process and destruction of architecture within the petrous apex. Treatment consists of intravenous antibiotics combined with myringotomy/tube placement as well as mastoidectomy.

Intracranial Complications

The spread of infection from suppurative ear disease can occur through a number of routes. It can occur through the blood vessels including direct extension along venules traveling through the temporal bone. Direct spread through bone erosion, or via the labyrinth, endolymphatic ducts, congenital or traumatic malformations and defects can also occur *(25,26)*. Despite a low overall incidence, intracranial complications from otitis media can be life-threatening and pose a high risk of mortality and morbidity in children. Therefore, early suspicion confirmed by radiological imaging leading to early surgical intervention is essential *(27)*. In a 15-year review of 33 cases of intracranial complications from acute and chronic otitis media, Penido et al. *(10)* found that headache, persistent fever, and purulent otorrhea were the most common presenting symptoms.

Meningitis

Meningitis is defined as an inflammatory process affecting the meninges, the protective membranes enveloping the brain and spinal cord. It is the most frequent intracranial complication associated with acute otitis media *(8,28)*. The following symptoms and signs are associated with meningitis: lethargy, altered mental status, nuchal rigidity, Kernig's sign (hip flexion with knee extension inciting pain), Brudzinski's sign (neck flexion causing flexion of the child's hip and knee), rash, and seizures. However, in a quarter of children with meningitis secondary to otitis media, the most common early symptoms are headache and fever, with an unremarkable otoscopic examination *(27)*. Infants often manifest nonspecific symptoms of irritability and poor feeding and often lack clear meningeal signs *(29)*.

The rapid development of meningeal signs in a child with suppurative otitis media is typically associated with *S. pneumoniae* or *H. influenza* *(28)*. Other bacteria including *S. aureus*, *P. aeruginosa*, and Proteus species may also be implicated in intracranial complications of acute otitis media *(29)*. In the case of rapid onset of meningitis, the child may have an associated inner ear malformation, including Mondini deformity which allows the middle ear bacteria access to the cerebrospinal fluid through the stapes footplate or round window *(28)*.

Early diagnosis of meningitis is vital in order to effectively treat this life-threatening complication. A detailed history and thorough physical examination, including an ophthalmic examination is mandatory. A CT scan of the brain should be performed prior to lumbar puncture, which remains the gold standard for diagnosis of meningitis. Myringotomy with or without tube placement is recommended for drainage of the source of the infection as well as for culture, especially in the present era of increasing antibiotic resistance *(30)*.

Management of a child with suspected meningitis includes emergent admission for appropriate intravenous antibiotics, initiating therapy with broad spectrum antibiotics like ceftriaxone which have excellent cerebrospinal fluid penetration *(28)*, myringotomy with or without tube placement, and possible concomitant steroids. The latter may decrease the inflammatory changes caused by the infection and reduce the potential neurologic sequelae, especially deafness *(31,32)*. Without appropriate treatment, patients may progress to develop altered mental status, neurological deficits, and possibly death.

Intracranial Abscess

An intracranial abscess from otitis media occurs by direct extension from the middle ear, often via valveless emissary veins. This abscess is almost exclusively located adjacent to the temporal bone, at the junction of the temporal lobe and cerebellum *(10,29,33)*. Intracranial abscesses are more frequently encountered as a complication of chronic otitis media with cholesteatoma rather than as a complication of acute otitis media.

Intracranial abscesses may localize above the dura (epidural), below the dura but above brain parenchyma (subdural), or within the brain parenchyma itself (intraparenchymal). Epidural abscesses often present with vague symptoms of headache, fever, and symptoms indistinguishable from the primary disease process. In contrast, subdural empyemas often progress rapidly and cause significant mass effect and swift neurological deterioration.

Intraparenchymal abscesses have four recognized clinical stages of development: invasion, localization, enlargement, and termination *(28)*. During the invasion stage (initial encephalitis/cerebritis), the patient may present with a low-grade fever, lethargy/malaise, decreased concentration, and headache. The symptoms are subtle and nonspecific, and can spontaneously resolve over 3–5 days. Local inflammation, vascular dilation, microthrombosis, small vessel rupture, and edema can be found in the brain *(34)*. The localization stage is asymptomatic, and may last for weeks. In the third stage, the inflamed area liquefies and the expansion of the fluid collection causes mass effect, focal neurological deficits, seizure, and possibly loss of consciousness. The late stage of the abscess involves capsule formation to contain the abscess. During the latter two stages, the fluid collection may cause a rise in intracranial pressure leading to brain herniation, and if rupture occurs death may be imminent *(34)*.

Diagnosis rests on a careful history and physical examination as well as imaging. Lumbar puncture is contraindicated as brainstem herniation from the sudden release of pressure may occur. CT and MRI imaging are especially helpful in the primary diagnosis of the abscess as well as for following the disease progression. MRI with gadolinium has greater soft tissue resolution and is superior especially early in the course of the disease *(35)*. Typical organisms responsible for intracranial abscesses include mixed anaerobic/aerobic organisms, with *Pseudomonas aeruginosa*, various streptococcal and staphylococcal organisms, Gram-negative enteric bacilli, and *Bacteroides fragilis* *(35)*.

Primary treatment of the intracranial abscess consists of intravenous antibiotics for a minimum of 4–6 weeks and surgical drainage often through a burrhole craniotomy. Myringotomy and tube placement may also be warranted. Seizures may continue after surgery, so anticonvulsive therapy may be used as prophylaxis for at least 3 months following the procedure.

Lateral and Sigmoid Sinus Thrombosis

The proximity of the otitic infection adjacent to the dura overlying the sigmoid and lateral venous sinuses may result in inflammation and thrombosis of these sinuses. Thrombus blocks the venous drainage system, thereby elevating intracranial pressure and dilating the ventricle. This may also lead to disseminated emboli, internal jugular vein thrombosis, and retrograde thrombosis of the cerebral vein, leading to neurological deficits, and possibly stroke. In children, the most common signs and symptoms of lateral sinus thrombosis include intermittent spiking "picket fence" fevers, headaches, otalgia, vomiting, vertigo, diplopia, chills, and neck pain *(36)*. Children with hypercoagulabe states including Protein C and S deficiency are predisposed to developing this complication *(37,38)*. MRI or magnetic resonance venography (MRV) scans are generally preferred to definitively establish the diagnosis.

Treatment focuses on eliminating the source of the infection and inflammation with myringotomy or mastoidectomy and appropriate intravenous antibiotics for a 6-week period. Early surgical intervention seems to improve overall prognosis that is superior in children compared to adults ***(36,39,40)***. Anticoagulation use is controversial as there are reports of hemorrhagic complications in children ***(41)***. Internal jugular vein ligation and surgical evacuation of clot are rarely used ***(36,41)***.

Otitic Hydrocephalus

Otitic hydrocephalus involves increased intracranial pressure without signs of hydrocephalus, and without ventricular dilation or focal neurologic deficit ***(42)***. Symptoms include headaches, lethargy, blurred vision, nausea, and vomiting. The majority of patients with otitic hydrocephalus have bilateral papilledema, and some have ipsilateral abducens nerve palsy. The typical presentation is often nonspecific and the diagnosis may be a challenge.

Definitive diagnosis is based on elevated opening pressure (>240 mmH_2O) during lumbar puncture, with normal cerebrospinal findings ***(42,43)***. MRI/MRV scans are helpful by demonstrating thrombus in the sigmoid sinus. Treatment involves mastoidectomy for the appropriate disease process, prolonged intravenous antibiotics, steroids, diuretics, and possibly anticoagulants ***(42)***. A lumbar drain or ventricular shunt may be necessary in the intervening time while the elevated pressure is treated medically. It is important to monitor vision throughout the period of treatment ***(5)***. If the condition is not recognized or treated, blindness, stroke, or brain herniation leading to death may occur.

References

1. Berman S. Otitis media in developing countries. Pediatrics 1995 Jul;96(1 Pt 1):126–131.
2. Bahadori RS, Schwartz RH, Ziai M. Acute mastoiditis in children: an increase in frequency in Northern Virginia. Pediatr Infect Dis J 2000 Mar;19(3):212–215.
3. Ghaffar FA, Wordemann M, McCracken GH, Jr. Acute mastoiditis in children: a seventeen-year experience in Dallas, Texas. Pediatr Infect Dis J 2001 Apr;20(4):376–380.
4. Bach KK, Malis DJ, Magit AE, et al. Acute coalescent mastoiditis in an infant: an emerging trend?. Otolaryngol Head Neck Surg 1998 Nov;119(5):523–525.
5. Leskinen K, Jero J. Complications of acute otitis media in children in southern Finland. Int J Pediatr Otorhinolaryngol 2004 Mar;68(3):317–324.
6. Kvaerner KJ, Bentdal Y, Karevold G. Acute mastoiditis in Norway: no evidence for an increase. Int J Pediatr Otorhinolaryngol 2007 Oct;71(10):1579–1583.
7. Goldstein NA, Casselbrant ML, Bluestone CD, et al. Intratemporal complications of acute otitis media in infants and children. Otolaryngol Head Neck Surg 1998 Nov;119(5):444–454.
8. Dhooge IJ, Albers FW, Van Cauwenberge PB. Intratemporal and intracranial complications of acute suppurative otitis media in children: renewed interest. Int J Pediatr Otorhinolaryngol 1999 Oct;49(Suppl 1):S109–S114.
9. Ho D, Rotenberg BW, Berkowitz RG. The relationship between acute mastoiditis and antibiotic use for acute otitis media in children. Arch Otolaryngol Head Neck Surg 2008 Jan;134(1):45–48.
10. Penido NO, Borin A, Iha LC, et al. Intracranial complications of otitis media: 15 years of experience in 33 patients. Otolaryngol Head Neck Surg 2005 Jan;132(1):37–42.
11. Roddy MG, Glazier SS, Agrawal D. Pediatric mastoiditis in the pneumococcal conjugate vaccine era: symptom duration guides empiric antimicrobial therapy. Pediatr Emerg Care 2007 Nov;23(11):779–784.
12. Scott TA, Jackler RK. Acute mastoiditis in infancy: a sequela of unrecognized acute otitis media. Otolaryngol Head Neck Surg 1989 Dec;101(6):683–687.
13. Luntz M, Keren G, Nusem S, et al. Acute mastoiditis – revisited. Ear Nose Throat J 1994 Sep;73(9):648–654.
14. Pelton SI. New concepts in the pathophysiology and management of middle ear disease in childhood. Drugs 1996;52(Suppl 2):62–66.
15. Gliklich RE, Eavey RD, Iannuzzi RA, et al. A contemporary analysis of acute mastoiditis. Arch Otolaryngol Head Neck Surg 1996 Feb;122(2):135–139.
16. Harley EH, Sdralis T, Berkowitz RG. Acute mastoiditis in children: a 12-year retrospective study. Otolaryngol Head Neck Surg 1997 Jan;116(1):26–30.
17. Faye-Lund H. Acute and latent mastoiditis. J Laryngol Otol 1989 Dec;103(12):1158–1160.
18. Kvestad E, Kvaerner KJ, Mair IW. Acute mastoiditis: predictors for surgery. Int J Pediatr Otorhinolaryngol 2000 Apr;52(2):149–155.
19. Rosen A, Ophir D, Marshak G. Acute mastoiditis: a review of 69 cases. Ann Otol Rhinol Laryngol 1986 May;95(3 Pt 1): 222–224.
20. Nadal D, Herrmann P, Baumann A, et al. Acute mastoiditis: clinical, microbiological, and therapeutic aspects. Eur J Pediatr 1990 May;149(8):560–564.
21. Makeham TP, Croxson GR, Coulson S. Infective causes of facial nerve paralysis. Otol Neurotol 2007 Jan;28(1):100–103.
22. Baxter A. Dehiscence of the fallopian canal. An anatomical study. J Laryngol Otol 1971 Jun;85(6):587–594.
23. Chole RA, Donald PJ. Petrous apicitis. Clinical conside-rations. Ann Otol Rhinol Laryngol 1983 Nov;92(6 Pt 1):544–551.
24. Contrucci RB, Sataloff RT, Myers DL. Petrous apicitis. Ear Nose Throat J 1985 Sep;64(9):427–431.

25. Gower D, McGuirt WF. Intracranial complications of acute and chronic infectious ear disease: a problem still with us. Laryngoscope 1983 Aug;93(8):1028–1033.
26. Bento R, de Brito R, Ribas GC. Surgical management of intracranial complications of otogenic infection. Ear Nose Throat J 2006 Jan;85(1):36–39.
27. Albers FW. Complications of otitis media: the importance of early recognition. Am J Otol 1999 Jan;20(1):9–12.
28. Head and Neck Surgery-Otolaryngology, 4th edition. Bailey BJ, editor. 2006. Philadelphia: Lippincott Williams & Wilkins.
29. Kangsanarak J, Fooanant S, Ruckphaopunt K, et al. Extracranial and intracranial complications of suppurative otitis media. Report of 102 cases. J Laryngol Otol 1993 Nov;107(11):999–1004.
30. Zapalac JS, Billings KR, Schwade ND, et al. Suppurative complications of acute otitis media in the era of antibiotic resistance. Arch Otolaryngol Head Neck Surg 2002 Jun;128(6):660–663.
31. McIntyre PB, Berkey CS, King SM, et al. Dexamethasone as adjunctive therapy in bacterial meningitis. A meta-analysis of randomized clinical trials since 1988. JAMA 1997 Sep;278(11):925–931.
32. Greenwood BM. Corticosteroids for acute bacterial meningitis. N Engl J Med 2007 Dec;357(24):2507–2509.
33. Kurien M, Job A, Mathew J, et al. Otogenic intracranial abscess: concurrent craniotomy and mastoidectomy – changing trends in a developing country. Arch Otolaryngol Head Neck Surg 1998 Dec;124(12):1353–1356.
34. Saez-Llorens X. Brain abscess in children. Semin Pediatr Infect Dis 2003 Apr;14(2):108–114.
35. Hafidh MA, Keogh I, Walsh RM, et al. Otogenic intracranial complications. A 7-year retrospective review. Am J Otolaryngol 2006 Nov;27(6):390–395.
36. Garcia RD, Baker AS, Cunningham MJ, et al. Lateral sinus thrombosis associated with otitis media and mastoiditis in children. Pediatr Infect Dis J 1995 Jul;14(7):617–623.
37. Carvalho KS, Bodensteiner JB, Connolly PJ, et al. Cerebral venous thrombosis in children. J Child Neurol 2001 Aug;16(8):574–580.
38. Ram B, Meiklejohn DJ, Nunez DA, et al. Combined risk factors contributing to cerebral venous thrombosis in a young woman. J Laryngol Otol 2001 Apr;115(4):307–310.
39. Manolidis S, Kutz JW, Jr. Diagnosis and management of lateral sinus thrombosis. Otol Neurotol 2005 Sep;26(5):1045–1051.
40. Ooi EH, Hilton M, Hunter G. Management of lateral sinus thrombosis: update and literature review. J Laryngol Otol 2003 Dec;117(12):932–939.
41. Shah UK, Jubelirer TF, Fish JD, et al. A caution regarding the use of low-molecular weight heparin in pediatric otogenic lateral sinus thrombosis. Int J Pediatr Otorhinolaryngol 2007 Feb;71(2):347–351.
42. Kuczkowski J, Dubaniewicz-Wybieralska M, Przewozny T, et al. Otitic hydrocephalus associated with lateral sinus thrombosis and acute mastoiditis in children. Int J Pediatr Otorhinolaryngol 2006 Oct;70(10):1817–1823.
43. Andrews JC, Canalis RF. Otogenic pneumocephalus. Laryngoscope 1986;96(5):521–528.

Complications of Sinusitis

Rodney Lusk

Key Points

- Complications of sinusitis are best described as an extension of the infection into the orbit or cranium. These infections are almost always secondary to an acute sinusitis. A history of recurrent or chronic sinusitis is frequently absent.
- The infection is usually caused by a streptococcal or staphylococcal species which is frequently highly resistant to antibiotics. These infections can have significant morbidity and mortality if not recognized and treated early.
- Failure to recognize complicated sinusitis may result in blindness, permanent diplopia, seizures, hemiparesis, mental retardation, and death. The longer the delay in the diagnosis the greater the chance of developing these sequelae or possibly death.
- These patients must be aggressively managed via a team approach involving primary care, infectious disease, otolaryngology, neurosurgery, and ophthalmology.
- If aggressive medical management including broad-spectrum antibiotics that cross the blood–brain barrier does not result in prompt resolution of the symptoms, surgical intervention to drain the sinusitis and extension of the infection is warranted. The surgical intervention is dictated by the location and severity of the complication and frequently involves multiple surgical specialties.

Keywords: Acutesinusitis • Chronicsinusitis • Subperiosteal abscess • Orbital abscess • Orbital cellulitis • Brain abscess • Subdural abscess

R. Lusk
Boys Town ENT Institute, Boys Town National Research Hospital, Omaha, NE, USA
e-mail: luskr@boystown.org

Complications of sinusitis are almost always secondary to acute infections. The infections most frequently extend into the orbit but may also extend into the intracranial compartment. These acute complications are associated with significant morbidity and possible mortality if not treated early and aggressively. Clinicians must be aware of their manifestations and act quickly to prevent permanent sequelae or death.

Definition

Any infection extending beyond the confines of the sinus cavity, most commonly the orbit or cranium, would by definition be considered a complication. Orbital complications are much more common than intracranial complications and are most frequently associated with ethmoiditis, while intracranial complications are generally associated with frontal sinusitis and occur in older patients. During the pre-antibiotic era 17–20% of the patients with orbital cellulitis died from meningitis or had permanent loss of vision in the affected eye *(1)*. One of the key factors in the pathogenesis of orbital cellulitis is the thinness of the lamina papyracea separating the ethmoid sinus from the orbit (Fig. 1) *(2)*. The lamina papyracea is actually thicker in pediatric patients and more likely to be thin or dehiscent in adults. However, children have an immature immune system that predisposes them to infection particularly with resistant bacteria. It is important to remember that most intraorbital complications are the result of an acute not a chronic ethmoiditis. The ipsilateral ethmoid sinus is involved in almost all cases of orbital cellulitis and abscess. Extension into the orbit is thought to occur by four potential methods (Fig. 2):

R.B. Mitchell and K.D. Pereira (eds.), *Pediatric Otolaryngology for the Clinician*,
DOI: 10.1007/978-1-60327-127-1_30, © Humana Press, a part of Springer Science + Business Media, LLC 2009

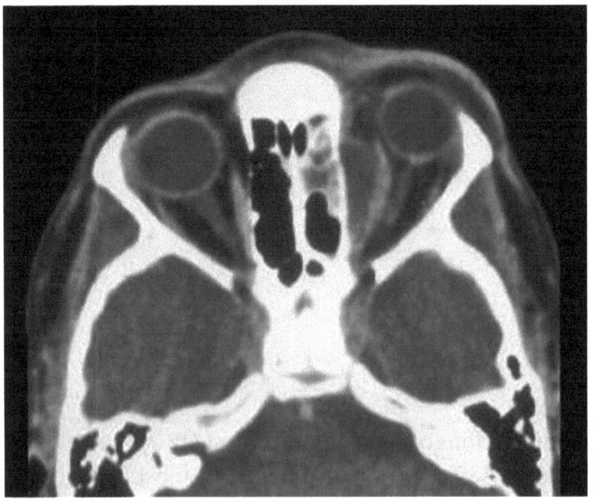

Fig. 1 Patient with left subperiosteal abscess, note adjacent ethmoid disease

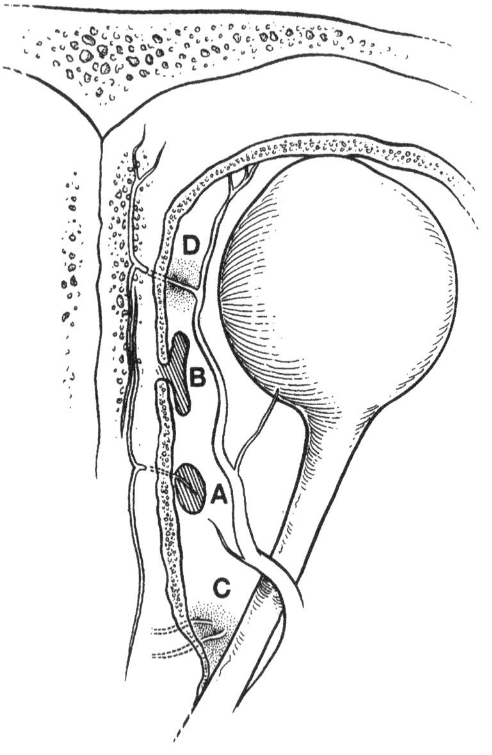

Fig. 2 Potential paths of orbital bacterial invasion

1. Venous: Venous channels without valves, also known as diploic veins, connect the orbital cavity with the ethmoid, frontal, and maxillary sinuses. Infections can involve the veins and extend directly into the orbit.
2. Direct extension: Bony dehiscences are most likely to occur in the lamina papyracea. For reasons that are unclear, orbital abscesses are more likely to occur on the left *(3)*. Extension from the frontal sinus is much less likely to occur in younger children because the frontal sinus has not developed.
3. Lymphatic seeding: There are no lymph vessels within the orbit and therefore lymphatic seeding is theoretically possible but unlikely *(2)*.
4. Arterial: Infection extending along arteries is possible but again not likely to be an important cause *(2)*.

Intracranial complications are more likely to occur in adolescent or adult patients and include: meningitis, epidural, subdural, and brain abscess *(4)*. These are frequently a direct intracranial extension of sinus disease, usually in the frontal sinus. Although ear disease was the most common predisposing factor for intracranial sepsis in the past, sinusitis is currently the most common etiologic factor *(5)*.

Prevalence

Orbital cellulitis is the most common complication of acute sinusitis and is associated with ethmoiditis in 98% of the cases *(6)*. Although a lot less common, intracranial complications are always life-threatening and tend to be more common in adolescent males *(7)*. Orbital and intracranial infections may occur simultaneously *(7)*.

Diagnosis

Orbital complications: Most children with sinusitis and orbital cellulitis have a temperature greater than 38.5°C, an elevated white count of greater than 15,000, and lethargy. Differentiation between an orbital cellulitis and abscess is a difficult but crucial first diagnostic step. This differentiation may not be possible on clinical grounds alone, and further diagnostic or surgical intervention may be required to correctly stage the infection. Staging the extent of an intraorbital infection is clinically useful. The classification developed by Chandler has gained the widest acceptance *(2)*.

Figure 3 is a representation of Chandler's different subgroups.

Group 1: Preseptal cellulitis – edema and erythema of the upper and/or lower lids occurs without limitation of ocular motility, no visual loss, and usually no chemosis.

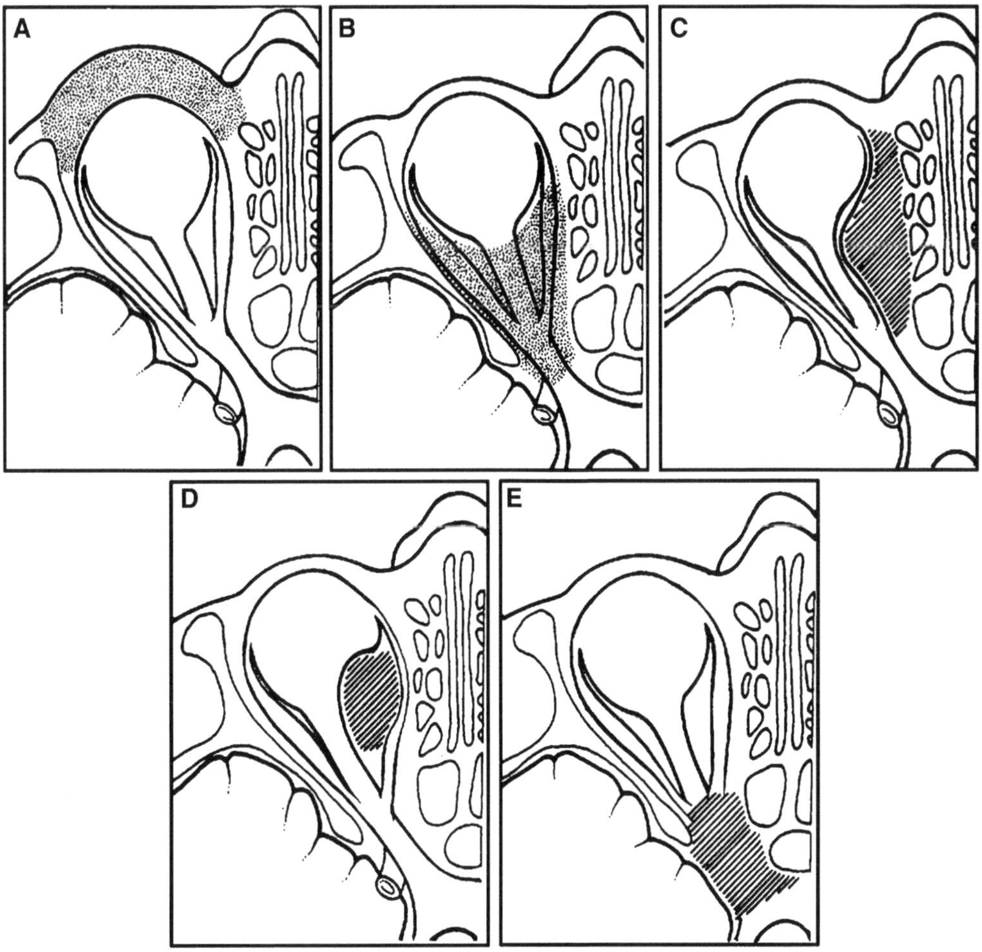

Fig. 3 Axial diagram of progressive stages of inflammation of the orbit. (**A**) Preseptal inflammation; (**B**) Orbital cellulitis, involving the fat within the orbit; (**C**) Subperiosteal abscess formation; (**D**) Orbital abscess formation within fat and muscle cone; (**E**) Cavernous sinus thrombosis

Group 2: Orbital cellulitis without abscess – diffuse edema of the adipose tissue within the orbit but no abscess formation and symmetrical axial proptosis

Group 3: Orbital cellulitis with subperiosteal abscess – abscess formation between the orbital periosteum and orbital bone; the abscess frequently displaces the globe and points to the location of the abscess.

Group 4: Orbital cellulitis with abscess in the orbital adipose tissue – proptosis is usually severe with orbital displacement. Ophthalmoplegia and visual loss may ensue without prompt treatment.

Group 5: Cavernous sinus thrombosis – spread of orbital infection into the cavernous sinus may result in bilateral disease and blindness.

Proptosis is frequently a good differentiator between preseptal and orbital infections. Preseptal cellulitis is generally associated with inflammation and edema of the lids but may involve the conjunctiva. Involvement of the conjunctiva cannot however differentiate between an orbital cellulitis or abscess. Any expanding mass within the orbit can be associated with conjunctival swelling (chemosis) (Fig. 4) and ophthalmoplegia. Proptosis (Figs. 5 and 6) may be associated with ophthalmoplegia and/or diminished vision in 73% of children *(6)*; both are alarming signs and require immediate and accurate assessment. The direction of displacement of the globe may point to the location of the abscess. It is important to understand that in general, the greater the proptosis the more severe the inflammation and the larger the abscess.

If there is progression to an abscess, antibiotics are much less likely to cure the infection and surgical

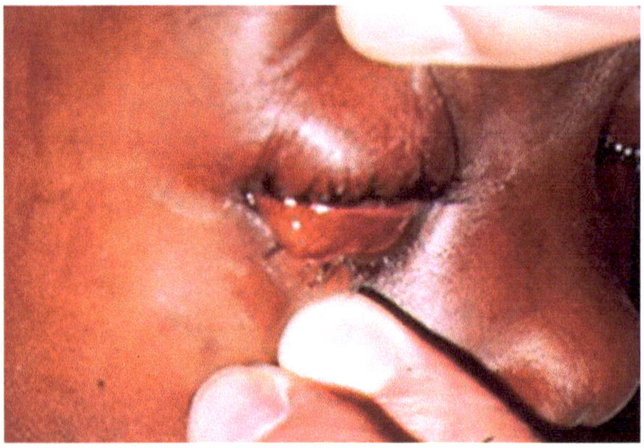

Fig. 4 Chemosis of conjunctiva

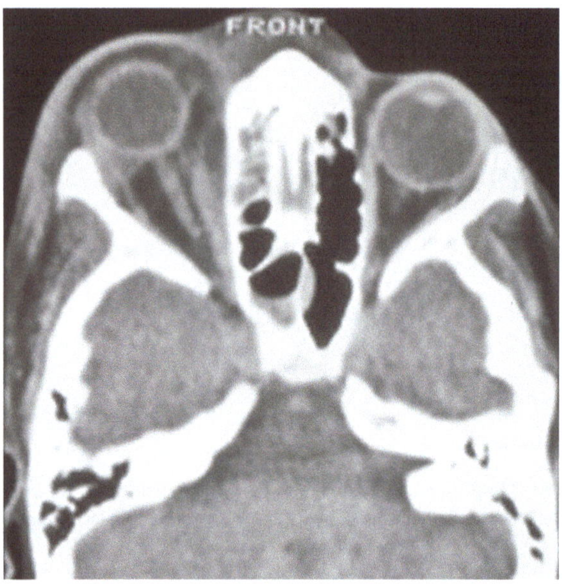

Fig. 5 CT scan of proptosis with right subperiosteal abscess

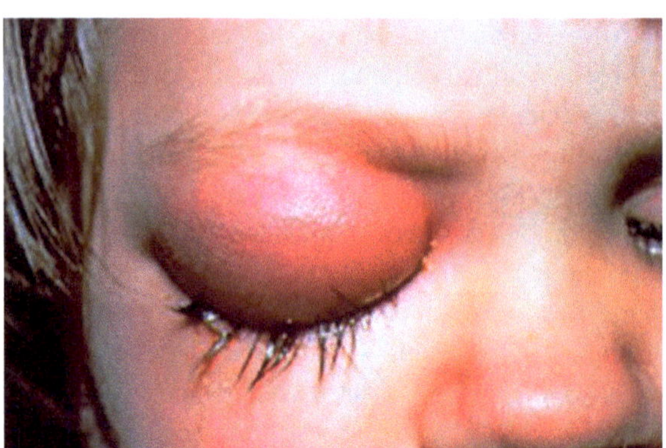

Fig. 6 Proptosis of orbit

drainage will probably be required. Significant chemosis may limit testing of visual acuity and examination of the eye. An immediate ophthalmology consultation is always warranted if a decrease in visual acuity is suspected. This can occur in an alarming number of patients with orbital cellulitis *(8)* and any delay in diagnosis increases the chances of a permanent visual impairment *(9)*. Decreasing vision in both eyes is indicative of cavernous sinus thrombosis, a very serious and life-threatening complication.

Brain abscesses are most likely to occur in the frontal lobes and diagnosis can be difficult as symptoms are often silent *(10, 11)*. Cellulitis and orbital abscess formation may result in increased intracranial pressures which would manifest with bradycardia, papilledema, a stiff neck, hypertension, nausea, vomiting, and decreased consciousness. A dilated pupil is an ominous sign suggesting transtentorial herniation *(12)*. Intracranial abscesses typically present with fever, headaches, seizures, nuchal rigidity, focal neurological signs, and occasionally photophobia *(13)*. Patients with an epidural abscess generally present with dull headaches, sudden elevation of temperature, and a normal cerebrospinal fluid (CSF) *(14)*. Patients with subdural abscesses are usually toxic with mental status changes, severe headaches, nuchal rigidity, papilledema, cloudy CSF, and focal neurologic changes *(14)*.

Diagnostic Tests

Clinically it may be very difficult to distinguish between an orbital cellulitis and an orbital abscess *(15)*. The axial CT scan (Figs. 1 and 5) with contrast remains the single best test to differentiate between a subperiosteal abscess and an orbital abscess *(15)*. A CT scan is appropriate if the patient is treated with intravenous antibiotics and not improving over a 24-h period. CT scans will also help find the location and extent of acute sinusitis and are required for surgical intervention. MRI scans are not particularly useful in the assessment of orbital infections but are very helpful in defining intracranial extension of the disease (Fig. 7). When intracranial signs or symptoms are present, it is extremely important to obtain a CT or MRI scan prior to lumbar puncture to decrease the

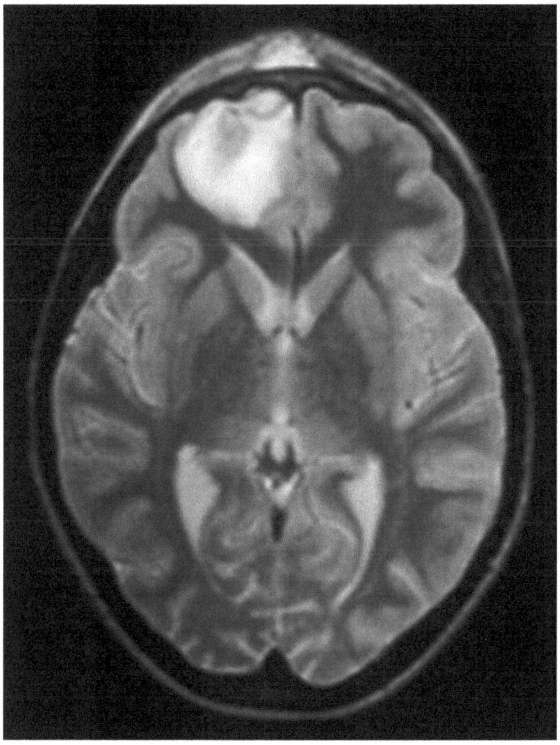

Fig. 7 MRI of brain abscess

chance of brain stem herniation. It should be noted however that the initial staging of the complications of sinusitis may have to be revised after surgical intervention. Blood cultures are not particularly helpful and are positive in only 4% *(9)*.

High-Risk Groups

Children are at a significantly higher risk for complications of acute sinusitis and orbital cellulitis has been reported even in neonates *(16)*. Preseptal cellulitis accounts for approximately 80% of all the periorbital infections. Approximately 20% of children have orbital cellulitis or abscesses and a much smaller subgroup will have intracranial complications *(17)*. Younger children are more likely to have orbital cellulitis than older children but adolescent males are more likely to have intracranial complications *(18)*. Swimmers also appear to have a higher incidence of sinusitis and orbital cellulitis *(18)*. There is an increased risk of sinusitis in children who are intubated or comatose. Of children who develop an orbital abscess and intracranial complications, 87% are secondary to staphylococcal or streptococcal species *(7,9,19)*. Community-acquired methicillin-resistant staphylococcus aureus has been reported as a particularly progressive infection associated with blindness *(20, 21)*.

Frontal sinus infections can invade the marrow of both the anterior and posterior tables. If this happens, the diploic veins transfer infection into the CNS and cause subdural empyemas or brain abscesses *(22)*. The signs and symptoms of complicated frontal sinusitis may be nonspecific rendering the infection difficult to diagnose without a CT scan. Subtle extension into the frontal lobe may at times only be seen on a MRI scan. CT scans should be obtained with the necessary information for image-guided surgery.

Treatment

Cellulitis: In general, medical management is more successful in younger rather than older children. If the infection is clinically a preseptal cellulitis it is quite acceptable to initiate therapy with intravenous antibiotics *(17)*. Older children are much more likely to require surgical intervention *(23)*. If intravenous antibiotics are used as an initial management, they should be broad spectrum given the high incidence of polymicrobial infections *(7)*. If the child does not show significant improvement in 24 h, a CT scan of the sinuses, or if an intracranial complication is suspected, a MRI is indicated. Lack of improvement suggests that the orbital cellulitis has developed into an abscess and will likely require surgical intervention.

Most investigators now feel that endoscopic ethmoidectomy with drainage through the lamina papyracea is the most efficacious way to treat a medial subperiosteal orbital abscess (*24,25*). Axial and coronal CT scans will help define precisely the location of the abscess. Precise identification of the abscess intraoperatively is possible utilizing image-guided endoscopic techniques. Invariably there is bilateral involvement of the ethmoid sinuses but since this is an acute infection, surgical intervention of the opposite side must be based on the clinical history and findings. If there is a significant history of recurrent infections then it would be reasonable to proceed with bilateral endoscopic sinus surgery. If not, it is quite reasonable to treat only the affected side surgically and manage the ethmoiditis on the opposite side with intravenous antibiotics. Clinical studies now indicate that endoscopic sinus surgery in the pediatric age group is not associated with interruption of facial growth *(26,27)*.

Intracranial: Medical management should include intravenous antibiotics with broad spectrum that readily cross the blood–brain barrier such as penicillin/chloramphenicol, cefotaxime, nafcillin, vancomycin, or ceftazidime. The antibiotic used is determined by the most likely infecting organism and the patient's known allergies. Medical management of intracranial abscesses has met with variable success. Surgical intervention includes craniotomy and endoscopic ultrasound-guided needle aspiration *(28)*. The choice of procedure is dictated by the location and extent of the lesion. If the frontal sinus and frontal lobe are both involved, the craniofacial approach may be required to address both sites. Increasingly, the frontal sinus is drained from below through an endoscopic approach unless there is clear osteitis of the anterior or posterior table of the frontal sinus.

Outcome

Orbital cellulitis: Preseptal cellulitis rarely leads to visual impairment. Orbital abscess, if not treated immediately and aggressively, can lead to visual impairment. Cavernous sinus thrombosis can lead to bilateral blindness and can be fatal. Up to 11% of cases of orbital cellulitis result in visual loss.

Intracranial complications: Sequela from intracranial complications of sinusitis include seizures, blindness, hemiparesis, and death. The older the patient the more likely is a fatal outcome *(29)*. An early diagnosis and expedited medical and surgical intervention will reduce significant long-term disability and fatality.

References

1. Gamble RC. Acute inflammation of the orbit in children. Arch Ophthalmol 1933; 10:483–497.
2. Chandler JR, Langenbrunner DJ, Stevens ER. The pathogenesis of orbital complications in acute sinusitis. Laryngoscope 1970; 80:1414–1428.
3. Ritter FN. The maxillary sinus. In: Ritter FN, editor The Paranasal Sinuses: Anatomy and Surgical Technique. St. Louis: Mosby, 1973.
4. Johnson DL, Markle BM, Wiedermann BL, Hanahan L. Treatment of intracranial abscesses associated with sinusitis in children and adolescents. J Pediatr 1988; 113:15–23.
5. Hoyt DJ, Fisher SR. Otolaryngologic management of patients with subdural empyema. Laryngoscope 1991; 101:20–24.
6. Nageswaran S, Woods CR, Benjamin DK, Jr., Givner LB, Shetty AK. Orbital cellulitis in children. Pediatr Infect Dis J 2006; 25(8):695–699.
7. Reynolds DJ, Kodsi SR, Rubin SE, Rodgers IR. Intracranial infection associated with preseptal and orbital cellulitis in the pediatric patient. J AAPOS 2003; 7(6):413–417.
8. Beech T, Robinson A, McDermott AL, Sinha A. Paediatric periorbital cellulitis and its management. Rhinology 2007; 45(1):47–49.
9. Chaudhry IA, Shamsi FA, Elzaridi E, et al.. Outcome of treated orbital cellulitis in a tertiary eye care center in the Middle East. Ophthalmology 2007; 114(2):345–354.
10. Pennybaker J. Abscess of the Brain in Modern Trend in Neurology. London: Butterworth, 1951.
11. Bradley PJ, Manning KP, Shaw MD. Brain abscess secondary to paranasal sinusitis. J Laryngol Otol 1984; 98:719–725.
12. Dawes JDK. The management of frontal sinusitis and its complications. J Laryngol Otol 1961; 75:297–354.
13. Johnson DL, Markle BM, Wiedermann BL, Hanahan L. Treatment of intracranial abscesses associated with sinusitis in children and adolescents. J Pediatr 1988; 113:15–23.
14. Parker GS, Tami TA, Wilson JF, Fetter TW. Intracranial complications of sinusitis. South Med J 1989; 82:563–569.
15. Moloney JR, Badham NJ, McRae A. The acute orbit. Preseptal (periorbital) cellulitis, subperiosteal abscess and orbital cellulitis due to sinusitis. J Laryngol Otol Suppl 1987; 12:1–18.
16. Cruz AA, Mussi-Pinhata MM, Akaishi PM, Cattebeke L, Torrano dS, Elia J, Jr. Neonatal orbital abscess. Ophthalmology 2001; 108(12):2316–2320.
17. Sobol SE, Marchand J, Tewfik TL, Manoukian JJ, Schloss MD. Orbital complications of sinusitis in children. J Otolaryngol 2002; 31(3):131–136.
18. Mills RP, Kartush JM. Orbital wall thickness and the spread of infection from the paranasal sinuses. Clin Otolaryngol 1985; 10(4):209–216.
19. Haddadin A, Saca E, Husban A. Sinusitis as a cause of orbital cellulitis. East Mediterr Health J 1999; 5(3):556–559.
20. Anari S, Karagama YG, Fulton B, Wilson JA. Neonatal disseminated methicillin-resistant Staphylococcus aureus presenting as orbital cellulitis. J Laryngol Otol 2005; 119(1):64–67.
21. Rutar T, Zwick OM, Cockerham KP, Horton JC. Bilateral blindness from orbital cellulitis caused by community-acquired methicillin-resistant Staphylococcus aureus. Am J Ophthalmol 2005; 140(4):740–742.
22. Feder HM, Jr., Cates KL, Cementina AM. Pott puffy tumor: a serious occult infection. Pediatrics 1987; 79:625–629.
23. Ritter FN. The Paranasal Sinuses, Anatomy and Surgical Technique. St. Louis, MO: C.V. Mosby Co., 1973.

24. Manning SC. Endoscopic management of medial subperiosteal orbital abscess. Arch Otolaryngol Head Neck Surg 1993; 119(7):789–791.
25. Arjmand EM, Lusk RP, Muntz HR. Pediatric sinusitis and subperiosteal orbital abscess formation: diagnosis and treatment. Otolaryngol Head Neck Surg 1993; 109(5):886–894.
26. Senior B, Wirtschafter A, Mai C, Becker C, Belenky W. Quantitative impact of pediatric sinus surgery on facial growth. Laryngoscope 2000; 110(11):1866–1870.
27. Bothwell MR, Piccirillo JF, Lusk RP, Ridenour BD. Long-term outcome of facial growth after functional endoscopic sinus surgery. Otolaryngol Head Neck Surg 2002; 126(6):628–634.
28. Yamamoto M, Fukushima T, Hirakawa K, Kimura H, Tomonaga M. Treatment of bacterial brain abscess by repeated aspiration--follow up by serial computed tomography. Neurol Med Chir (Tokyo) 2000; 40(2):98–104.
29. Rosenbaum GS, Cunha BA. Subdural empyema complicating frontal and ethmoid sinusitis. Heart Lung 1989; 18:199–202.

Index

W

Z

MIX
Papier aus verantwortungsvollen Quellen
Paper from responsible sources
FSC® C105338

If you have any concerns about our products,
you can contact us on
ProductSafety@springernature.com

In case Publisher is established outside the EU,
the EU authorized representative is:
Springer Nature Customer Service Center GmbH
Europaplatz 3, 69115 Heidelberg, Germany

Printed by Libri Plureos GmbH
in Hamburg, Germany